Environmental Sustainability and Green Technology in Pharmaceutical Research

This timely volume explores the relationship between environmental responsibility and pharmaceutical innovation, providing insights into how sustainable methods are already changing pharmaceutical research, as well as discussing their impact on medical science and healthcare in the future.

Highlighting a range of cutting-edge topics such as green chemistry, waste reduction, energy efficiency and the development of eco-friendly pharmaceuticals, this book provides a comprehensive overview of how the pharmaceutical industry is being revolutionized by sustainable practices. Readers will also learn about biocatalysis, renewable feedstocks and environmentally benign solvents, spotlighting their roles in reducing the environmental footprint of drug production. Featuring case studies that offer practical insights and lessons learned, this book addresses the multidisciplinary nature of environmental sustainability by bridging the gaps between pharmaceutical science, environmental science, engineering and policymaking.

This will be a valuable resource for researchers, students and professionals alike.

Rajnish Srivastava is a professor at the Chitkara University School of Pharmacy, Chitkara University, Himachal Pradesh, India, with distinguished expertise in regulatory toxicology, nanostructured drug delivery systems, and preclinical pharmacology. He has successfully led multiple consultancy projects funded by national agencies and pharmaceutical industries, focusing on dermal and neurodegenerative disorders. His research primarily centers on the development of advanced nanostructured drug delivery systems using low-energy approaches, along with the identification of novel molecular targets and biomarkers for neurological, metabolic, and dermatological diseases. He has made notable contributions to hybrid therapeutic strategies for diabetes and its associated complications, including diabetic neuropathy, reflecting a strong translational research approach. Srivastava possesses extensive experience in experimental protocol design and in vivo pharmacological evaluations, with a focus on developing and validating preclinical screening models. He also has strong expertise in regulatory toxicology and safety pharmacology, ensuring compliance with established research standards. He has published over 50 research papers in reputed international journals and holds 5 patents. Additionally, he has authored more than 30 international book chapters and 4 books in pharmaceutical sciences. He serves as a reviewer for over

30 internationally recognized journals and has been associated with the Committee for the Control and Supervision of Experiments on Animals (CCSEA) for more than 14 years. He was awarded the Best Faculty Facilitation Award (2015) by the Madhya Pradesh Council for Science and Technology (MPCST) for his excellence in teaching and academic contributions.

Nitin Verma currently serves as a professor and principal at the Chitkara University School of Pharmacy, Chitkara University, Himachal Pradesh, India. He is a member of the Board of Studies, Academic Council, and coordinator of the Academic–Industry Partnership Programme with Reddy's Laboratories, Zydus Healthcare, Mankind Pharma, Abbott, etc. He has executed projects worth more than ₹ 4.5 crores with government agencies and industry. His biography is included in *Who's Who in Medicine and Healthcare 2011–2012* (8th Edition) based on outstanding achievements in medicine and healthcare around the world, and he has been recognized by the International Biographical Centre (IBC), Cambridge, England, with The Cambridge Certificate for Outstanding Medical Achievement 2012. Verma is a member of various professional societies and serves on the reviewer board of multiple journals. Verma is actively engaged in research, with a special focus on toxicology, risk assessment of chemicals and their impact on the environment and human health, computational toxicity studies, and natural products. He is the recipient of several prestigious awards such as the Global Senior Scholar Exchange Program Award (USA), ToxScholar Outreach Award (USA), IUTOX Award (USA), ASIO Scientist of Indian Origin, and Global Initiative Funding by the Society of Toxicology (SOT), USA. He has presented his research at various international conferences and congresses held in the USA, Greece, Rome, Slovakia, Australia, Japan, Switzerland, Singapore, and Spain. Based on his extensive expertise in research, academics, and administrative leadership, Verma's dedicated efforts are directed toward enhancing students' careers, strengthening their professional growth, and fostering a culture of excellence and innovation.

Amit Chaudhary is a professor at the Chitkara University School of Pharmacy, Chitkara University, Himachal Pradesh, India, and a distinguished researcher in the field of targeted drug delivery systems. He is widely recognized for his innovative contributions toward the design, development, and optimization of advanced drug delivery platforms aimed at enhancing therapeutic efficacy, solubility, bioavailability, and patient compliance. His research integrates modern pharmaceutical approaches with translational outcomes, significantly contributing to the advancement of drug delivery science. Chaudhary has been honored with several prestigious awards, including the Innovative Researcher Award (2025) and the Prof. M. L. Schroff Pharma Recognition Award (2025) by Pharmalok, in recognition of his exceptional contributions to pharmacy education and research. His other accolades include the Best Academician Award (2024), Star Debutant of the Year (2023), Best Principal Award (2021), and Best Researcher Award (2019–20), reflecting his excellence across academic leadership, teaching, and research. An accomplished mentor, he has supervised over 80 postgraduate and doctoral students (M.Pharm and Pharm.D) in their research projects. He actively contributes to academic and professional development through participation in more than 65 national and international conferences, seminars, and faculty development programs, and has delivered 19 invited lectures as a resource person. Chaudhary has published over 100 research and review articles in peer-reviewed journals of repute, holds 21 patents (including 11 granted), and has an H-index of 10 with around 1000 citations. He has also authored book chapters and a book titled *Enhancement of Solubilization and Bioavailability of Poorly Soluble Drugs*. Additionally, he serves as the state secretary of the Society of Pharmaceutical Education and Research (SPER), Himachal Pradesh

Gagandeep Kaur is a professor at the Chitkara University School of Pharmacy, Chitkara University, Himachal Pradesh, India, and a distinguished researcher in the field of medicinal chemistry and drug discovery. She earned her Ph.D. in Pharmaceutical Sciences in 2018 from Maharishi Markandeshwar (Deemed to be) University, Mullana. Kaur is widely recognized for her contributions to the synthesis of medicinal compounds and their pharmacological evaluation, with a strong emphasis on translating chemical innovations into therapeutic applications. Her research expertise encompasses the design and synthesis of heterocyclic compounds, molecular docking, computational drug design, and natural product chemistry. Over the years, she has made significant contributions to the development of novel bioactive molecules with promising pharmacological potential, reflecting a robust integration of synthetic and in silico approaches. An accomplished academician, Kaur has actively participated in over 25 national and international conferences, seminars, and faculty development programs, demonstrating her commitment to continuous learning and academic excellence. She has published more than 35 research and review articles in reputed peer-reviewed journals and has contributed 15 book chapters to Scopus-indexed publications. Her strong inclination toward innovation is reflected in her intellectual property achievements, with over 10 patents filed, including 5 granted by the Indian Patent Office. In addition to her research accomplishments, Kaur is known for her student-centric approach and academic leadership, fostering a dynamic and research-oriented learning environment. Through her sustained efforts, she continues to advance the frontiers of pharmaceutical chemistry and drug discovery.

Dhriti Verma currently serves as an assistant professor at the Chitkara University School of Pharmacy, Chitkara University, Himachal Pradesh. She earned her Ph.D. in Pharmaceutical Sciences from Shoolini University, Solan. With a strong academic foundation and a deep interest in pharmaceutical innovation, Verma has established herself as a promising researcher and educator. Her scholarly contributions include over eight research and review publications and book chapters, reflecting her active engagement in the areas of novel drug delivery systems and phytopharmaceuticals. Complementing her academic pursuits, she has also filed six patents, underscoring her commitment to translating research into impactful innovations. Driven by curiosity and a passion for discovery, Verma continues to inspire students and peers through her dedication to teaching, research excellence, and her vision for advancing pharmaceutical sciences.

Environmental Sustainability and Green Technology in Pharmaceutical Research

Current Issues and Future Directions

Edited by
Rajnish Srivastava, Nitin Verma, Amit Chaudhary, Gagandeep Kaur and Dhriti Verma

Routledge
Taylor & Francis Group
LONDON AND NEW YORK

First published 2027
by Routledge
4 Park Square, Milton Park, Abingdon, Oxon OX14 4RN

and by Routledge
605 Third Avenue, New York, NY 10158

Routledge is an imprint of the Taylor & Francis Group, an informa business

British Library Cataloguing-in-Publication Data
A catalogue record for this book is available from the British Library

ISBN: 978-1-041-07432-8 (hbk)
ISBN: 978-1-041-07431-1 (pbk)
ISBN: 978-1-003-64048-6 (ebk)

DOI: 10.4324/9781003640486

Typeset in Times New Roman
by codeMantra

Contents

Figures

Tables

Contributors

Shikha Aggarwal, Guru Gobind Singh College of Pharmacy, Yamuna Nagar, Haryana, India.

Snigdha Bhardwaj, Department of Pharmaceutics, KIET School of Pharmacy, KIET Group of Institutions, Ghaziabad, Delhi-NCR, India.

Amit Chaudhary, Chitkara University School of Pharmacy, Chitkara University, Himachal Pradesh, India.

Kanupriya Chauhan, Moradabad Educational Trust Faculty of Pharmacy, Moradabad, Uttar Pradesh, India.

Bhawna Chopra, Guru Gobind Singh College of Pharmacy, Yamuna Nagar, Haryana, India.

Dev Prakash Dahiya, School of Pharmacy, Abhilashi University, Mandi, Himachal Pradesh, India.

Manisha Dhiman, Shiva Institute of Pharmacy, Bilaspur, Himachal Pradesh, India.

Kamal Dua, Discipline of Pharmacy, Graduate School of Health, University of Sydney, Sydney, Australia.

Sushil Giri, Axis Institute of Pharmacy, Kapur, Uttar Pradesh, India.

Kapil Kumar Goel, Pharmaceutical Chemistry Division, Department of Pharmaceutical Sciences, Gurukul Kangri Deemed to be University, Haridwar, India.

Diksha Gulati, Guru Gobind Singh College of Pharmacy, Yamuna Nagar, Haryana, India.

Mandeep Kumar Gupta, Amity Institute of Pharmacy, Amity University, Lucknow Campus, Uttar Pradesh, India.

Shalini Juglan, Pharmaceutical Chemistry Division, Department of Pharmaceutical Sciences, Gurukul Kangri Deemed to be University, Haridwar, India.

Neha Kanojia, Chitkara University School of Pharmacy, Chitkara University, Himachal Pradesh, India.

Gagandeep Kaur, Chitkara University School of Pharmacy, Chitkara University, Himachal Pradesh, India.

Hurmat, Chitkara University School of Pharmacy, Chitkara University, Himachal Pradesh, India.

Anil Kumar, Department of Pharmaceutical Science, Geeta University, Naultha, Panipat, Haryana, India.

Anu Kumar, Department of Biotechnology, Chandigarh University, Punjab, India.

Jatin Kumar, Chitkara University School of Pharmacy, Chitkara University, Himachal Pradesh, India.

Lalit Kumar, Shiva Institute of Pharmacy, Bilaspur, Himachal Pradesh, India.

Geetanjali Mehara, Moradabad Educational Trust Faculty of Pharmacy, Moradabad, Uttar Pradesh, India.

Devika Rana, School of Pharmacy, APG Shimla University, Himachal Pradesh, India.

Anchal Sharma, Shiva Institute of Pharmacy, Bilaspur, Himachal Pradesh, India.

Aruna Sharma, Chitkara University School of Pharmacy, Chitkara University, Himachal Pradesh, India.

Karan Sharma, Shiva Institute of Pharmacy, Bilaspur, Himachal Pradesh, India.

Nitin Sharma, Department of Pharmaceutics, Amity Institute of Pharmacy, Amity University, Noida, Uttar Pradesh, India.

Shivam Sharma, Guru Gobind Singh College of Pharmacy, Yamuna Nagar, Haryana, India.

Vikas Sharma, Guru Gobind Singh College of Pharmacy, Yamuna Nagar, Haryana, India.

Akriti Singh, Chitkara University School of Pharmacy, Chitkara University, Himachal Pradesh, India.

Peeush Singhal, Pharmaceutical Chemistry Division, Department of Pharmaceutical Sciences, Gurukul Kangri Deemed to be University, Haridwar, India.

Vikas Solanki, Chitkara University Institute of Engineering and Technology, Chitkara University, Punjab, India.

Parul Sood, Chitkara University School of Pharmacy, Chitkara University, Himachal Pradesh, India.

Rajnish Srivastava, Chitkara University School of Pharmacy, Chitkara University, Himachal Pradesh, India.

Somesh Thapliyal, Department of Pharmaceutical Sciences, Hemvati Nandan Bahuguna (HNB) Garhwal University, Srinagar, Garhwal, Uttarakhand, India.

Suraj Tyagi, Pharmaceutical Chemistry Division, Department of Pharmaceutical Sciences, Gurukul Kangri Deemed to be University, Haridwar, India.

Dhriti Verma, Chitkara University School of Pharmacy, Chitkara University, Himachal Pradesh, India.

Ritu Vishnoi, Pharmaceutical Chemistry Division, Department of Pharmaceutical Sciences, Gurukul Kangri Deemed to be University, Haridwar, India.

1 Optimizing Healthcare Management through Sustainability

Anchal Sharma, Anu Kumar, Manisha Dhiman, Karan Sharma, Amit Chaudhary, and Lalit Kumar

1 Introduction

Sustainability across different sectors is increasingly prioritized because of the demands of urgent climate change addressing, and thus zero-order targets are met by 2050 (Verdonck & Verniers, 2023). Operational innovation and patient-centered approaches are the major goals of healthcare management for patient outcome enhancements and hence maximum efficacy. To use predictive analytics and to improve the workflow and resource allocation effectively, various technologies such as telemedicine, artificial intelligence, and electronic healthcare records are widely used (g training, 2024). To overcome the negative consequences of global issues such as aging of population, climatic changes, and thus environmental degradation, sustainable development has followed the future prediction of 2030 for the development of sustainability, which was adopted by United Nations Member States in 2015 and is specific to healthcare. Gender equity, good health and well-being, clean water and sanitation, and affordable and clean energy are the specific issues where healthcare teams are directly involved in the key process of development of sustainable goals (Mostepainuk et al., 2023).

Healthcare administration involves the major and essential components such as analyzing varied patient demands using cultural competency, having good verbal communication, and treatment planning for personalized care, in which patient-centered care cornerstones are usually involved. Various programs of preventive care, group buying, and value-based models are included by an organization or industry as cost containment tactics without reducing the standards or measures. For the development of staff as an investment, different well-designed programs, reward systems, and ongoing training sessions are added for outstanding care using a competent, dedicated, and motivated team (Kwame & Petrucka, 2021).

To obtain an effective and excellent result from patients, healthcare administration works as a milestone for all the tactics. Problems for maintaining the industry standards and thus proactively facing the problems of actual dashboard decisions can be accessed using data-driven endeavors using the assessment of KPIs (Adekugbe et al., 2024).

In the current era, medical buildings are being optimized by the researchers to explore the advanced technology potential, thus enhancing the deep learning

DOI: 10.4324/9781003640486-1

technology development, usually by graph convolutional networks (GCN). Building design can be more accurately optimized using GCN, which is effective for maintaining the complex spatial and functional relationship and thus able to distinguish the influence pattern and dependencies of learning using different facilities (Hu et al., 2024). This includes the functional interdependency and spatial connectivity between the examination rooms, waiting areas, and also the medical facilities. For example, the protocol for infection control must be considered proximity to reduce the delay of diagnostic areas while aligning with the design of efficient examination rooms. Graph convolutional networks can be used to model these multi-dimensional relationships; thus, intelligence as well as accuracy of architectural design can be improved. These approaches ensure operational excellence as well as resilience; thus, the future needs can be adopted for the revolutionization. There is generally a lot of difference between the designs of healthcare buildings, as well as commercial or residential buildings. Patient flow design is the first healthcare building that must be considered. Complex healthcare equipment or configurations or emergency situations must be rapidly responded to, and these come under second-tier healthcare buildings. Functional requirements and structural characteristics of the buildings can be analyzed using reduction in energy consumption and thus can be optimized using the Complex Grid Network (CGN) model as a complex building model for energy consumption. Lighting systems, air conditioning systems, and equipment operations can be affected by the energy demand of medical buildings; thus, CGN model optimization not only accounts for the functional area layout but also, by configuring and optimizing the equipment rooms, leads to more energy consumption of the overall building.

Industrialization and the pharmaceutical sector increased day by day, and with this, the impact on the environment also increased due to industrial waste and pollution. The ecological effects of conventional medication production, which frequently entails dangerous chemicals, large amounts of waste, and excessive energy consumption, are putting continuous pressure on the pharmaceutical sector to embrace sustainable techniques (Kumar & Maurya, 2024).

In the pharmaceutical sector, sustainability is crucial for lowering pollution levels in the environment, enhancing resource efficiency, and shielding public health. It supports long-term economic growth and regulatory compliance while guaranteeing moral, low-waste production. Green chemistry and eco-friendly production are important areas of focus (Sah et al., 2025).

Green technology in pharmaceutical sciences and research is an essential and vital sector that fosters the demands of environmentally sustainable methods in drug research. The aim of green chemistry is to minimize the usage and manufacturing of chemicals that are hazardous to the environment. It offers a sustainable solution by minimizing pollution in industries and protecting both human health and our ecosystem (Msingh et al., 2021).

Green technology, which is commonly referred to as sustainable or environmentally friendly innovation, is now a vital pursuit in the area of pharmaceutical sciences because the ecological impact of drug manufacture, use, and disposal is growing. As the world is becoming increasingly aware of the importance of environmental health and the need to be more regulated, the field of pharmaceutical research is experiencing a paradigm shift in the sense that it is trying to become cleaner, safer, and more sustainable. This part explains the existing difficulties in the pharmaceutical industry in using green technology and provides future guidelines to reach the sustainability of the environment in drug development and pharmaceutical research.

1.1 Importance of Sustainability in Healthcare

To improve public health and thus to save lives, the healthcare sector possesses significant environmental impacts, such as:

- a Greenhouse gas emissions
- b Resource consumption
- c Waste generation
- d Air and water pollution
- e Supply chain impacts
- f Deforestation and land use

1.1.1 Greenhouse Gas Emissions

For population health, climatic change is the largest threat (Romanello et al., 2022). From the beginning of the 21st century, there has been a significant rise in the temperature, and it is in the continuous process of accelerating speed. Earth's mean global temperature is recorded as the highest since 2023, 0.6° higher as compared to 1950–2020; the critical level of pre-industrial temperature approximately reached 1.5°C (Copernicus In., 2023). The ecosystem, water and food production, and healthcare well-being of the population have been affected by global warming all over the world (Roberts et al., 2022). Around 5% of global greenhouse gas emissions are affected by the healthcare sector, which includes carbon dioxide, methane, and ozone (Pichler et al., 2019). The greenhouse gas emissions in the healthcare sector involve various sectors.

1.1.1.1 ENERGY USE

Hospital and healthcare facilities are energy-intensive, relying on electricity and heating and cooling systems that often use fossil fuels. Optimizing healthcare management through sustainability involves reducing overall energy consumption via energy-efficient upgrades, implementing renewable energy solutions like solar and geothermal, and leveraging smart technologies such as IoT and BMS to monitor and control energy use. These strategies, when integrated, will lead to the reduction of operational costs while also promoting the facility's resilience, but most importantly, this will reduce the health sector's massive carbon footprint toward promoting environmental sustainability.

1.1.1.2 MEDICAL SUPPLY CHAIN

The manufacture, transportation, and end-of-life cycle of medical supplies/equipment form part of the supply chain and contribute to environmental impact.

1.1.1.2.1 Strategies for Energy Efficiency and Sustainability

Upgrade Infrastructure: Replace inefficient lighting with LEDs and improve building insulation to regulate the temperature rather than relying on heating, ventilation, and air conditioning (HVAC) systems.

Energy-Efficient Equipment: Invest in energy-efficient medical devices, boilers, and equipment for a reduction in power usage.

Implement Smart Technologies: Building management systems can maintain the building's HVAC, lighting, and power systems with predictive control and real-time adjustments that minimize energy wastage. The IoT-enabled sensors will monitor and control lighting, temperature, and equipment usage to ensure proper deployment of resources.

Embrace Renewable Energy: Installing on-site solar panels, wind turbines, and geothermal systems from various sources of renewable energy will offset reliance on the grid and generate clean power. Following are the measures to be taken in order to embrace the sustainable operational use of renewable energy:

- i **Conduct Energy Audits**: Analyze energy usage to detect the improvement areas.
- ii **Promote Energy-Conscious Behavior**: Educate staff on energy-saving practices to develop a sustainable culture in the organization.
- iii **Improve Data Management**: Utilization of cloud computing services in managing data from an offsite, thus reducing energy requirements from data management devices.
- iv **Sustainable Procurement**: Choosing suppliers and products based on certain environmentally friendly attributes to mitigate the whole energy supply chain footprint.

1.1.1.2.2 Benefits of Sustainable Energy in Healthcare

Reduced Operational Costs: Savings in electricity and gas charges can result in substantial savings.

Environmental Impact: Reduced levels of greenhouse gas emissions, which in turn helps in the moderation of the effects of global warming on the environment.

Enhanced Resilience: More independence from other grids to provide reliable power to critical care devices.

Improved Environment: Better air quality and effective temperature control help in maintaining a healthful and comfortable working environment.

Positive Public Image: He/she demonstrates an enthusiasm for environmentalism that is highly valued by the public and investors.

1.1.2 Resource Consumption

The healthcare sector uses a lot of natural resource consumption. It is an area of major significant achievement in sustainability in healthcare departments. It includes efficient use of energy. It also includes efficient use of energy and water, medical supplies, and many other resources in a bid to reduce the impact on the environment as well as cost. Most effective utilization refers to more efficient use of energy.

1.1.3 Waste Generation

To protect the environment and public health, medical waste management is considered a critical global imperative. All the healthcare activities are generated from this complex waste stream and thus composed of different materials, including personal protective equipment (PPE) and medical devices to pharmaceuticals, radioactive substances, and chemicals. In medical waste management there were unprecedented crises during the COVID-19 pandemic worldwide, exposing significant systemic vulnerabilities. Environmental and health implications have become substantial using medical waste management (Karimi, 2024; Liang, 2021).

1.1.4 Air and Water Pollution

Medical waste management treatment, particularly using thermal methods, leads to air emissions that may lead to health issues as well as environmental risks (Singh & Ogusritan, 2022). Primary pollutants include dioxins and furans from the incineration of chlorinated plastics, heavy metals from various medical devices and materials, particulate matter from combustion processes, and acid gases from chemical waste treatment (Bolan et al., 2023). Emissions can be reduced significantly using control systems that manage modern air pollution as per the recommendations and demonstrations of researchers. Fabric filters lead to particulate matter removal up to 99%, while 90–99% of dioxin reactions can occur using activated carbon injection. Ninety-five percent of acid gases can be removed effectively using wet scrubbers (Kaushal et al., 2024).

1.1.5 Supply Chain Impact

To derive different social responsibilities and thus ensure the economy of the medical supply chain, there is also a need to address the environmental issues for which today's healthcare sector can be critically managed using sustainable supply chain management (Das, 2017). The medical history demonstrates the challenges, such as the complex network of suppliers, manufacturers, distributors, and healthcare providers while meeting the demand of patient quality (Sarkis et al., 2021). The healthcare sector plays a pivotal role in society, aiming to promote well-being and preserve human health. However, the delivery of healthcare services is not devoid of environmental, social, and economic impacts. As such, the importance of sustainability in healthcare supply chains cannot be overstated. In the light of the supply chains of the healthcare industry, the concept of sustainability comes into play for several valid reasons. To begin with, sustainability in the supply chains of the healthcare industry is of the essence and of vital significance so as to reduce the adverse effects of the same on the environment to the maximum possible extent (Duque-Uribe et al., 2019). This is because supply chains of the healthcare industry are found to affect the environment significantly due to large volumes of wastes generated pertaining to medicines that have to be disposed of or the energy used in the operation of different hospitals and clinics. Moreover, the greenhouse effect has also started impacting the environment due to large quantities of greenhouse gases emanating out of the operations of various clinics and hospitals. To sum up, the supply chains of the same can reduce the negative impact on the environment to a maximum possible extent so as to save the environment from damage (Kanokphanvanich et al., 2023).

1.2 Key Components of Sustainable Supply Chain Management in the Medical Sector

The definition of a sustainable supply chain in the medical industry embraces a general approach geared toward managing the movement of services or products and information groups from supply organizations to healthcare providers with sustainability in mind. Some of the key elements that contribute to sustainable development and further continuous improvement within a medical supply chain are as follows. Ethical sourcing refers to the process of selecting suppliers or partners based on priorities such as corporate social responsibility, fair labor standards, and environmental conservation. In the medical industry, such ethics in procurement means ensuring safety, efficiency, and quality in drugs, healthcare products, and consumables. Screening suppliers for their compliance with international standards and regulations thus enables healthcare organizations to cut various associated risks related to environmental degradation, child labor, and forced labor (Sampson, 2021). Environmental sustainability refers to the contribution of medical supply chains to minimizing environmental impacts through waste reduction, energy efficiency, and pollution prevention. Medical facilities generate loads of wastes, including hazardous medical waste, pharmaceuticals, and single-use plastics. These healthcare organizations reduce their potential harm to the natural environment and further contribute to nature conservation through the implementation of recycling programs, adoption of reusable medical devices, and minimization of packaging wastes (Sousa et al., 2021; Elabed et al., 2019). Stakeholder collaboration and engagement create mutual partnerships and alliances across the medical supply chain. Healthcare organizations need to respond closely to the issue of sustainability challenges and driving collective action from suppliers, manufacturers, distributors, regulators, and other stakeholders. Together with stakeholders, joint procurement, supplier development, and industry-wide standards development provide a different array of opportunities for stakeholders to leverage their combined influence in order to effect positive change and drive sustainable practices.

Continuous improvement and innovation involve ongoing pursuits of excellence and the exploration of new approaches to sustainability within the medical supply chain. The emerging technologies and best practices currently need to be embraced by the healthcare organizations that lead to learning and encourage innovation from stakeholders. It was expected that a culture of continuous improvement within a healthcare organization may help them to adapt quickly to changing market dynamics, regulatory requirements, and stakeholder expectations while driving progress toward sustainability goals.

1.3 Key Strategies for Sustainability in Healthcare

The healthcare sector needs to adopt sustainable practices to reduce the environmental footprint while maintaining high-quality care. A multifaceted approach addressing energy use, waste management, procurement, and infrastructure is essential. Below are the key strategies in healthcare:

- i Transition of Renewable Energy
- ii Improve Waste Management
- iii Sustainable Procurement
- iv Optimize Water Use
- v Design and Build Green Facilities
- vi Promote Sustainable Transportation
- vii Incorporate Education and Culture Chains
- viii Invest in Digital Solutions
- ix Monitor and Report Sustainability Progress

1.3.1 *Transition of Renewal Energy*

To formulate a hospital design using sustainability, a renewable energy transition plays a major role. Various renewable energy sources available online are adopted by different hospitals, such as solar panels, wind turbines, and geothermal systems, so that the use or demand of conventional power grids may get reduced (Kyriakarakos & Dounis, 2020). Installing solar panels on the rooftops of hospitals leads to the conversion of electricity from sunlight and can be used as a power source for different hospital functions. Energy or power demand of hospitals can be fulfilled by solar power installation as per recent studies, but factors to be considered are space availability, climate, and location (Guerrero & Ramos, 2023). This leads to improvement of healthcare facilities by reducing the fluctuations in energy costs and also leads to reduction of greenhouse gas emissions; thus, long-term operational savings can be enhanced (Elam Cheren & Ashok Kumar, 2022).

1.3.2 *Improve Waste Management*

Healthcare waste management is the waste produced by healthcare activities. It is commonly known as hospital waste, medical waste, or infectious waste. The major sources include hospitals, health posts, emergency medical care services, healthcare centers, and dispensaries. Other sources are dental clinics, psychiatric hospitals, and illegal drug users. The waste management improvements mainly involve pathological waste, chemical waste, and hazards from infectious waste. Pathological waste includes human tissues, including placentas, body parts, and blood. Anatomical waste is the subgroup of pathological waste and consists of recognizable body parts. Sharp needles, infusion sets, scalps, blades, and broken glasses. Pharmaceutical waste: expired or no longer needed pharmaceuticals, items contaminated by or containing pharmaceutical bottles and boxes. Genotoxic waste: substances with genotoxic properties, meaning they can cause genetic damage, such as certain drugs and genotoxic chemicals (Tilley et al., 2021).

1.3.3 Sustainable Procurement

Sustainable procurement of goods and services for healthcare must address the entire lifecycle of healthcare delivery, spanning the manufacture and supply of goods such as pharmaceutical products and medical devices, the actual delivery of healthcare with efficient and sustainable procurement of services for resources like water and energy, and appropriate disposal of used products at the end of life, including waste, packaging materials, and food waste. The incorporation of appropriate technical specifications in tender documents for the sustainable procurement of goods is a strategic way to create demand for the production of such goods. The Sustainable Procurement in Health Care Guide, a useful resource recently released by Health Care Without Harm, provides a step-by-step guide to sustainable procurement in healthcare (HCWH & GGHH, 2020).

1.3.4 Optimize Water Use

Optimizing water use in healthcare requires understanding it as a critical system input, intrinsically linked to energy consumption, waste streams, and overall ecological health. The theoretical underpinning for water conservation in healthcare is based on ecological principles, systems thinking, and an understanding of the interrelation between resource management and operational resilience.

In its essence, the conservation of water in this sector operates behind the principle that water is indeed a limited and very important resource whose use needs to be optimized to meet both short-term operational imperatives and long-term ecological sustainability. This approach looks at a healthcare facility not in isolation but as a complicated system within a greater socio-ecological environment. The theoretical basis informally leans heavily on ecological science, given the understanding that water forms a crucial part of biogeochemical cycles. Healthcare facilities, due to their design and function, create considerable demands on regional and local water cycling.

This consumption not only affects the quantity of freshwater availability for ecosystems and other human uses but also influences energy use, as the treatment, transport, and heating/cooling of water all involve significant energy inputs. In effect, therefore, reducing the water use naturally contributes to energy conservation and greenhouse gas emission reductions, aligning with broader climate action goals. Systems thinking is the analytical frame within which these interdependencies become more understandable. It underscores feedback loops, emergent properties, and nonlinear interactions across the entire water footprint in facilities. For example, low-flow fixtures contribute to lowered direct water demands but might also decrease wastewater loads and demands for hot water heating—a benefit cascade. Conversely, losses due to unchecked leaks or inefficient processes lead to systemic inefficiencies that increase resource waste and heighten operational costs.

This shifts the focus from a simple model of inputs versus outputs in the direction of dynamics and interlinkages behind the water use within the complex environment of a healthcare institution. The theory posits that by meticulously managing water as a critical system input, facilities can enhance their operational efficiency, reduce their environmental impact, and build greater resilience against water scarcity and associated risks (https://term).

1.3.5 Design and Build Green Facilities

"Green building" refers to good design and practices of management in various building construction phases, and thus, using this operation, energy and a healthy environment can be promoted. To develop and promote the green building principles, the leading organization in the United States is the US Green Building Council, a broad coalition including representation from the construction industry, the financial sector, government, and public interest organizations.

The Green Guide of Healthcare (GGHC) simultaneously includes the green building and healthcare. Various environmental health principles and practices such as planning, construction of designs, operations, and healthcare facility maintenance can be improved using these healthcare kits. For the development of healthcare building design and healthcare industries, this guide played a major role in healthier building materials, and leadership goals have been achieved by the healthcare industries for bringing the health issues to green design (https://term).

Construction industry representation, the financial sector, government, and public interest organizations, along with green building principles, in a US board coalition are being developed and promoted by the US Green Building Council (USGBC). The USGBC and GGHC are working cooperatively to integrate the principles developed in the Green Guide into a healthcare-specific version of the USGBC's third-party certified LEED program.

Healthcare Business Network is a national network of professionals that include green building professionals, environmental and health activists, socially responsible investment advocates, and persons who are interested in preserving the global environment and thus leads to improvement of public health by providing healthier building materials.

1.3.6 Promote Sustainable Transportation

Sustainable transportation promotion is important for health researchers, policymakers, and transportation planners. Prevention of disease, prolongation of life, and health equity promotion, as well as social, physical, and mental well-being, are the major concerns for population health. Population health for sustainable transportation can be improved using transportation choices and neighbor walkability as well as by increasing the exposure of green spaces. Population choice can have an impact on sustainable transportation policies. Important evidence using fruitful research on these topics can lead to transportation planners, policy developers, community officials, and public health experts (Menon, 2022).

1.3.7 Incorporate Education and Culture Chain

Education directly impacts health literacy, socioeconomic status, and health behaviors, which in turn influence overall health.

- **Knowledge and skills**: Education provides individuals with the skills to understand complex health information and navigate the healthcare system. A strong educational foundation is associated with better health literacy, using which informed decisions can be chosen by people for their well-being.
- **Healthy behaviors**: People with higher education led to practicing healthier behaviors, such as avoiding smoking and obesity. This is often because education encourages and fosters an appreciation of health-enhancing lifestyle choices.
- **Socioeconomic status**: Educational attainment is positively related to higher income and job security. This gives the person access to better resources that determine health, such as quality housing, nutritious food, and health insurance.
- **Community and policy**: On a larger scale, higher national education levels come under better public health conditions, including lower infant mortality and higher vaccination rates. Education is also used by public health professionals to implement health promotion programs and campaigns.

Culture influences every aspect of human behavior, including beliefs about health, illness, and treatment. Ignorance of cultural contents leads to misunderstandings, distrust, and poor health outcomes.

- **Perceptions of health and illness**: A person's culture can shape their perception of health and wellness, including their beliefs about the causes of disease. For example, a patient may attribute their illness to supernatural forces, while a provider might rely on biomedical science.
- **Healthcare decisions**: Culture affects when, where, and how patients seek help. Some cultures may prefer traditional healing practices before resorting to Western medicine, while others may require the consent of extended family members for treatment.
- **Health promotion activities**: Health promotion strategies that are not associated with cultural beliefs may be rejected by a community. Culturally sensitive health education materials, however, are more likely to be accepted and acted upon.
- **Communication barriers**: Cultural differences can lead to communication challenges between patients and healthcare providers. For example, a patient

might avoid direct eye contact as a sign of respect, while a provider might misinterpret this behavior.

- **Integrating education and culture for healthcare**: The effective integration of education and culture is a cyclical process that promotes better health outcomes. This is often accomplished through cultural competency and safety training for healthcare professionals.

1.4 Key Educational Strategies for Healthcare Professionals

- **Cultural competency training**: This training equips healthcare providers with the skills and knowledge to effectively work with patients who are from different cultural backgrounds. It is vital for all health workers to receive education on the specific needs of their patients.
- **Experiential learning**: Educational experiences such as cultural immersion or community-based training provide a deeper understanding of patients' living environments and circumstances.
- **Simulation-based education**: Using tools like role-playing with standardized patients allows students to practice communication skills in a safe environment.
- **Community involvement**: Partnering with community leaders, advocates, and patients helps ensure health education and promotion materials are culturally relevant and acceptable to the intended audience. By incorporating both educational tools and cultural awareness, healthcare systems can create an inclusive environment that builds trust and ultimately leads to improved health outcomes and reduced health disparities (Amran et al., 2019; Balabel & Alwetaishi, 2021).
- **Invest in digital solutions**: In the 1990s, as the 'e-health' term was coined, various healthcare organizations started using healthcare technologies. As per the suggestions, in the last two decades, there was more relevancy in digital transformation in healthcare. A recent study shows that digital transformation is the research area of the future, which is similar to industry topic 4.0. All the new healthcare treatments, including digital transportation or its applications to develop new research for the treatment purpose, are termed Healthcare 4.0. (H4.0) (Hariharan & Kumar, 2025). Both the administrative support processes and patient care come under these consequences. The COVID-19 pandemic accelerated the digital transformation of healthcare organizations, leading approximately 75% of healthcare organizations to increase the adoption of digital transformation as a way to provide enhanced assistance to patients (Aittasalo et al., 2017).
- **Monitor and report sustainability progress**: An essential social challenge for social healthcare services and consumers is to maintain sustainable healthcare using high-quality, safe, and effective healthcare. In fact, in the healthcare system, cost-saving potential for efficient use of energy and other sources is clear, but it may take a longer time for environmentally friendly hospitals, healthcare structures, and clinical laboratories to be stable as per norms. These goals can be achieved using a common vision for future actions and the European Union healthcare system. These goals can be achieved using the implementation of the European Union policies and a visionary plan for future action. All the social

implementers must be responsible and accountable for the true cost and risk of polluting nature, which leads to serious consequences for public health and the environment. Individual efforts may remain insufficient; thus, the entire society should be responsible for reducing the environmental issues for waste management. Public health and environmental risks may lead to serious consequences if it is too late to take action for reducing the environmental footprints. Various recommendations and solutions involving reduction of waste during collection and recycling, thus avoiding different environmental issues, can be raised and implemented only if healthcare individuals as well as stakeholders are accountable for actions and environmental impacts (Ferrigno et al., 2023).

2 Green Technology in Pharmaceutical Sciences and Research

2.1 Principles of Green Chemistry in Pharmaceuticals

Green chemistry principles emphasize the use of safe and renewable raw materials and nontoxic chemicals and processes to improve energy efficiency by conducting reactions at room temperature, using biodegradable material, reducing the use of hazardous solvents and auxiliaries, and avoiding waste rather than its treatment

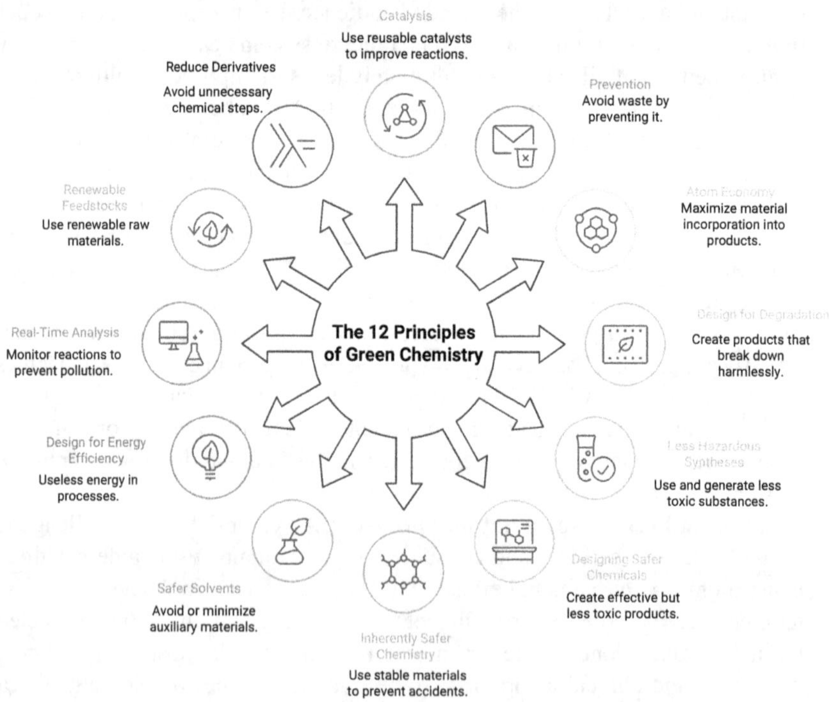

Figure 1.1 Principle of green chemistry.

(Figure 1.1). The ultimate goal is to make drug manufacturing and testing safe, sustainable, and environmentally friendly (Tang et al., 2005; Al-Shatti et al., 2023).

2.2 Green Synthesis and Drug Development

In the context of drug development, "Green synthesis" refers to the use of green technology in chemistry concepts to manufacture pharmaceutical molecules and create drug evaluation methods in such a way that is safe, affordable, and environmentally beneficial (Figure 1.2) (Kar et al., 2021; Mishra et al., 2021).

2.2.1 Biocatalysis and Enzyme-Based Synthesis

Biocatalysis is a potent tool to make processes sustainable and safe due to its numerous advantages in green technology. Nowadays, this technique is adopted by many pharmaceutical and food industries. Examples of biocatalysis, like enzymes, can work under neutral pH and room temperature; due to their high specificity, they

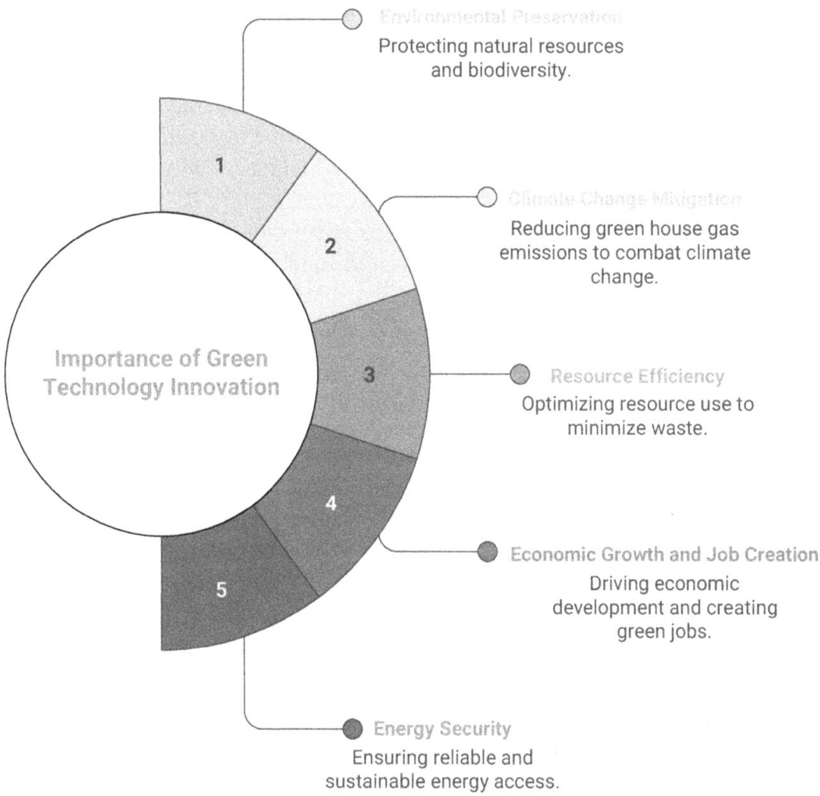

Figure 1.2 Importance of green technology innovation.

produce less waste, and due to their biodegradable nature, they are environmentally friendly (Kim et al., 2024; O'Connell et al., 2024).

2.2.2 *Solvent-Free and Aqueous-Phase Reactions*

In chemical operations, solvents are the significant source of waste and causes of environmental contamination. By reducing or eliminating the usage of solvents, green chemistry aims to lessen their harmful, combustible, and non-renewable effects. Green technology emphasizes replacing toxic chemicals, solvent-free synthesis, and solid-state reactions (Tickner et al., 2021; Aljuboori et al., 2022).

2.3 ***Green Analytical Techniques***

Analytical chemistry is one of the important branches of science that play a crucial role in quality control and product development. Various analytical techniques like chromatography and spectroscopy generate a large quantity of organic solvent as waste. These volatile solvents create a harmful impact on individual health and the environment, so there is a need to develop such techniques that are environmentally friendly and safe during human exposure. The development of green technology attracts many pharmaceuticals by means of eliminating or reducing organic solvents, replacing existing ones with ethanol and water and with other green alternatives without hampering the quality of the test or the performance of the analytical instrument. These techniques are budget-friendly, energy-efficient, and sustainable (Yang et al., 2015; Kaya et al., 2022).

Microscale analysis, energy-efficient instrumentation (e.g., UV-LED spectroscopy), recyclable columns in chromatography, and techniques for green sample preparation like solid-phase microextraction (SPME) are a few examples of green analytical practices (Sajid & Płotka-Wasylka, 2022).

2.4 ***Sustainable Formulation Development***

Active pharmaceutical ingredients (APIs) are essential to protect human life and well-being, but these APIs, their metabolites, and transformation products also pollute the environment and pose risks to human and ecological health. A sustainable solution is to design greener APIs with reduced environmental impact. This includes integrating ecological considerations into the drug investigation and development process.

The active pharmaceutical ingredients' (APIs') and excipient whole life cycle is planned holistically using a green chemistry strategy to minimize their environmental impact (Puhlmann et al., 2024; Ganesh et al., 2021).

Industries are now adopting the principles of green chemistry to develop sustainable green formulation techniques. In order to improve atom economy and decrease waste, one-pot reactions, process strengthening, and green solvents are used in pharmaceutical synthesis and formulation development by implementing the concepts of green chemistry, like biodegradable excipients, melt granulation techniques, and nanotechnology for drug targeting to minimize side effects (Kar et al., 2021).

2.5 Waste Reduction and Its Management

Pharmaceutical manufacturing must use a number of sustainability techniques and efficient waste management techniques to be environmentally friendly. Additionally, research is being done on recoverable and reusable precious metal catalysts from pharmaceutical waste streams. Eco-friendly packaging materials like bioplastic and recycled packaging materials in pharmaceutical packaging are initiatives to reduce waste and its environmental impact. Pharmaceutical residues in wastewater must be successfully and economically removed by advanced wastewater treatment technologies, particularly in solutions appropriate for smaller treatment facilities and less developed nations. Life cycle assessment is another strategy in green technology to assess environmental impact (Misszento & Amofah, 2024; Srivastava et al., 2021).

3 Environmental Sustainability in Pharmaceutical Research

Pharmaceutical research is developing new therapies that improve health outcomes. Standard laboratory practices can lead to heavy environmental burdens; they include high energy and water use, as well as toxic waste and air emissions. To build sustainability into this field is not just a regulatory obligation; it is a strategic process for preserving ecosystems while delivering safe and effective medicines. This chapter reviews methods for implant sustainability in research pipelines and the advantages that result for both the environment and the research enterprise.

3.1 Importance of Environmental Sustainability in Pharmaceutical Research

In the pharmaceutical industry, research and development are energy- and material-intensive. Laboratories consume electricity and heating, use purified water in large volumes, depend on rare and hazardous substances, and generate liquid and solid waste streams. Environmental sustainability seeks to cut these burdens through measures like resource equipment, green chemistry, and closed-loop waste management. Environmental impact of pharmaceutical research assessments shows that research environments can account for a large fraction of an organization's scope emissions, while laboratory solvents, residues, and packaging can contaminate water and landfills (Kümmerer, 2010). Regulatory and societal pressures are strict on environmental legislation and increasing public expectation for responsible practices and urge both research institutions and industry to fuse sustainability into their operations (Wang et al., 2020).

3.2 Sustainable Practices in Pharmaceutical Research

Sustainability requires coordinated innovation across laboratory infrastructure, reagent supervision, reaction pathway design, and life waste management.

3.2.1 Green Chemistry Principles

Green chemistry depends on engineering chemical processes that minimize or eliminate hazardous substances. In pharmaceutical research, core strategies comprise

a Selection of solvents and reagents
b Design of syntheses with reduced energy intensity
c Decrease of by-product formation

3.2.2 Energy and Resource Efficiency

Deployment of energy-efficient instrumentation, optimization of thermal control systems, and use of renewable energy sources collectively decrease the overall environmental burden (Clark & Tavener, 2007).

3.2.3 Waste Management

Systematic recycling and treatment of hazardous waste, combined with the reduction of single-use plastic and disposable laboratory items, are important for reinforcement of the sustainability agenda (Lundberg et al., 2019).

3.2.4 Sustainable Procurement

Choosing suppliers who are used to sustainable practices and who provide renewable or recycled materials reinforces the principles of a green supply chain (Kaplan & Ramachandran, 2018).

3.3 Technological Innovations Supporting Sustainability

Recent advancements in technology are driving the pursuit of sustainability in pharmaceutical research.

3.3.1 Automation and Digitalization

Automation decreases the errors and also the quantity of materials consumed, while digitalization increases experimental design and streamlines data management (Mackenzie et al., 2019).

3.3.2 Microreactor and Flow Chemistry

These two approaches are useful for more efficient chemical reactions, generating less waste and also consuming less energy than conventional batch processes (Gutmann et al., 2015).

3.3.3 *Biocatalysis*

It is an enzymatic process that provides a more environmentally friendly substitute for chemical catalysts in synthetic pathways (Hollmann et al., 2017).

3.4 *Challenges in Implementing Sustainability*

While the advantages are evident, there are numerous hindrances to their wide applicability:

3.4.1 *Cost and Investment*

In small research institutes, the cost of sustainable instruments may be higher, and the re-engineering of the processes can deter adoption since both have heavy expenses associated with them.

3.4.2 *Complexity of Regulation*

This involves the incorporation of new sustainable practices into already strict pharmaceutical regulations that require vigorous validation and continuous compliance as well.

3.4.3 *Cultural and Behavioral Factors*

Adoption may be slowed by researchers' resistance to change and ignorance of sustainability (Jones et al., 2020).

3.5 *Case Studies and Best Practices*

Case Study 1: Pfizer's Green Chemistry Initiative

In order to reduce waste production and improve overall process efficiency, Pfizer provides green chemistry concepts for synthesis pathways (Anastas et al., 2019).

Case Study 2: University Research Labs

According to Ruiz-Gonzalez (2025), certain university laboratories have implemented sustainable methods for managing chemical inventories and recycling solvents, resulting in reduced environmental impacts and operational expenses.

3.6 *Future Directions and Recommendations*

3.6.1 *Integration of Sustainable Metrics*

Targeted process improvements will be possible if pharmaceutical research adopts standardized measures for assessing environmental performance.

3.6.2 *Cross-Sector Collaboration*

Working together with business, academia, and government organizations will promote creative thinking and make it easier to share best practices.

3.6.3 Education and Training

Incorporating ideas into professional development and academic curricula will encourage a shift in the field's culture.

3.6.4 Investment in Sustainable Technologies

Long-term progress in sustained funding still depends on the development of green chemistry and sustainable manufacturing techniques.

4 Current Challenges and Future Directions in Green Technology and Environmental Sustainability in Pharmaceutical Sciences and Research

4.1 Current Challenges in Green Pharmaceutical Practices

4.1.1 Environmental Contamination and Waste Management

Among these, perhaps the most pressing issue is that of environmental discharge of active pharmaceutical ingredients (API) and intermediates. These drug substances can enter aquatic systems via pharmaceutical industry waste discharge and inappropriate waste disposal methods, as well as patient excretion. These drugs have potential harmful effects on aquatic ecosystems, including antimicrobial drugs, hormones, and analgesics.

The management of pharmaceutical wastes remains an inefficient process in both low and middle-income countries. Current wastewater treatments are not able to properly break down complex compounds originating from pharmaceuticals.

4.1.2 Energy-Intensive Manufacturing Processes

Conventional pharmaceutical production methods use a lot of energy and non-renewable resources. In certain situations, high energy consumption reduces the competitiveness of green alternatives by increasing manufacturing costs and the carbon footprint.

4.1.3 Use of Hazardous Solvents and Reagents

In the synthesis and formulation of drugs, organic solvents are widely utilized. Many of these solvents are dangerous to the environment, poisonous, and volatile. Solubility, yield, reaction rate, and scalability problems impede efforts to replace them with more environmentally friendly solvents.

4.1.4 Regulatory and Economic Barriers

Technological advancements frequently outpace regulatory systems. It is challenging to encourage environmentally friendly methods in pharmaceutical regulation due to the absence of green chemistry measures. Additionally, a major financial barrier is the high cost of switching to green technologies, particularly for small firms and academic research labs.

4.1.5 Limited Awareness and Training

The lack of knowledge and instruction on sustainable procedures among pharmaceutical experts is another issue that is often disregarded. The culture of pharmaceutical research and teaching still does not sufficiently incorporate green chemistry concepts.

4.2 Emerging Trends and Innovations in Green Pharmaceutical Research

4.2.1 Green Chemistry and Catalysis

Green chemistry is changing the synthetic pathways by maximizing atom economy and minimizing the use of hazardous chemicals. The development of green solvents and biocatalysts (such as water-based systems, supercritical CO_2, and ionic liquids) is leading to cleaner processes.

4.2.2 Continuous Manufacturing and Process Analytical Technology

Process Analytical Technology (PAT) and continuous production systems help with real-time process tracking, which leads to better goods, less waste, and more effective use of resources. These technologies have a significant impact on green production and align with the Quality by Design (QbD) methodology.

4.2.3 Cell-Based Production and Biopharmaceuticals

The pharmaceutical industry is increasingly becoming biologically based with the emergence of biologics such as monoclonal antibodies and RNA-based therapeutics. These are usually more sustainable (renewable inputs and less hazardous waste when compared to conventional chemical synthesis).

4.3 Continuous Manufacturing and Process Analytical Technology

Implementation of PAT and continuous manufacturing systems assists in monitoring processes in real time, resulting in improved utilization of resources, minimization of waste, and enhancement of product quality. These technologies are in line with the QbD strategy, and they play a major role in green manufacturing. Green manufacturing using QbD can be implemented using various software such as DesignExpert, SigmaStat, and GraphPad Prism.

4.4 Cell-Based Production and Biopharmaceuticals

The rise of biologics, such as monoclonal antibodies and RNA-based drugs, is causing the pharmaceutical industry to transition to biologically based manufacturing. They tend to be more sustainable, since they can utilize renewable resources and generate less harmful waste than conventional chemical synthesis.

4.5 Drug Delivery Green Nanotechnology

The application of nanotechnology in drug delivery is gaining popularity in order to increase efficacy and decrease dosage. Plant extracts or microbial synthesis of nanoparticles are more sustainable alternatives to traditional methods that use toxic chemicals and energy-intensive processes.

4.6 Environmental Risk Assessment (ERA) and Life Cycle Assessment (LCA)

LCA and ERA are currently being used by pharmaceutical companies to assess the environmental effects of drugs during their entire life cycle, including extracting materials and final disposal. The evidence-based creation of more ecologically friendly formulations and packaging is encouraged by these assessments.

4.7 Future Directions for Sustainability in Pharmaceutical Sciences

4.7.1 Integration of Circular Economy Principles

Resource consumption and waste production can be significantly decreased by putting circular economy ideas into practice, such as solvent recycling, waste valorization, and sustainable procurement. To close the loop, collaborations throughout the pharmaceutical supply chain are essential.

4.7.2 Green Drug Design and Degradable Pharmaceuticals

It is possible to reduce environmental contamination by creating "benign-by-design" medications that break down into nontoxic compounds after usage. This necessitates a fundamental change in the way that environmental persistence and pharmacological efficacy are assessed during the development process.

4.7.3 Policy Reforms and Incentives

Stronger regulations and financial incentives for sustainable pharmaceutical practices must be established by governments and international regulatory organizations. Mandatory environmental disclosures, tax breaks, and green certifications may encourage innovation and compliance.

4.7.4 Education and Capacity Building

It is essential that pharmacy and pharmaceutical science courses include green chemistry and sustainability modules. A culture of environmental responsibility will be developed through workshops and training programs for researchers, industry professionals, and regulators.

4.7.5 Collaboration and Open Innovation

Green technology adoption will be accelerated through cross-sector cooperation between industry, academics, environmental organizations, and legislators.

Open innovation platforms and public–private partnerships can foster scalable solutions and reduce redundancy in research efforts.

5 Conclusion

Environmental sustainability and green technology are no longer a choice in the pharmaceutical industry. sciences—they are essential. Although there are a number of challenges such as waste management, solvent toxicity, and regulatory inertia that are still very daunting, novel approaches like green synthesis, biopharmaceuticals, and continuous manufacturing are showing the way (Kate et al., 2022; Cannon et al., 2024). The future of pharmaceutical research is in the integration of therapeutic progress with the ecological equilibrium. A systemic change, which is backed by policy, education, and collaborative innovation, is required. Make sure that the advances in the pharmaceutical industry are not achieved at the expense of global health (World Resources Institute, 2020; Karliner et al., 2019).

Green technology is encouraging safer, cleaner, and more sustainable methods, which significantly modify the way drugs are developed (Fields et al., 2021). Improved efficiency and less environmental impact are being achieved through innovations. Solvent substitution, flow chemistry, biocatalysis, AI for optimizing green synthesis, and green nanotechnology for eco-friendly drug delivery are a few examples of strategies toward environmental safety. The goals of green chemistry are further supported by renewable feedstocks and waste reduction strategies. In general, the future of drugs will be more environmentally friendly and accountable (Möller et al., 2020; Chatterjee & Kar, 2020; Ali, 2021). Environmental sustainability in pharmaceutical research is safeguarding public health and the environment (Rasulev et al., 2020). Through adopting green chemistry principles, it increases technological advances and overcomes implementation challenges. Sustainable healthcare management can also benefit from the pharmaceutical industry. All the work and cooperation will guarantee continued innovation while reducing environmental impacts (Liu et al., 2020).

Bibliography

Adekugbe, A., & Ibeh, C. (2024). Utilizing comprehensive data dashboards to improve service delivery: Insights from U.S. case studies. *International Journal of Frontiers in Engineering and Technology Research*, 6, 008–018. https://doi.org/10.53294/ijfetr.2024.6.2.0030.

Aittasalo, M., Tiilikainen, J., Tokola, K., Seimela, T., Sarjala, S.M., Metsapuro, P., Hynynen, A., Suni, J., Sievanen, H., Vaha-Ypya, H., et al. (2017). Socio-ecological intervention to promote active commuting to work: Protocol and baseline findings of a cluster randomized controlled trial in Finland. *International Journal of Environmental Research Public Health*, 14, 1257.

Ali, B.J. (2021). Impact of consumer animosity, boycott participation, boycott motivation, and product judgment on purchase readiness or aversion of Kurdish consumers in Iraq. *Journal of Consumer Affairs*, 55(2), 504–523.

Aljuboori, S.B., Abdulrahim, N.A., Yassen, S., & Khaleel, H.H. (2022). Solvent role in organic chemistry in comparison with organic synthesis under solvent-free condition (green chemistry): A mini literature review. *Al-Rafidain Journal of Medical Sciences* (ISSN 2789-3219), 17(3), 109–115.

Al-Shatti, B.J., Alsairafi, Z., & Al-Tannak, N.F. (2023) Green chemistry and its implementation in pharmaceutical analysis. *Reviews in Analytical Chemistry*, 42(1), 20230069.

Amran, M.E., Muhtazaruddin, M.N., Bani, N.A., & Kaidi, H.M. (2019). Optimal distributed generation of green building assessment towards line loss reduction for Malaysian public hospital. *Bulletin of Electrical Engineering and Informatics*, 8(4), 1180–1188.

Anastas, P.T., et al. (2019). *Case Studies in Green Chemistry and Green Engineering*. ACS Publications.

Balabel, A., & Alwetaishi, M. (2021). Toward sustainable healthcare facilities: An initiative for development of Mostadam-HCF rating system in Saudi Arabia. *Sustainability*, 13(2), 6742.

Bolan, S. (2023). Review on distribution, fate and management of potentially toxic elements in incinerated medical waste. *Environmental Pollution*, 321, 121080.

Cannon, A.S., Warner, J.C., Vidal, J.L., O'Neil, N.J., Nyansa, M.M., Obhi, N.K., & Moir, J.W. (2024). A promise to a sustainable future: 10 years of the green chemistry commitment at beyond benign. *Green Chemistry*, 26(12), 6983–6993.

Chatterjee, S., & Kar, A. K. (2020). Why do small and medium enterprises use social media marketing and what is the impact: Empirical insights from India. *International Journal of Information Management*, 53, 102103.

Clark, J., & Tavener, S. (2007). Alternative solvents: Technology and applications. *Green Chemistry*, 9(9), 954–960.

Copernicus In: The 2023 Annual Climate Summary: Global climate highlight 2023. Copernicus, 18–27.

Das, D. (2017). Development and validation of scale for measuring sustainable supply chain management practices and performance. *Journal of Cleaner Production*, 164, 1344–1362.

Duque-Uribe, V., Sarache, W., & Gutiérrez, E.V. (2019). Sustainable supply chain management practices and sustainable performance in hospitals: A systematic review and integrative framework. *Sustainability*, 11(21), 5949.

Elabed, S., Belal, A., & Shamayleh, A. (2019). October. Sustainability of medical equipment in the healthcare industry: An overview. In *2019 Fifth International Conference on Advances in Biomedical Engineering (ICABME), Tripoli, Lebanon* (pp. 1–4). IEEE.

Elam Cheren, S., & Ashok Kumar, L. (2022). Optimization techniques for improving the performance of solar photovoltaic system in conjunction with health informatics and the hospital Energy Management System. *Journal of Medical Imaging and Health Informatics*, 11(12).

Ferrigno, G., Del Sart, N., Piccaluga, A., & Barmocelli, A (2023). Industry-based technologies and business models: a bibliometric analysis. *European Journal of Innovation Management*, 26(7), 502–526.

Fields, Z., Abdullah, Z.M., Musisi, A.N., & Mitchley, N.K. (2021). Using collective creativity and industry 4.0 technology to reduce the negative impact of a pandemic on entrepreneurs. In Z. Fields & Z. M. Abdullah (Eds.), *Handbook of Research on Using*

Global Collective Intelligence and Creativity to Solve Wicked Problems (pp. 133–155). IGI Global.

g training.2 (2024) Lastly, data-driven decision-making backs up these endeavors by keeping an eye on KPIs, comparing them to industry standards, and using real-time dashboards to proactively tackle problems. Seen as a whole, these tactics provide a cutting-edge method of healthcare administration that guarantees effectiveness and excellent results for patients, 7, 12.

Ganesh KN, Zhang D, Miller SJ, Rossen K, Chirik PJ, Kozlowski MC, Zimmerman JB, Brooks BW, Savage PE, Allen DT, Voutchkova-Kostal AM. (2021) Green chemistry: A framework for a sustainable future. *ACS Omega*, 6(25):16254–8.

Guerrero, G., & Ramos, A. (2023). Techno-economic assessment of solar technologies to meet hospitals energy needs. *International Journal of Applied Power Engineering*, 12(2), 162–178.

Gutmann, B., Cantillo, D., & Kappe, C.O. (2015). Continuous-flow technology—a tool for the safe manufacturing of active pharmaceutical ingredients. *Angewandte Chemie International Edition*, 54(23), 6688–6728.

Hariharan, R., & Kumar, R. S. (Eds.). (2025). *Recent Research in Management, Accounting and Economics (RRMAE)*. Taylor & Francis Group.

HCWH and GGHH. (2020). *Sustainable Procurement in Health Care Guide*. Practice Greenhealth.

Hollmann, F., et al. (2017). Biocatalysis for green chemistry: Past, present and future. Chemistry & Sustainability, Energy & Materials, 10(21), 4211–4227. https://term.sustainability-directory.com/term/water-conservation-in-healthcare. https://www.hercenter.org/facilitiesandgrounds/greenbuilding.php.

Hu, Danping, et al. (2024). Application of artificial intelligence technique in optimization and prediction of the stability of the walls against wind loads in building design. *Mechanics of Advanced Materials and Structures*, 31(19), 4755–4772.

Jones, C., et al. (2020). Overcoming barriers to sustainability in pharmaceutical research. *Journal of Cleaner Production*, 258, 120693.

Kanokphanvanich, C., Rattanawong, W., & Vongmanee, V. (2023). A new model for a sustainable healthcare supply chain prioritizes patient safety: Using the fuzzy Delphi method to identify healthcare workers' perspectives. *Sustainability*, 15(9), 7123.

Kaplan, M., & Ramachandran, S. (2018). Sustainable procurement in the pharmaceutical supply chain. *Journal of Supply Chain Management*, 54(2), 45–59.

Kar, S., Sanderson, H., Roy, K., Benfenati, E., & Leszczynski, J. (2021). Green chemistry in the synthesis of pharmaceuticals. *Chemical Reviews*, 122(3), 3637–710.

Karimi, H. (2024). Optimizing COVID-19 medical waste management using goal and robust possibilistic programming. *Engineering Applications of Artificial Intelligence, 1*:131:107838

Karliner J., Slotterback, S., Boyd, R., Ashby, B., & Steele, K. (2019). Health care's climate footprint: How the health sector contributes to the global climate crisis and opportunities for action. *Health Care Without Harm and ARUP*.

Kate, A., Sahu, L.K., Pandey, J., Mishra, M., & Sharma, P.K. (2022). Green catalysis for chemical transformation: The need for the sustainable development. *Current Research in Green and Sustainable Chemistry*, 5, 100248.

Kaushal, R., Rohit, & A.K., Dhaka. (2024). A comprehensive review of the application of plasma gasification technology in circumventing the medical waste in the post-COVID-19 scenario. *Biomass Conversion and Biorefinery*, 14(2), 1427–1442.

Kaya, S.I., Cetinkaya, A., & Ozkan, S.A. (2022). Green analytical chemistry approaches on environmental analysis. *Trends in Environmental Analytical Chemistry*, 33, e00157.

Kim, S., Ga, S., Bae, H., Sluyter, R., Konstantinov, K., Shrestha, L.K., Kim, Y.H., Kim, J.H., & Ariga, K. (2024). Multidisciplinary approaches for enzyme biocatalysis in pharmaceuticals: Protein engineering, computational biology, and nanoarchitectonics. *EES Catalysis*, 2(1), 14–48.

Kumar, R., & Maurya, A. (2024). Green chemistry, techniques for sustainable pharmaceutical synthesis. *Journal of Drug Discovery and Health Sciences*, 30;1(04), 187–200.

Kümmerer, K. (2010). *Pharmaceuticals in the Environment: Sources, Fate, Effects and Risks*. Springer.

Kwame, A., & Petrucka, P.M. (2021). A literature-based study of patient-centered care and communication in nurse-patient interactions: Barriers, facilitators, and the way forward. *BioMed Central Nursing*, September 3; 20(1), 158. https://doi.org/10.1186/s12912-021-00684-2. PMID: 34479560; PMCID: PMC8414690.

Kyriakarakos, G., & Dounis, A. (2020). Intelligent management of distributed energy resources for increased resilience and environmental sustainability of hospitals. *Sustainability (Switzerland)*, 12(18), 1–4.

Liang, Y. (2021). Repercussions of COVID-19 pandemic on solid waste generation and management strategies. *Frontiers of Environmental Science & Engineering*, 15(6), 1–18.

Liu, H.Y., Chang, C.C., Wang, I.T., & Chao, S.Y. (2020). The association between creativity, creative components of personality, and innovation among Taiwanese nursing students. *Thinking Skills and Creativity*, 35, 100629.

Lundberg, J., et al. (2019). Implementing sustainability in academic chemical laboratories: A case study. *Sustainability*, 11(16), 4321.

Mackenzie, C.F., et al. (2019). Automation and digitization of chemical synthesis: Intelligent laboratories for green chemistry. *ACS Sustainable Chemistry & Engineering*, 7(19), 16279–16291.

Martínez-Peláez, R., Ochoa-Brust, A., Rivera, S., Félix, V.G., Ostos, R., Brito, H., Félix, R.A., & Mena, L.J. (2023). Role of digital transformation for achieving sustainability: Mediated role of stakeholders, key capabilities, and technology. *Sustainability*, 15(14), 11221.

Menon, R.R. (2022). *Strategic fit of service supply chains* (Doctoral dissertation, Monash University).

Mishra, M., Sharma, M., Dubey, R., Kumari, P., Ranjan, V., & Pandey, J. (2021) Green synthesis interventions of pharmaceutical industries for sustainable development. *Current Research in Green and Sustainable Chemistry*, 4, 100174.

Misszento, J.A., & Amofah, A.D. (2024). Implementing eco-friendly practices in the manufacturing, distribution, and disposal of medications, *International Journal of Research Publication and Reviews, 5*(11), 6677–6685.

Möller, K., Nenonen, S., & Storbacka, K. (2020). Networks, ecosystems, fields, market systems? Making sense of the business environment. *Industrial Marketing Management*, 90, 380–399.

Mostepainuk, A., Akalin, T., & Parish Reza, M. (2023). Practices pursuing the sustainability of a healthcare organization: A systematic review. *MDPI*, 15, 2353.

Msingh, R., Pramanik, R., Hazra, S., & Uni, J. (2021). Role of green chemistry in pharmaceutical industry: A review. *Journal of University Shanghai for Science and Technology*, 23, 291–299.

O'Connell, A., Barry, A., Burke, A.J., Hutton, A.E., Bell, E.L., Green, A.P., & O'Reilly, E. (2024). Biocatalysis: Landmark discoveries and applications in chemical synthesis. *Chemical Society Reviews*, 53(6), 2828–2850.

Pereno, A., & Eriksson, D. (2020). A multi-stakeholder perspective on sustainable healthcare: From 2030 onwards. *Futures*, 122, 102605.

Pichler, P.P., Jaccard, I.S., & Weisz, H. (2019). International comparison on healthcare carbon footprints. *Environmental Research Letters*, 14(6), 064004.

Puhlmann, N., Vidaurre, R., & Kümmerer, K. (2024). Designing greener active pharmaceutical ingredients: Insights from pharmaceutical industry into drug discovery and development. *European Journal of Pharmaceutical Sciences*, 192, 106614.

Rasulev, A., Yakhshieva, M., Yusupov, R., Abdullaeva, M., & Otaboev, F. (2020). The role of Islamic banking in the transformation of international corporations as a reflection of modern globalization and migration. *Архив научных исследований*, (20), 1–10.

Roberts, D.C., Tignor, M., Polokzanska, E.S., Mintenbeck, K., Alegria, A., Criag, M., Langdort, S., Loschke, S., Moller, V., Okem, A., Rama, B. (2022). Editors Climate Change 2022. Impacts, Adaptation, Vulnerability. Contribution of Working Group II of the Sixth Assesment Report of Intergovernmental Pannel on Climate Change, Cambrige UK and New York, NY, USA, Cambrige University Press.

Romanello, M., Di Nepoli, C., Drummond, P., Green, C., Kennard, H., & Lempard, P. (2022). The 2022 report of Lacent Countdown on health and climatic change, health at the mercy of fossil fuels. *Lancet*, 400(10363), 1691–1654.

Ruiz-Gonzalez, A. (2025). AI-driven chemical design: Transforming the sustainability of the pharmaceutical industry. *Future Pharmacology*, 5(2), 24.

Sah, M.K., Ettarhouni, Z.O., Pathak, R., Gawad, J., Bonde, C., Arya, S.P., & Bhattarai, A. (2025). Green chemistry: Strategies and sustainable approaches for bridging UN SDGS. *Chemistry Select*, 10(25), e00847.

Sajid, M., & Płotka-Wasylka, J. (2022). Green analytical chemistry metrics: A review. *Talanta*, 238, 123046.

Sampson, S. (2021). Good people doing bad things: Compliance regimes in organisations. *Journal of Legal Anthropology*, 5(1), 110–134.

Sarkar, B., & Singh, A. (2021). Economic challenges in adopting green chemistry in pharmaceutical industries. *Journal of Environmental Management*, 284, 112040.

Sarkis, M., Bernardi, A., hah, N., & Papathanasiou, M.M. (2021). Emerging challenges and opportunities in pharmaceutical manufacturing and distribution. *Processes*, 9(3), 457.

Singh, N., & Ogusritan, O.A. (2022). Medical waste current challenges and future opportunities for sustainable management. *Critical Reviews in Environmental Science and Technology*, 52(1), 52–60.

Sousa, A.C., Veiga, A., Maurício, A.C., Lopes, M.A., Santos, J.D., & Neto, B. (2021). Assessment of the environmental impacts of medical devices: A review. *Environment, Development and Sustainability*, 23, 9641–9666.

Srivastava, A., Dutta, S., Ahuja, S., & Sharma, R.K. (2021). Green chemistry: Key to reducing waste and improving water quality. *Handbook of Water Purity and Quality*, (2nd ed., 359–407).

Tang, S.L., Smith, R.L., & Poliakoff, M. (2005). Principles of green chemistry: PRODUCTIVELY. *Green Chemistry*, 7(11), 761–762.

Tickner, J.A., Simon, R.V., Jacobs, M., Pollard, L.D., & van Bergen, S.K. (2021). The nexus between alternatives assessment and green chemistry: Supporting the development and adoption of safer chemicals. *Green Chemistry Letters and Reviews*, 2;14(1), 23–44.

Tilley, E., Ulrich, L., Lüthi, C., Reymond, Ph., & Zurbrügg, C. (2021). *Compendium of Sanitation Systems and Technologies*. 2nd Revised Edition. Swiss Federal Institute of Aquatic Science and Technology (Eawag), Duebendorf, Switzerland.

Verdonck, P., & Verniers, I. (2023). "Enviornmental Sustainability in Healthcare: Managerial Concerns and Solutions", "Best Practice & Research Clinical Anaes.

Wang, Z., et al. (2020). Environmental sustainability in pharmaceutical manufacturing: A review. *Journal of Cleaner Production*, 254, 120095.

World Resources Institute. (2020). *Greenhouse gas protocol*. www.ghgprotocol.org.

Yang, T.T., Yuan, F.Q., Jin, R.Q., & Wang, Y. (2015). Advances in green analytical techniques and their applications in pharmaceutical analysis. *Chinese Journal of Pharmaceutical Analysis*, 35(12), 2070–2075.

2 Explore Telemedicine and Remote Healthcare Delivery Model

A Pathway to Lower Carbon Emissions

Amit Chaudhary, Nitin Sharma, Dev Prakash Dahiya, Kamal Dua, Vikas Solanki, and Jatin Kumar

1 Introduction

Telemedicine and remote healthcare delivery models—concluding synchronous and asynchronous services and associated use cases—positively affect health outcomes, cost-efficiency, and access to care. Although these benefits are well established, their potential to reduce health sector carbon emissions has received little attention (Vudathaneni et al., 2024). The prevailing health delivery model, dominated by in-person ambulatory clinic visits, accounts for approximately one-fifth of a nation's carbon footprint. A pathway toward lower carbon emissions within healthcare must therefore encompass telemedicine and remote delivery of healthcare services—technologies and associated clinical process paradigms that can meaningfully reduce the environmental toll of ambulatory care (Liu et al., 2024).

Healthcare services delivered remotely through information and communication technologies are known as telemedicine or sometimes connected health. Telemedicine enables clinical and non-clinical services to be provided in a more streamlined and convenient way and has become an important source for delivering healthcare internationally (Mehrolhassani et al., 2025). Appropriately designed and implemented telemedicine builds on major technological advances that can support patients' and professionals' needs when carried out on a remote basis. Telemedicine requires parity of esteem with in-person services, the regulatory environment to support their operation, and information governance policies to protect patients (Muzzamil et al., 2025). Adopting telemedicine in various industries can reduce transportation; therefore, as an approach to medical data-sharing, it can reduce greenhouse gas emissions. During the outbreak of COVID-19, the number of travelers decreased, and wider use of telemedicine was implemented with a positive attitude and increasing technology contributions (Addor et al., 2025).

The healthcare landscape has undergone a significant transformation through the integration of digital technologies, with telemedicine emerging as a pivotal innovation in medical service delivery. The convergence of advanced telecommunications and healthcare has created new pathways for patient care, particularly

DOI: 10.4324/9781003640486-2

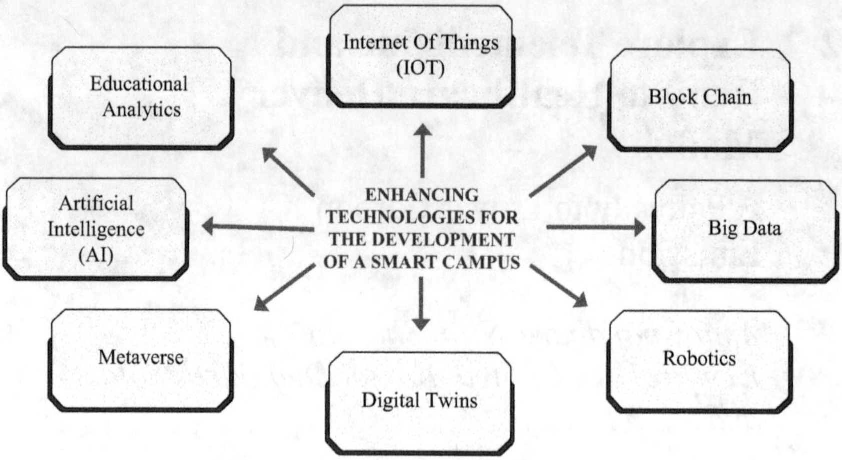

Figure 2.1 Telemedicine and remote healthcare delivery model: a pathway to lower carbon emissions.

beneficial for populations facing geographical or economic barriers to traditional healthcare access (Ezenwaji et al., 2025). Telemedicine represents the systematic application of telecommunications technology to provide clinical care from a distance. Its origins can be traced to the late 1950s, but recent technological advancements have dramatically expanded its capabilities and applications (Othman et al., 2025). The technology enables healthcare providers to evaluate, diagnose, and treat patients remotely, utilizing various digital platforms and tools that facilitate real-time communication and data exchange (Adeloduna & Anyanwub, 2025). The COVID-19 pandemic catalyzed widespread telemedicine adoption, accelerating what might have otherwise taken years of gradual implementation. Healthcare systems worldwide rapidly adapted their service delivery models to incorporate virtual care options, ensuring continuity of care while minimizing infection risks (Olowoyo et al., 2025). This rapid transition demonstrated telemedicine's potential to maintain healthcare accessibility during crises while highlighting the need for robust digital infrastructure and standardized protocols (Huda et al., 2025). Modern telemedicine encompasses various modalities, including synchronous video consultations, asynchronous communication, remote patient monitoring, and mobile health applications (Figure 2.1). These technologies enable healthcare providers to extend their reach beyond traditional clinical settings, offering services ranging from routine check-ups to specialized consultations. The integration of artificial intelligence and machine learning algorithms further enhances diagnostic capabilities and treatment planning, marking a new era in healthcare delivery (Saleh et al., 2025; Ghaderzadeh, 2025).

1.1 Overview of Telemedicine

Telemedicine is the practice of providing medical treatments remotely through the use of information and communication technology, enabling patients and doctors to communicate without being in the same physical location (Gamus et al., 2025). Recent external pressures have accelerated the growth of telemedicine and other remote healthcare delivery models. These delivery models provide patients with convenient access to healthcare services while also reducing carbon emissions.

Detailed analyses of the environmental effects of telemedicine and remote healthcare delivery models, therefore, speak to how these carbon emission changes are produced. Nevertheless, although a variety of remote healthcare delivery and telemedicine-related research continues to provide long-term forecasts of carbon emissions reductions, the existing literature overemphasizes the double-reduction factor (Adirim, 2025). Studies focus heavily on direct travel displacement while generally ignoring the more complex interactions that characterize the innovative nature of remote service delivery and its integrated role in conventional settings (Choi, 2025).

By combining telemedicine with other services and traditional medical treatment, it is possible to provide full care remotely and can increase convenience without raising carbon emissions. In general, availability and convenience are key determinants of the mode by which healthcare is delivered (Ismail & Ebinezar, 2025). The observed (and anticipated) reductions in environmental impact associated with the extensive use of telemedicine reflect both the reduced need for travel and the substitution of low-carbon remote care for otherwise high-carbon conventional care (Ghaderzadeh, 2025).

The discussion synthesizes and integrates the existing telemedicine literature and develops a conceptual-legal framework for the effective delivery of remote healthcare services (Chauhan et al., 2024). It is argued that the inherent merit of telemedicine stems from its innovative ability to enhance accessibility and provide care directly within patients' residences. Three remote care plans serve as points of reference: (1) an immediate reactive plan, which synchronously treats or triages users on demand; (2) a scheduled planned-reactive plan, which follows up with users based on known health states and clinical histories; and (3) a chronic care model, which proactively engages users through asynchronous monitoring, prevention, and management (Armstrong & Tanaka, 2025).

1.2 Definition and Scope

Telemedicine has experienced significant growth, supported by information and communication technologies and augmented by advances in remote monitoring technologies and the continued miniaturization of sensors (Bianchi & Gutierrez, 2025). The Centers of Disease Control and Prevention defines telemedicine as "the use of electronic information and telecommunication technologies to support long-distance clinical healthcare, patient and professional health-related education, public health, and health administration."

Remote healthcare delivery models extend telemedicine offerings with patient-centric solutions, such as remote patient monitoring, assistive living, and mobile workers. These models provide continuous access to care anywhere and anytime through either synchronous or asynchronous processes (Ta et al., 2025).

Synchronous/Remote Care involves real-time consultations via phone, webcam, or videoconferencing, establishing live communication that extends traditional care beyond physical health facilities and ensures immediate response and direct advice (Kumar & Ganesh, 2024).

Asynchronous/Store and Forward is based on the periodic collection and transmission of data stored on a central server, whose processing results in signs and patterns that can inform diagnosis and therapy when abnormal values occur. This mode can be viewed as continuous, routine, healthy monitoring capable of converting primary into secondary care when medical staff are alerted to emerging needs (Swati et al., 2025).

Telemedicine supports the conventional healthcare system by facilitating remote interventions through the Internet, mobile communication, and computer networks, utilizing telemedicine-enabled examination devices, such as stethoscopes, microscopes, ECG monitors, and X-ray or ultrasonic devices (Booker et al., 2025).

1.3 Fundamentals of Telemedicine: Essential Elements

Telemedicine systems' infrastructure consists of a number of essential parts that work together to provide remote healthcare delivery. The technical infrastructure comprises secure servers, encrypted communication pathways, and specialized software platforms custom-built for healthcare purposes (Dalimunthe et al., 2025; Kumar et al., 2025). The hardware requirements normally consist of high-resolution cameras, quality microphones, and other medical equipment modified for remote use. The devices vary from simple vital sign monitors to complex diagnostic devices that can send real-time patient information (Jagatheesaperumal et al., 2025). Figure 2.2 depicts a schematic representation of the core components of telemedicine.

1.4 History and Evolution

Increasing demand for healthcare worsens the sector's environmental impact. Telemedicine and Remote Healthcare Delivery Models (RHM) reduce that impact by lowering patients' carbon emissions. Telemedicine enables clinical healthcare

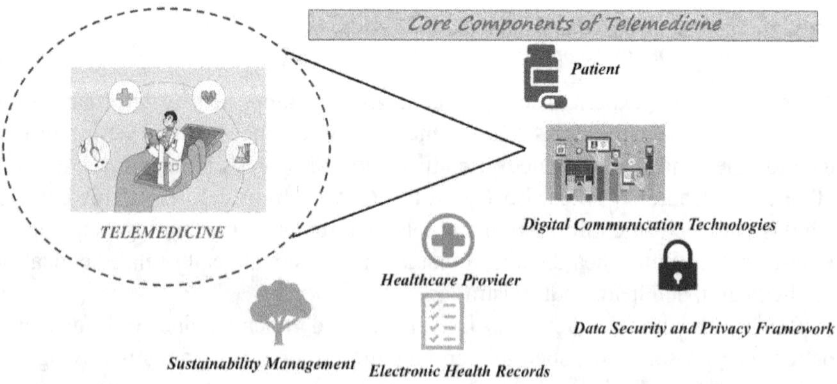

Figure 2.2 Schematic representation of core components of telemedicine.

when providers and patients are not collocated through electronic exchange of information (Rafi et al., 2025). Real-time, synchronous RHM services connect patients and health professionals directly through telecommunications; asynchronous services, which encompass visits and remote monitoring, collect relevant health data for subsequent review by providers, and currently receive wider adoption. High equipment costs originally limited adoption, but the ongoing digital revolution expands possibilities for remote care (Mazziotti et al., 2025).

Remote healthcare delivery refers to systems that allow patients to interact with clinicians, provide personal health data, and receive care without the constraints of time and place. The term encapsulates technologies and processes designed to remove the traditional constraints of synchronous and collocated medical services (Muralidhar et al., 2025). Three distinctions characterize RHM: (1) synchronous versus asynchronous care; (2) provided in addition to, or in place of, traditional services; and (3) patient-centric versus institution-centric delivery.

Widely promised efficiency and convenience promote RHM adoption, particularly when diagnostic and management protocols such as those for laboratory testing support remote care.

Emissions from patient travel represent a substantial part of healthcare's carbon footprint. A combination of telecommunications, remote monitoring, and home- or community-based care offers a potent sustainability strategy (Ratheesh et al., 2025).

1.5 Types of Telemedicine

Telemedicine describes any healthcare provision that transcends geographical, temporal, or social barriers.

1. Traditional diagnosis and treatment entail a patient's travel to a healthcare center.

Modern telemedicine replaces such journeys through direct communication with providers or maintenance of records when a direct interaction is impossible. Generation and transmission of potentially large amounts of data via communication networks often demand complex infrastructure, such as videoconferencing systems, electronic patient records, and transmission networks (SHI et al., 2025).

Differences in the timing of events establish the arrival of the request and the response, distinguishing between remote consultations conducted synchronously or asynchronously. Both modalities have applications across specialties and use cases, and asynchronous telemedicine services have evolved rapidly on their own. A third form derives from continuous or near-real-time monitoring of patients' health status, with data transmitted for interpretation and prompt intervention if necessary. One example involves remote monitoring of cardiac activity (Tshiamala & Tartibu, 2025).

1.5.1 Synchronous Telemedicine

Synchronous telemedicine is a category of telemedicine featuring real-time, simultaneous engagement between patients and healthcare providers, typically enabled by video communication platforms. Incorporating this modality into healthcare enables remote evaluation, diagnosis, and treatment while actively accommodating patients' questions and concerns (Zhang & Feng, 2025).

The broader field of telemedicine focuses on surmounting geographical and temporal barriers that hinder traditional in-person care. The high global penetration levels of fast and reliable telecommunication services render telemedicine a highly integrable means of delivering equitable care at reasonable costs, while simultaneously preserving and often improving quality. The evolutionary lineage of medicine, telecommunication, and networks collectively empowers modern telemedicine as an exceptionally patient-centric and flexible mode of healthcare provision, readily adaptable to different clinical and environmental circumstances (Sebai et al., 2025).

1.5.2 Asynchronous Telemedicine

It promotes remote diagnostic discussions between specialists and primary care physicians and aids sophisticated decision-making. This type of method provides static information, including medical images, laboratory results, and patient history, for evaluations, allowing clinicians to transfer information without the need for real-time interaction (Chen et al., 2025).

2 Remote Patient Monitoring

Vital indicators include blood pressure, heart rate, respiration rate, body temperature, blood glucose, and general health state. Monitoring integrates the application of specialized devices and remote access software to retrieve, store, and analyze patients' data remotely (Dziuba et al., 2025). Numerous medical conditions, including asthma, congestive heart failure, diabetes, hypertension, and renal failure, benefit from patient monitoring devices. Patient monitoring is particularly beneficial for chronic illnesses like heart disease, hypertension, diabetes, and asthma, where ongoing measurements and data are essential for the clinical, economic, and environmental success of the healthcare system. Remote patient monitoring is a form of telemedicine that employs mobile/online health technologies for the collection of patient information outside of the conventional healthcare environments. Wearable technology to track blood pressure, blood sugar, oxygen saturation, body temperature, weight, and heart rate is one example of the technologies (Gonzales & Zhang, 2025). This type of telemedicine can benefit older patients who live in remote communities or require ongoing care for chronic illnesses. Nurses provide home-based remote patient monitoring services to communicate symptoms, measurements, and requests with healthcare providers via email, phone calls, or a proprietary clinic portal. The collected data are reviewed by qualified healthcare professionals, who can make clinical decisions related to symptom management, scheduling, and medication adjustment (Aisyah et al., 2025).

2.1 Benefits of Telemedicine for Patients

The telemedicine process provides patients with convenient access to medical care without the necessity for travel: (1) synchronous, asynchronous, and remote patient monitoring (RPM) telemedicine services enable health interventions to occur outside the walls of traditional healthcare settings; (2) conducting health services remotely is important for increasing healthcare accessibility and efficiency in many settings; (3) traditional healthcare systems possess a large carbon footprint and utilize natural resources at unsustainable levels; healthcare delivery accounts for 4.4% of global net emissions (Ch et al., 2025). It is therefore crucial to identify less carbon-intensive alternatives. Telemedicine can reduce the carbon footprint of the health sector, particularly by replacing travel-based clinical appointments with technology that facilitates synchronous communication. Considering the adverse impacts of a high-carbon healthcare system and the importance of remote care in many markets, identifying low-carbon opportunities to provide remote healthcare services is a worthwhile contribution to mitigating carbon emissions (Rizzo et al., 2024).

2.2 *Benefits of Telemedicine for Healthcare Providers*

Telemedicine offers healthcare providers operational benefits that translate to sustainability gains. The capacity to manage more patients remotely can result in reduced clinical space requirements, thereby lowering the resources invested in heating, cooling, and powering physical facilities (Bolcato et al., 2024). Concurrently, the implementation of a telehealth infrastructure diminishes reliance on paper records and disposable medical supplies, contributing to decreased environmental impact. Furthermore, telemedicine can yield increased revenue streams for providers while facilitating work-life integration through increased flexibility (Ivanova et al., 2024).

Telemedicine can reduce the carbon emissions of healthcare delivery by offering an environmentally friendly mode of communication that can obviate the need for physical visits. Based on variables like appointment length, bandwidth usage, and usage rates, the carbon footprint of a telemedicine consultation is generally 40–70 times less than that generated by an in-person visit (Khondakar et al., 2024). To achieve the significant greenhouse gas reductions necessary to counter climate change, telemedicine might have to be made standard fare for healthcare routines instead of being limited to underserved populations (Jones-Esan et al., 2024).

A durable healthcare system needs to serve all segments of the population, including those residing in remote rural communities. Providing healthcare in rural regions can be challenging due to various issues: insufficient primary care services, specialist shortages, an aging population, and increased medical expenditures (Obisesan et al., 2024).

Telemedicine provides a means of extending clinical healthcare services from a distance using information-communication technologies. Rapid telemedicine developments reduce the risk of cross-infections during the COVID-19 pandemic while guaranteeing the continuous provision of medical services (Saeed et al., 2024). Due to the numerous benefits associated with telemedicine, a number of successful examples illustrate a significant reduction of emissions while enabling additional positive outcomes and mitigating further spread of viruses that cause illness (Mercier et al., 2024).

A one-year analysis for a single health system in the United States indicated that telemedicine appointments saved nearly 87,000 kg of CO_2 emissions, a reduction equivalent to taking 45 coal-fired power plants offline for a day 1. Shift of appointments from in-person to telemedicine further saves an estimated 80,000 kg of CO_2. With the highest rates of usage associated with early adoption of telemedicine, continued federal investments in supporting infrastructure will only enhance the ability to expand the availability of virtual visits (Atnang et al., 2024).

A cross-sectional assessment of 1,438 new patient visits in a large cancer network revealed that telemedicine visits reduced an estimated 8,711 metric tons of CO_2 emissions in the specific oncology context. The main challenges to broader implementation of telemedicine in oncology were the quality and extent of Internet service, limitations of workflow, and user ability and preference (Shrivastava & Shrivastav, 2024).

3 Telemedicine and Carbon Emission Reduction

By reducing carbon emissions, telemedicine not only improves patient care and healthcare accessibility but also makes a substantial contribution to environmental sustainability. Frequent patient travel to clinics or hospitals is a common component of traditional healthcare delivery, which raises vehicle emissions and fuel consumption. Telemedicine lessens the need for in-person commutes by facilitating digital follow-ups, remote monitoring, and virtual consultations. For instance, it has been demonstrated that the widespread use of telemedicine reduces patient travel by thousands of kilometers per year, which results in significant reductions in greenhouse gas emissions (van der Zee et al., 2024).

Additionally, telemedicine lessens the need for actual hospital infrastructure for standard consultations, which lowers energy costs for heating, cooling, and lighting in medical facilities. The carbon-saving potential of telemedicine is much more evident in rural and isolated areas, where travel distances are lengthy and public transportation options are scarce. Thus, by promoting more environmentally friendly healthcare practices, telemedicine supports global sustainability goals in addition to its medical and financial benefits. Per-consultation carbon savings reported in the literature range widely (about 0.7–372 kg CO_2e per consultation), according to a systematic review, with travel reduction accounting for the majority of savings (Ciaralo et al., 2025).

For example:

- According to a national cancer dataset research, patients who would have otherwise driven more than 60 minutes would have saved an average of 98.6 kg of CO_2 every visit, with high-use subgroups saving millions of kilograms of CO_2 over time. This study demonstrates how savings increase with specialization and travel distance (Jin et al., 2025).
- In certain outpatient groups, cardiology telehealth programs have reported saving approximately 19.1 kg of CO_2 every visit; in bigger programs, these savings amount to hundreds of thousands of kilograms over several years.

- According to research on cancer care modeling from academic institutions in the United States, decentralizing clinical care—that is, replacing in-person visits with remote ones when clinically appropriate—could cut national greenhouse gas emissions from cancer care by about 33% for the clinical components of the model (Umpierre et al., 2025; Li et al., 2025).

3.1 Telemedicine and Sustainability

Sustainability in healthcare encompasses social, economic, and environmental factors in addition to clinical efficacy. Telemedicine is a key component of sustainable healthcare systems because it radically changes the way health services are provided, directly supporting each of these pillars (Samal & Samantaray, 2024).

3.2 Environmental Sustainability

By reducing the need for travel for both patients and providers, telemedicine lowers fuel consumption and greenhouse gas emissions, hence reducing the carbon footprint of healthcare delivery. Additionally, it reduces the need for actual hospital infrastructure for routine visits, which lowers the energy needed for heating, ventilation, and lighting. Telemedicine also lessens medical waste and paper use by moving medications, consultations, and medical data online. Telemedicine improves healthcare's alignment with international climate goals when combined with digital infrastructure powered by renewable energy sources (Savoldelli et al., 2024).

3.3 Social Sustainability

From a societal standpoint, telemedicine improves healthcare access equity and inclusivity. Reduced travel burdens assist older folks, people with mobility impairments, and people living in rural and distant areas. In order to guarantee that vulnerable people receive necessary services, this model also permits continuity of care during emergencies like pandemics, natural disasters, or conflict situations. Telemedicine promotes work-life balance for patients and healthcare professionals by facilitating more flexible care delivery (Özen et al., 2024; Arora et al., 2025).

3.4 Economic Sustainability

By reducing travel expenses, time away from work, and childcare costs related to hospital visits, telemedicine helps patients pay less out of pocket. Through more efficient utilization of infrastructure, more efficient deployment of personnel, and improved chronic condition management through remote monitoring, it can save operating costs for healthcare institutions. Long-term savings from these efficiencies increase the cost-effectiveness and resilience of healthcare (Delarmente et al., 2025; Conte et al., 2025).

4 Challenges and Barriers to Implementation

Widespread adoption of telemedicine faces several obstacles related to technology, regulation, engagement, and literacy. Persistent barriers include poor infrastructure, complex or incompatible software, restrictions on licensing and reimbursement, insufficient high-quality digital content, limited broadband access, underdeveloped business models, low digital literacy, and lack of leadership and planning. Inadequate access to necessary equipment constitutes another frequently reported difficulty. Consequently, telemedicine often suffers from fragmentation and underutilization and lacks sufficient incentives and sources of support for adoption and sustainability (Chu et al., 2025; Zurl et al., 2025).

According to a health policymakers' survey in Iran, telemedicine presently accounts for only a small fraction of healthcare delivery. Geographic characteristics, therefore, trickle down as an additional layer of challenge (Gaebe et al., 2025). The dense population and limited availability of medical centers in mountainous and desert regions, coupled with impassable roads, hinder in-person care and facilitate instead the spread of infectious diseases. The dispersion of small population centers only accentuate that difficulty and diverts the costs of development and health promotion. Healthcare systems in such countries would therefore benefit considerably from alternative methods to gain access and communicate with hospitals and medical centers located in distant cities (Weppner et al., 2025).

4.1 Challenges and Limitations

4.1.1 Technical Challenges

Telemedicine systems have numerous technical issues that impair the quality and delivery of services. In telemedicine, network connectivity is a major concern, particularly for underserved and rural communities whose infrastructure may be unstable or lack Internet (Zito et al., 2025). Technical issues during a virtual consultation may have an impact on the patient's satisfaction and the standard of care. System integration issues occur in trying to integrate telemedicine platforms with current electronic health records and other healthcare information systems (Galts et al., 2025).

4.1.2 Limitations

Some medical treatments and illnesses require a physical inspection or intervention that cannot be completed efficiently via the virtual platform. Because in some circumstances, the incapacity to do physical examinations can limit the accuracy of the diagnosis. Clinicians will need to assess carefully which clinical situations are suited for telemedicine and which demand a face-to-face visit. Lack of physical contact could influence the relationship between healthcare providers and patients in certain specialties (Akgun & Palamar, 2025). Table 2.1 depicts challenges and solutions in telemedicine implementations.

Table 2.1 Challenges and solutions in telemedicine implementations

Challenge	*Specific Issues*	*Proposed Solutions*
Technical	Connectivity issues, system integration	Redundant systems, standardized protocols
Regulatory	Licensing, privacy compliance	Interstate compacts, enhanced security
Financial	Infrastructure costs, reimbursement	Grant funding, policy advocacy

4.2 *Legal Issues*

Interstate licensure rules pose major hurdles for healthcare professionals interested in practicing telemedicine across state lines. Liability issues and malpractice insurance implications must be handled with great care while rolling out telemedicine services (Parker et al., 2025). Regulations of privacy and data security need to be met through strong technical measures and organizational policies. The changing landscape of telemedicine regulations demands the flexibility of healthcare organizations in their implementation approach (Hendrix et al., 2025).

4.3 *Financial Barriers*

The significant upfront infrastructure costs associated with telemedicine implementation can be a barrier for small healthcare institutions. Government programs and insurance firms have different reimbursement plans, which affect how profitable telemedicine services are (Mainer-Pearson et al., 2025). There may be a prolonged return on investment time, requiring careful resource and financial planning. Financial strategies ought to account for the expenses of ongoing technical support and maintenance (Lathan et al., 2025).

4.4 *Social and Cultural Barriers*

The use of telemedicine by patients varies by population group, with certain populations being resistant to receiving care virtually. In virtual settings, linguistic and cultural barriers may be exacerbated, necessitating additional support services (Eldeeb et al., 2025). The efficient use of telemedicine technologies can be influenced by the degree of digital literacy among patients and healthcare professionals. For older and underprivileged groups, the digital gap presents unique difficulties (Yahia et al., 2025).

4.5 *Healthcare Quality*

It can be especially difficult to guarantee the constant quality of treatment across virtual delivery. The creation of quality measures for telemedicine services requires ongoing evaluation and modification (Shokoohi et al., 2025). It could be necessary to modify satisfaction surveys and outcome tracking for use in virtual care settings. The technological and clinical aspects of telemedicine service delivery must be the main focus of quality improvement initiatives (Sugawara et al., 2025).

4.6 Development of the Workforce

For healthcare workers to deliver treatment effectively via virtual methods, they require specialized training and skill development. Integration of telemedicine into training programs and medical colleges is still lacking. Implementation may be hampered by healthcare workers' inertia. To support telemedicine services, enterprises must address staffing structures and process modifications (Aldawoodi et al., 2025).

4.7 Issues with Interoperability

When telemedicine platforms are not compatible with one another, it can cause problems for healthcare companies that use different systems. Technical incompatibilities may hinder data interchange between different healthcare systems and providers (Van Rhee et al., 2025). Carefully thought-out and technically sound system integration with current healthcare information systems is required. The need for seamless information flow across various platforms and providers remains a significant challenge (Vanaria et al., 2025).

5 Emerging Trends in Telemedicine

5.1 Artificial Intelligence and Machine Learning

Integration into telemedicine platforms of artificial intelligence and machine learning increases the capability of diagnostic assessments and treatment planning (Table 2.2). Beyond a patient's immediate care setting, sophisticated algorithms allow for pattern detection and clinical decision assistance in the creation of more precise diagnoses (Zhang et al., 2025). Improved remote monitoring tools continue to expand the scope of virtual care delivery. Applications of virtual reality and augmented reality in medical education and some therapeutic settings show promise (Schmidt et al., 2025).

Table 2.2 Emerging trends in telemedicine

Trend	*Timeline*	*Expected Impact*	*Barriers for Implementation*
AI integration	2023–2025	Enhanced diagnostics	Technical complexity
IoMT expansion	2024–2026	Improved monitoring	Cost, standardization
5G implementation	2023–2027	Reduced latency	Infrastructure requirements
VR applications	2024–2028	Enhanced training	Technology adoption
Blockchain	2025–2030	Improved security	System complexity

5.2 Integration of Internet of Medical Things (IoMT)

End-to-end patient monitoring and care delivery are becoming more feasible thanks to the proliferation of networked medical equipment. Advances in wearable technologies offer real-time insights and continuous health data production (Liu et al., 2025). More sophisticated RPM is made possible by intelligent medical gadgets with enhanced connectivity features. The integration of IoMT devices with telemedicine platforms enables more precise and proactive healthcare delivery (Harris et al., 2025).

5.3 Mobile Health Apps

Applications for mobile health are becoming more complex, providing more features and greater integration potential. Artificial intelligence is being used more and more for preliminary symptom screening and triage. The potential to provide remote care is further enhanced by the development of mobile-based diagnostic capabilities. Formal healthcare systems are increasingly combining with mobile healthcare apps (Shinde et al., 2025).

5.4 Preventive Care and Predictive Analytics

Predictive modeling for healthcare delivery is becoming increasingly complex thanks to advanced data processing capabilities. Combinations of several data sources allow for a more thorough evaluation of patients' risks. By examining patterns in each patient's unique health data, preventive care treatments are being tailored to each patient. Real-time analytics allow for more timely interventions and care plan modifications (Li & Ci et al., 2025).

5.5 Virtual Reality in Medical Practice

Medical education and healthcare delivery are seeing new uses for virtual reality technologies. Virtual reality therapy has the potential to improve mental healthcare and pain management. Virtual reality is being used more and more in medical education programs to teach skills and practice procedures. More captivating patient education encounters are improved by the technology (Verdonck & Verniers, 2025).

5.6 Blockchain Technology

Blockchain technology may find use in the safe administration and sharing of medical records. The technology can improve the privileging and credentialing procedures for healthcare providers. Claims management and insurance processing can be made more efficient with smart contracts. Applications of blockchain technology can improve pharmaceutical supply chains' security and transparency (Al-Battat & Iyer, 2025).

5.7 5G Networks' Effects

The introduction of 5G networks, which offer improved connectivity and reduced latency, is expected to unleash the promise of telemedicine. More sophisticated real-time healthcare applications will be supported by larger bandwidth capacities. More extensive remote monitoring systems will be supported by more sophisticated mobile capabilities. Innovative telemedicine solutions will be able to be deployed more widely thanks to the technology (Mesteru et al., 2025).

5.8 Customized Healthcare

These days, telemedicine platforms incorporate genetic and molecular data into recommendations for patient care. More effective therapies are made possible by combining treatment planning, monitoring, and personalized medicine techniques. The availability of remote genetic counseling services is growing. More focused therapeutic involvement is possible when telemedicine and personalized medicine are coupled [88].

5.9 Global Health

Telemedicine technologies are opening up access to healthcare services in the developing world. The delivery of healthcare is enabled by international collaborations through virtual platforms. Telemedicine is increasingly being used in global health programs for education and service delivery. Cross-border provision of healthcare services is becoming possible through sophisticated telecommunication technologies (Seckam et al., 2025).

5.10 Technological Limitations

Telemedicine is a developing field with a strong potential for development and innovation. The level of technological maturity varies widely among telemedicine specialties. The availability of long-standing commercial solutions within certain telemedicine sub-specialties, such as teleradiology, demonstrates this technological maturity (Chaudhuri & Agarwal, 2025). Some services, such as telepathology, require niche expertise to handle digital diagnostics and streaming protocols and are still under commercial development. Telemedicine services need to be tailored to their target group and geographical location. Research is needed on a larger scale to evaluate the impact of different telemedicine solutions on carbon emissions as a fully integrated part of healthcare activity (Brusco et al., 2025).

5.11 Regulatory Issues

The effective development and deployment of telemedicine are strongly influenced by regulatory frameworks, yet these often lag behind technological advancements. State licensing procedures, for example, typically restrict physicians to practicing only within their licensed jurisdictions (Larsen et al., 2025). This creates complications for delivering telemedicine across state borders. Moreover, concerns about the quality of care add another layer of complexity. For instance, there is a proposition that each state should empower its medical licensing authority to require physicians engaged in telemedicine within the state to obtain registration from the respective licensing board. Registration criteria could include adherence to defined minimum practice standards. Enforcement mechanisms might rely on comity among states, complemented by coordinated multi-state credentialing requirements (Wong et al., 2025). Such standards would serve to exclude applicants lacking sufficient education or training, thereby protecting consumers. They would also help ensure that a physician registered to practice telemedicine in one state holds licenses and operates in states with comparable legal frameworks. Addressing reciprocal enforcement in this manner aligns with patients' best interests. Parallel to regulatory measures, telemedicine-focused organizations should collaborate with accreditation bodies such as Joint Commission on Accreditation of Healthcare Organizations and National Committee for Quality Assurance to establish credentialing standards, thereby alleviating the administrative burden associated with obtaining credentials at each location. Finally, for ethical reasons, physicians should consistently secure informed consent from patients before initiating telemedicine services (Duane et al., 2025).

5.12 Patient Acceptance and Engagement

Understanding the environmental impact of telemedicine is crucial for its role in climate change mitigation. While the technology itself requires resources, its implementation can lead to significant environmental benefits by reducing emissions from healthcare processes. Telemedicine generates far fewer carbon emissions than traditional care models, where patients and health workers travel to appointments. It enables a shift from intensive, travel-based care toward efficient, close-to-home service delivery (Godard et al., 2025). As a potent climate change mitigation strategy, broader adoption of telemedicine is necessary to reduce healthcare's contribution to greenhouse gas emissions and support a transition toward low-carbon, sustainable systems. However, realizing this potential depends on patient acceptance and engagement. Current knowledge in this area is limited, particularly regarding demographic differences in receptivity. Women, elderly patients, and individuals with disabilities or chronic conditions tend to be less receptive to telemedicine, underscoring the need for tailored approaches to enhance engagement. Even at a general level, agreement with screening for mental health conditions via telemedicine is below 50%. Low levels of acceptance and engagement may limit telemedicine's potential for reducing both expenditures and carbon emissions (Şenel Tekin & Bekar, 2025).

5.13 Case Studies of Successful Telemedicine Programs

Telemedicine is a well-documented method for reducing the carbon footprint associated with healthcare delivery. This is demonstrated by international examples, including the United Kingdom's "Digital First" program and Singapore's national telemedicine regulations, and national initiatives such as Australia's COVID-19 telehealth billing arrangements. In the oncology patient population, such schemes have established potential for broad benefit at low risk if appropriately supported (Nicksa et al., 2025).

6 Future Directions in Telemedicine

Telemedicine, emerging from a Boeing engineering technologist's 1950s vision and NASA-supported 1960s experiment, accelerated with telecommunications and consumer electronics advancement. Defined as delivery of clinical and preventive health services with two-way voice or visual communication technologies, telemedicine increasingly addresses both urgent and non-urgent care, particularly suited for rural and underserved areas. It mitigates long-distance travel by facilitating local service, thereby enhancing patient access to specialty care, reducing indirect costs, increasing visit frequency, and enabling effective follow-up and medication adherence (Ren et al., 2025).

Synchronous and asynchronous modes constitute principal delivery approaches. Mixed perspectives on telemedicine adoption reflect technological issues, high implementation investment, and political, regulatory, and educational barriers. Despite these challenges, telemedicine enhances cost-effectiveness and satisfaction when well developed and deployed. Bioethical considerations relative to human dignity and rights, including access equity and informed consent, underpin global cooperation initiatives (Verma et al., 2025).

Core principles of sustainability and sustainable development permeate theoretical and practical formulations. Environmental impact and carbon emissions considerations are fundamental, especially in the health sector, where challenges to low-carbon delivery have expanded in recent decades. The global community recognizes the necessity of timely, efficient, affordable access and service delivery. Telemedicine represents a highly promising technology to realize these objectives across regions (Di Spirito et al., 2025).

Analysis of healthcare-related carbon footprint identifies transportation as the predominant contributor, varying by healthcare system—emergency, elective, inpatient, and outpatient—and transportation mode—road, rail, and air. Healthcare provider and patient travel dominate estimates, corroborated by comparative data from Australia, Sweden, and the United States. While historic avoidance of this travel through telemedicine is difficult to separate from medical travel reductions, initial modeling indicates carbon emissions from telemedicine remain well below conventional outpatient visits. Successful telemedicine programs exist both internationally and nationally (Nunes et al., 2025).

7 Comparative Analysis of Telemedicine Models

Telemedicine encompasses the provision of clinical and diagnostic services over distance, enabling both patients and healthcare providers to be in separate

Table 2.3 Clinical applications across medical specialties

Specialty	*Applications*	*Implementation Level*	*Outcomes*
Primary care	Chronic disease management, follow-up visits	High	Improved access, reduced no-shows
Dermatology	Skin condition diagnosis, lesion monitoring	High	Comparable to in-person care
Psychiatry	Therapy sessions, medication management	High	High patient satisfaction
Cardiology	Remote monitoring, ECG interpretation	Medium	Early intervention capability
Neurology	Stroke assessment, movement disorders	Medium	Reduced time to treatment

locations during communication (Casalinuovo, 2025). The main components of a telemedicine solution include a computer with software, a telecommunication link, and peripheral devices enabling the transmission of specific examinations and findings (Table 2.3). Delivery models for telemedicine involve various combinations of synchronous and asynchronous elements, as well as different locations and participation modes of patients and healthcare personnel (AlHilali et al., 2025). The three fundamental delivery modes are synchronous, asynchronous, and remote health monitoring or mobile health (m-health). Synchronous telemedicine involves real-time, live interaction between individuals or groups using video communication technologies; it encompasses applications such as tele-mentoring, teleconsultations, and diagnostic services conducted through videoconferences (Jenifer et al., 2025). In the asynchronous mode, also known as store-and-forward, data is exchanged without the need for all participants to be present simultaneously. Electronic transmission of surveys, sonograms, and CT scans to other individuals or sites typifies this model, with the individual or group providing the service responding when able or when necessary. Mobile health utilizes wearable devices or portable language translation programs to allow continuous or real-time follow-up without requiring synchronous communication (Badanta et al., 2025).

7.1 Specialty Applications

7.1.1 Tele Dermatology

Dermatological disorders are especially enhanced by telemedicine sites' visual assessment ability. High-resolution imaging devices can allow for close-up skin examinations, and dermatologists are able to diagnose and follow up on several types of skin disorders. The store-and-forward feature is especially useful in monitoring long-term condition changes. Dermatologists can successfully treat chronic skin diseases, provide follow-up treatment, and provide consultative services to primary care physicians through virtual sites (Jensen, 2025).

7.1.2 Telepsychiatry

Mental healthcare services offered via telemedicine platforms have been extremely effective. Online sessions ensure privacy and convenience without compromising the therapeutics alliance. The medium allows psychiatrists to carry out routine therapy sessions, medication maintenance, and crisis intervention services. Telepsychiatry has made mental healthcare delivery widely available, especially where there is limited access to psychiatric care (DesRoche et al., 2025).

7.1.3 Telecardiology

Cardiologists can remotely monitor patients' heart rhythm, blood pressure, and other cardiovascular indicators using long-term monitoring equipment. Wearable virtual integration offers real-time data streams to facilitate early cardiac event diagnosis and prompt action. Post-operative monitoring and management of chronic heart failure have proved to be of specific value through telecardiology services (Lv & Cho, 2025).

7.1.4 Tele Neurology

Neurological tests conducted via telemedicine platforms support the diagnosis and treatment of stroke, the assessment of movement problems, and headache consultation. In emergency cases, the technology enables prompt specialist consultation, especially for remote hospitals without on-site neurologists. Teleneurology has improved acute stroke care through expeditious assessment and treatment decision protocols, dramatically enhancing patient outcomes (Tseng et al., 2025).

7.1.5 Emergency Care

Through remote triage evaluation and specialist consultation for more serious situations, telemedicine makes it possible for emergency medicine to play a crucial role. The technology is especially helpful to rural emergency departments, which can access expert decision-making in challenging situations. The system is extremely useful in disaster response situations, allowing coordination among assorted health facilities and practitioners. Management of mass casualty incidents has been facilitated through virtual command centers for coordinating patient dispersal and allocation of resources (Salemdeeb, 2025).

7.1.6 Public Health

7.1.6.1 Disease Surveillance

Because telemedicine systems provide real-time data gathering and processing, they are crucial to public health surveillance. During the COVID-19 pandemic, this feature was very helpful in enabling prompt action against the spread of the disease. The technology allows public health authorities to track disease patterns, detect clusters, and institute targeted interventions better (Al Zuheimi, 2025).

7.1.6.2 Health Education and Prevention

Virtual platforms have revolutionized the delivery of health education, allowing healthcare practitioners to provide preventive care information to larger groups of audiences. Telemedicine platforms allow for interactive sessions and workshops that promote patient engagement and comprehension. The technology enhances continuous patient education programs, chronic disease management training classes, and preventive care programs (Singh et al., 2025).

7.1.6.3 Rural Healthcare

Telemedicine improves access to specialists and home monitoring programs, thereby reducing major gaps in healthcare access in remote locations. Through virtual consultation with urban medical facilities, rural health centers can now offer cutting-edge medical care. Rural healthcare professionals can receive ongoing education thanks to the technology, giving them the most recent skills and information. In rural areas, virtual care coordination has enhanced patient outcomes by giving prompt access to specialized medical knowledge (Chandiramohan et al., 2025).

8 Implementation

8.1 Clinical Workflow

Close integration with current clinical workflows is required when using telemedicine. It is necessary to create organizational procedures for scheduling patients, recording virtual visits, and coordinating care. In order to provide seamless patient care delivery, the implementation process involves giving considerable thought to emergency protocols and follow-up procedures (Madan, 2025).

8.2 Provider Training

Healthcare providers must receive in-depth instruction on how to use technical platforms and virtual examination techniques. Training covers emergency responses, paperwork requirements, and remote patient evaluation techniques. A significant component of provider training is communication tactics specifically designed for virtual care delivery. Continuous training and support help providers stay proficient with changing telemedicine technology (Raz et al., 2025).

8.3 Measuring the Effectiveness of Telemedicine

Utilizing information and communication technology, telemedicine offers a novel approach to remote medical consultations, guidance, diagnosis, and treatment with the goals of quality control, efficient healthcare delivery, and service personalization. Cost, carbon savings, and clinical outcome are the main indicators of telemedicine's efficacy. There are three fundamental approaches to remote healthcare delivery: synchronous, asynchronous, and remote monitoring. The biggest advantage of synchronous telemedicine, which uses real-time interactive video conferencing or phone calls, is that it allows patients and physicians to travel to the medical center with less carbon footprint. Asynchronous telemedicine, also known as store-and-forward, reduces carbon emissions related to travel for the majority of services by gathering and sending medical data, such as digital pictures or biosignals, that the consulting physician can study whenever it is convenient for them (Peng et al., 2025).

Remote monitoring. An alternative approach is one in which mobile healthcare applications allow patient data to be collected and stored for later transmission the next time an opportunity arises to get online (Flynn et al., 2025).

9 Conclusion

Telemedicine, capable of saving energy and materials required to travel to a hospital, reduces carbon emissions with the added benefits of improving accessibility and lowering costs. Conversations with patients on medical issues can be conducted remotely through telephones, smartphones, or computers instead of requiring face-to-face communication. Other forms of expression such as holography or virtual reality are expected to be used in remote healthcare delivery. Asynchronous telemedicine delivers services to patients and doctors at different times, while synchronous telemedicine enables real-time interaction.

Oncology patients illustrate the advantages of telemedicine for clinical practice. Patients who were farther away from the hospital had greater carbon emissions, implying that the commuting necessary for face-to-face visits would be decreased only if off-site medical care increased. Telemedicine produces significantly less carbon pollution than do usual care patterns in which patients and health professionals drive to appointments. Wider use of telemedicine might have a notable contribution to lessening greenhouse gas emissions promoting climate change, which demands empirical evidence of clinical, economic, and environmental advantages and further research to compare the effect of various telemedicine solutions. Since telemedicine is closer to the environmental impact of walking to a local hospital than to Stevens and Scandurra's green healthcare pyramid, it offers a better reference for green healthcare and a new sustainability strategy.

Providing an appropriate communication tool is crucial for completing a remote appointment, and the procedure must be coordinated so that both parties are free simultaneously during synchronous telemedicine appointments. An appropriate model will continue to depend on the patient's condition and hospital resources. Telemedicine constitutes an effective and flexible model for delivering remote healthcare based on individual facility circumstances. The contents of appointments can begin simply with one-on-one conversations and move toward sharing medical images or multi-person connections. To overcome the challenges and limitations of telemedicine—such as the digital divide, technology costs, data security, and limited clinical applicability in complex cases—multifaceted strategies are required. Expanding broadband connectivity and ensuring affordable access to smartphones or computers can minimize inequity in remote care. Hospitals and governments should invest in user-friendly, secure platforms that comply with privacy regulations to build trust among patients and clinicians. In addition, training programs for both healthcare providers and patients can enhance digital literacy and confidence in using telemedicine tools. Hybrid care pathways, where routine check-ups are conducted remotely and complex assessments remain in-person, can strike a balance between efficiency and clinical quality. Finally, integrating renewable-powered data centers and promoting eco-efficient digital infrastructure will further reinforce telemedicine's sustainability advantages while addressing its technological and environmental limitations. Last but not least, incorporating data centers that run on renewable energy sources and encouraging environmentally friendly digital infrastructure will strengthen telemedicine's sustainability benefits while resolving its technological and environmental drawbacks.

References

Addor, V., Fragnière, E., Demartines, N., & Agri, F. (2025). What are the objective key elements for successful deployment of telemedicine in hospitals: A holistic approach after 2 years of using a connected tracking solution. *Journal of Hospital Administration*, 14(1), 10–19.

Adeloduna, M. O., & Anyanwub, E. C. (2025). Telehealth implementation: A review of project management practices and outcomes. *Matrix Science Medica*, 9(1), 1–5.

Adirim, T. (2025). Digital health technologies: Virtual health and remote Patient monitoring. In T. Adirim (Ed.), *Digital Health, AI and Generative AI in Healthcare: A Concise, Practical Guide for Clinicians* (pp. 11–26). Springer Nature Switzerland.

Aisyah, N., Wibowo, F., Sari, I. P., Yusof, Z. B., & Saputra, B. (2025) Evaluating the efficacy of telemedicine in the long-term monitoring of patients with inflammatory bowel disease: A multicenter randomized trial, Kern Public, pp. 1–17.

Akgun, Z., & Palamar, M. (2025). Sustainability and minimization of carbon footprint in ophthalmology: What can we change in the outpatient clinic routine? *Eye*, 39, 2363–2368.

Al Zuheimi, M. H. (2025). Development of new technologies and intellectual property regulations in the sultanate of Oman. In N. Naim, A. AlDebasi, & D. Price (Eds.), *Intellectual Property and Innovation: Contemporary Developments in the GCC Member States* (pp. 79–107). Springer Nature Singapore.

Al-Battat, K. R., & Iyer, S. S. (2025). Social media influence in telemedicine for online patient doctor consultation. *Edelweiss Applied Science and Technology*, 9(1), 692–705.

Aldawoodi, N. N., Turner, K., Patel, K., Coughlin, E., Mhaskar, R., Streitmatter, C., … & Ackerman, R. S. (2025). A randomized controlled trial comparing pre-anesthesia evaluation via telemedicine to in-person at an NCI-designated comprehensive cancer center. *Telemedicine and e-Health*, 31(12), 1432–1442.

AlHilali, S., Bin Helayel, H., & Al-Swailem, S. (2025). Advancing sustainability in ophthalmic surgeries and interventions: A narrative review of environmental impact and best practices. *Clinical Ophthalmology*, 19,713–720.

Armstrong, D., & Tanaka, Y. (2025). Boosting telemedicine healthcare assessment using internet of things and artificial intelligence for transforming Alzheimer's detection. *Global Journal of Medical Terminology Research and Informatics*, 3(1), 8–14.

Arora, J. S., Smith, R. W., Green, A., Hentz, V. R., Curtin, C., & Fox, P. M. (2025). Reducing health care's carbon footprint: The environmental impact of telephone clinic visits for hand surgery. *The Journal of Hand Surgery*, 51(3), 321.e1–321.e7.

Atnang, M., Samsidar, S., & Mustamin, S. B. (2024). A systematic review of telemedicine in pediatrics evidence from randomized controlled trials. *Journal of Scientific Insights*, 1(1), 33–42.

Badanta, B., Porcar Sierra, A., Fernández, S. T., Rodríguez Muñoz, F. J., Pérez-Jiménez, J. M., Gonzalez-Cano-Caballero, M., … & de-Diego-Cordero, R. (2025). Advancing environmental sustainability in healthcare: Review on perspectives from health institutions. *Environments*, 12(1), 9.

Bianchi, G., & Gutierrez, J. (2025). Telehealth in hospital medicine beyond the COVID-19 pandemic: Expanding access, enhancing efficiency, and transforming care, IntechOpen.

Bolcato, V., Basile, G., Bianco Prevot, L., Fassina, G., Rapuano, S., Brizioli, E., & Tronconi, L. P. (2024). Telemedicine in Italy: Healthcare authorization profiles in the modern medico-legal reading. *International Journal of Risk & Safety in Medicine*, 35(4), 337–343.

Booker, R. J., Hunter, A., Sharpe, D., Claydon, M., Bartels, O., & Naumann, D. N. (2025). Reach-back to subject matter experts improves healthcare quality, influences the decision to evacuate and reduces costs: An observational study of the UK Defence Medical Services Deployed Telemedicine System. *BMJ Mil Health,* 2024–002941.

Brusco, M., Trivellini, S., Cozzali, R., Brusaferro, A., Morelli, O., Simonte, R., … & Valitutti, F. (2025). *The environmental impact of pediatric celiac disease diagnosis and follow-up*. JPGN Reports.

Casalinuovo, S. (2025). Lab-On-Mask as a telemedicine device: Implementation of commercial and innovative textile sensors for breath analysis, Rome: Sapienza University of Rome.

Ch, A. S., Pervaiz, F., Nawaz, H., Rafiq, S., Bibi, Y., Almagharbeh, W. T., & Mobeen, M. (2025). Health equity in telemedicine: Addressing disparities in digital healthcare access-A narrative review-S. *Insights-Journal of Life and Social Sciences*, 3(2), 56–62.

Chandiramohan, A. J., Zahabi, S., Sowerby, L., You, P., Davidson, J., Dann, C., & Strychowsky, J. E. (2025). Environmental impact and provider satisfaction associated with ePrescriptions in otolaryngology: A quality improvement study. *Journal of Otolaryngology-Head & Neck Surgery*, 54, 19160216251328883.

Chaudhuri, S., & Agarwal, S. (2025). Telerehabilitation in physiotherapy practice: A boon or a bane?. *European Journal of Physiotherapy*, 1–3.

Chauhan, P., Bali, A., & Kaur, S. (2024). Breaking barriers for accessible health programs: The role of telemedicine in a global healthcare transformation. In M. B. Garcia & R. P. P. de Almeida (Eds.), *Transformative Approaches to Patient Literacy and Healthcare Innovation* (pp. 283–307). IGI Global Scientific Publishing.

Chen, X., Ma, X., Scheibe, K. P., & Johnson, N. (2025). Omnichannel in healthcare? Offline-to-online spillover effects and implications for telemedicine in treating chronic patients. *Journal of Management Information Systems*, 42(1), 273–309.

Choi, D. J. (2025). The role and prospects of telemedicine in the treatment of heart failure patients: A narrative review. *The Ewha Medical Journal,* 48(2), e26.

Chu, M., Jiang, B., Li, H., Teh, F., Quek, J., Tan, A., … & Wong, Y. J. (2025). Improving uptake of telemedicine (phone/video consult): Methods and lessons learnt. *BMJ Open Quality*, 14(2), e003179.

Ciaralo, P. P. D., Cardoso, P. F. G., Minamoto, H., Bibas, B. J., de Carvalho, C. R. R., & Pego-Fernandes, P. M. (2025). Estimated carbon emissions and support cost savings to telemedicine for patients with tracheal diseases. *International Journal of Medical Informatics*, 195, 105757.

Conte, L. E., Orsi, M., Peruzzi, A., Fantozzi, C., Campanelli, M., Benavoli, D., … & Gentileschi, P. (2025). Preoperative remote consultation for a green bariatric surgery: Can telemedicine be safe for patients and sustainable for the environment? *Frontiers in Surgery*, 12, 1604486.

Dalimunthe, W., Ismaidar, I., & Simarmata, M. (2025). Patient legal protection in the digital era and study of telemedicine services in Indonesia. *DE LEGA LATA: Jurnal Ilmu Hukum*, 10(1), 40–49.

Delarmente, B., Romanov, A., Cui, M., Tseng, C. H., Damberg, C. L., Fendrick, A. M., & Mafi, J. N. (2025). Impact of telemedicine use on outpatient-related CO. *The American Journal of Managed Care*, 31(9), 294–298.

DesRoche, C., Soulez, G., Boucher, L., Fohlen, A., & Menard, A. (2025). Steps toward environmental sustainability in interventional radiology. *Canadian Association of Radiologists Journal*, 76(4), 603–610.

Di Spirito, F., Giordano, F., Di Palo, M. P., De Benedetto, G., Aulisio, L., & Boccia, G. (2025). Sustainable dental and periodontal practice: A narrative review on the 4R-framework—reduce, reuse, rethink, recycle—And waste management rationalization. *Dentistry Journal*, 13(9), 392.

Duane, B., Larkin, J., Caiazzo, M. L., Arenas, M. D., Griffin, A., Audije-Gil, J., … & Ortiz, A. (2025). But how green is it actually? Calculating the environmental footprint of Kidney care environmental optimisations within haemodialysis. *Clinical Kidney Journal*, 18(9), sfaf220.

Dziuba, D. O., Khavryuchenko, O. V., Domoratskyi, O. E., Maruniak, S. R., Mazur, A. P., Sharikadze, O. V., & Viter, D. V. (2025). Telemedicine as a tool for the digitization of healthcare. *Emergency Medicine*, 21(2), 130–139.

Eldeeb, S., Chieng, A., Xu, C. T., & Prochaska, J. J. (2025). Quantifying the pro-environmental impacts of telehealth tobacco treatment. *Telemedicine Reports*, 6(1), 171–178.

Ezenwaji, C. O., Alum, E. U., & Ugwu, O. P. C. (2025). Bridging the gap: Telemedicine as a solution for HIV care inequities in rural and vulnerable communities. *International Journal for Equity in Health*, 24(1), 205.

Flynn, C. R., de Guzman, R., Ayodele, O., Schiller, J. H., Lichter, K., Hwang, E. S., … & O'Reilly, S. (2025). Climate change and cancer care: Impacts and implications for patients and healthcare professionals, *ecancer*, 19, 1973.

Gaebe, K., Ng, A., Spiegel, J. L., Le, T. N., Lin, V. Y. W., & Chen, J. M. (2025). Cost Benefit and Carbon Emission Saving Analysis of Remote Cochlear Implant Programming. *The Laryngoscope,* 135(10), 3877–3884.

Galts, C., Anvari, S., Kim, A., Leontiadis, G., & Armstrong, D. (2025). Sustainable practice in gastroenterology: Travel-related CO_2 emissions for gastroenterology clinic appointments in Canada. *Journal of the Canadian Association of Gastroenterology*, 8(1), 7–12.

Gamus, A., Chodick, G., Blachar, Y., & Shalom, T. (2025). Triadic model of assisted telemedicine: Review of adoption challenges globally and in Israel. *Telemedicine and e-Health.*

Ghaderzadeh, M. (2025). Perspective chapter: Integrating artificial intelligence into telemedicine–opportunities, challenges, and future directions for healthcare delivery, IntechOpen.

Godard, F., Oosthoek, J., Alexis, A., Léo, P., Fontaine, E., Dahmani, M., … & Drouet, C. (2025). Estimation of carbon footprint in nuclear medicine: Illustration of a french department. *European Journal of Nuclear Medicine and Molecular Imaging*, 52(9), 3455–3464.

Gonzales, A. L., & Zhang, C. (2025). First-level fundamentals: Computer ownership is more important for internet benefits than in-home internet service. *Journal of Computer-Mediated Communication*, 30(3), zmaf007.

Harris, M., Chin, A. G., Smith, J., & Baxi, C. (2025). A trust-based theoretical model to determine adoption of telemedicine services. *Journal of Computer Information Systems*, 1–15.

Hendrix, E. M. B., de Jong, D. C., de Jong, M. J., Becx, M. C. J. M., van Bodegraven, A. A., Dijkstra, G., ... & Duijvestein, M. (2025). P0027 The carbon footprint of remote monitoring of IBD patients–a green opportunity for sustainable outpatient care. *Journal of Crohn's and Colitis*, 19(Supplement_1), i368–i369.

Huda, R. K., Chowhan, R. S., Arora, S., Seervi, D., Verma, S., Singh, J., ... & Babu, B. V. (2025). Perceptions of healthcare workers and patients on the implementation of telemedicine in hard-to-reach areas: A qualitative study from rajasthan, India. *Digital Health*, 11, 20552076251331874.

Ismail, Y., & Ebinezar, S. G. (2025). A review of evolution and applications of telemedicine in healthcare. *Journal of Pharma Insights and Research*, 3(2), 043–052.

Ivanova, J., Wilczewski, H., Klocksieben, F., Cummins, M., Soni, H., Ong, T., ... & Bunnell, B. (2024). Patient preferences for direct-to-consumer telemedicine services: Replication and extension of a nationwide survey. *JMIR Human Factors*, 11, e51056.

Jagatheesaperumal, S. K., Barreto, A. G., & C. de Albuquerque, V. H. (2025). Metaverse platforms for immersive healthcare: A survey on telemedicine solutions. *ACM Computing Surveys*, 58(2), 1–31. https://doi.org/10.1145/3762180

Jenifer, R. D., Vettriselvan, R., Saxena, D., Velmurugan, P. R., & Balakrishnan, A. (2025). Green marketing in healthcare advertising: A global perspective. In K. Chaudhary (Ed.), *AI Impacts on Branded Entertainment and Advertising* (pp. 303–326). IGI Global Scientific Publishing.

Jensen, L. H. (2025). Video in the clinic: Advancing care for patients, professionals, and the planet. *The Lancet Digital Health*, 7(6), 100875.

Jin, Q., Tian, W., & Jin, Z. (2025). Digital empowerment and trade-embodied carbon intensity: Insights from value-added decomposition in services. *Humanities and Social Sciences Communications*, 12(1), 1–10.

Jones-Esan, L., Somasiri, N., & Lorne, K. (2024). Enhancing healthcare delivery through digital health interventions: A systematic review on telemedicine and mobile health applications in Low and Middle-Income Countries (LMICs). https://doi.org/10.21203/rs.3.rs-5189203/v1

Khondakar, K. R., Tripathi, D., Mazumdar, H., Ahuja, K., & Kaushik, A. (2024). Tailored MXenes and graphene as efficient telemedicine platforms for personalized health wellness. *Materials Advances*, 5(10), 4091–4111.

Kumar, A., Ahmad, F., & Alam, B. (2025). Towards real time Alzheimer's diagnosis: A PSO-GA-driven deep learning solution for telemedicine. *International Journal of Imaging Systems and Technology*, 35(5), e70180.

Larsen, S. M., Jessen, N. H., Friederichsen, B., Brodersen, J. B., & Árnadóttir, Á. (2025). How to approach sustainability in general practice: A workshop experience with a qualitative analysis amongst general practitioners in Denmark. *Scandinavian Journal of Public Health*, Advance online publication. https://doi.org/10.1177/14034948251333003.

Lathan, R., Hitchman, L., Walshaw, J., Ravindhran, B., Carradice, D., Smith, G., ... & Yiasemidou, M. (2025). Postoperative remote first care for financially and environmentally sustainable healthcare. *NPJ Digital Medicine*, 8(1), 299.

Li, F., & Ci, F. (2025). Spatiotemporal evolution and driving factors of coupling coordination among China's digital economy, carbon emissions efficiency, and high-quality economic development. *Sustainability*, 17(14), 6410.

Li, Z., Xiang, L., Ning, J., Li, W., Huang, Y., & Xiao, X. (2025). Pathways to sustainable health care development: Study on the carbon reduction potential of telemedicine in China. *Journal of Medical Internet Research*, 27, e63927.

Liu, X., Chen, L., Lu, Y., Chang, M., Xiao, Y., Yang, H., … & Zhang, L. (2025). Research on the impact of the digital economy on carbon emissions based on the dual perspectives of carbon emission reduction and carbon efficiency. *Scientific Reports*, 15(1), 3416.

Liu, Z., Brandon-Jones, A., & Vasilakis, C. (2024). Unpacking patient engagement in remote consultation. *International Journal of Operations & Production Management*, 44(13), 157–194.

Lv, D., & Cho, E. (2025). The unseen carbon cost of AI workforce: A behavioral theory perspective of environmental scalability. *Business Horizons*, 68(6), 759–776.

Madan, V. (2025). Trambulance-an innovate transport model, aligning healthcare delivery with sustainable development: A case study from the northern care alliance NHS foundation trust, UK. *Discover Sustainability*, 6(1), 271.

Mainer-Pearson, G., Stewart, K., Williams, K., Pawlovich, J., Graham, S., Riches, L., … & Ho, K. (2025). Estimating patient and family costs and CO_2 emissions for telehealth and in-person health care appointments in British Columbia, Canada: Geospatial mixed methods study. *Journal of Medical Internet Research*, 27, e56766.

Mazziotti, G., Pongiglione, B., Carrone, F., Meregaglia, M., Angelucci, A., Costantino, M. L., … & Compagni, A. (2025). Improvement of medication adherence in osteoporosis through telemedicine combined with email: A patient-reported experience and outcome measure-based prospective study. *BMJ Health & Care Informatics*, 32(1), e101338.

Mehrolhassani, M. H., Yazdi-Feyzabadi, V., Dehnavieh, R., Bahaadinbeigy, K., & Kargar, M. (2025). Barriers to telemedicine establishment in Iran: A systematic review. *Iranian Journal of Public Health*, 54(4), 739.

Mercier, O., Parpia, R., Presseau, J., Muldoon, K. A., & Sampsel, K. (2024). Telemedicine and virtual healthcare for survivors of sexual assault and intimate partner violence: A qualitative study. *Women's Health*, 20, 17455057241252958.

Mesteru, E. G. (2025). Sustainability in the management of the private medical sector in Romania: A European, USA and Japan comparison. *Sustainability*, 17(12), 5360.

Muralidhar, L. B., Swapna, H. R., Sathyanarayana, N., Nethravathi, K., Rahul, V., Pandey, D., & Dadheech, P. (2025). Quantum cryptography for biomedical image security in next-generation telemedicine networks. In P. K. Pattnaik, R. Kumar, & S. K. Bhoi (Eds.), *Advanced Secure Transmission of Telemedicine-Based Bio-Medical Images* (pp. 273–306). IGI Global Scientific Publishing.

Muzzamil, M., Karim, M., Khurram, S. S., Aga, I. Z., Hashmi, S., Hassan, H. G., & Younus, Y., 2025. Patient perspectives and utilization of telemedicine for chronic conditions in Pakistan barriers and facilitators towards its access. *Discover Public Health*, 22(1), p.30.

Nicksa, G. A., Chicoine, N., Li, L. T., Jamshidi, R., Lehane, A. J., Raval, M. V., King, S. D., & Greenberg, S. 2025. 'Protecting our patients' future through perioperative sustainability: Action and advocacy for the pediatric surgeon'. *Seminars in Pediatric Surgery*, 35. https://doi.org/10.1016/j.sempedsurg.2025.151518.

Nunes, A. R., Karaba, F., Geddes, O., Bickerton, A., Atherton, H., Dahlmann, F., … & Dale, J. (2025). Implementation of decarbonisation actions in general practice: A systematic review and narrative synthesis. *BMJ Open*, 15(2), e091404.

Obisesan, O. O., Aidonojie, P. A., Onwubiko, K. J., & John, D. J. (2024). Intimate partner violence (IPV), the culture of silence: Telemedicine as panacea and its challenge in Nigeria. *NIU Journal of Humanities*, 9(2), 21–32.

Olowoyo, K. S., Esan, D. T., Olowoyo, P., Oyinloye, B. E., Fawole, I. O., Aderibigbe, S., … & Adeyanju, B. T. (2025). Treatment adherence and outcomes in patients with tuberculosis treated with telemedicine: A scoping review. *Tropical Medicine and Infectious Disease*, 10(3), 78.

Othman, Z. K., Musa, S. S., Ahmed, M. M., Okesanya, O. J., Alhammadi, O. A. S., & Eliseo III, D. L. P. (2025). Digital health technologies in Kurdistan region of Iraq: A narrative review of enhancing healthcare accessibility and quality. *Discover Public Health*, 22(1), 227.

Kumar, M. S., & Ganesh, D. (2024). Improving telemedicine through IoT and cloud computing: Opportunities and challenges. *Advances in Engineering and Intelligence Systems*, 30;3(03), 123–135.

Özen, F., Kaynar, A. H., Korkut, A. K., Teker Açıkel, M. E., Kaynar, Z. D., & Kaynar, A. M. (2024). The role of telemedicine towards improved sustainability in healthcare and societal productivity in Turkey. *PloS One*, 19(12), e0314986.

Parker, E. B., Young, C. C., Bluman, E. M., & Smith, J. T. (2025). The carbon footprint of in-person versus virtual orthopaedic care. *JAAOS Global Research & Reviews*, 9(7), e25.

Peng, K., Muhammad, M., Feng, Y., Ren, J., & Mejri, M. (2025). Dynamic connectedness in FinTech and sustainability: Unraveling risk spillovers across environmental governance, green finance, clean energy, and digital innovations. *Green Finance, Clean Energy, and Digital Innovations,* SSRN Working Paper / Preprint, 1–26.

Rafi, Z., Khan, S., Ahmad, S., & Kaur, K. (2025). The synergy of nanomedicine and telemedicine. *Telemedicine and E-Health Essentials*, 28–50.

Ratheesh, N., Jain, E., & Lakshmi, D. (2025). Advancing healthcare for travelers: The integration of mobile health applications in telemedicine. In *Navigating Innovations and Challenges in Travel Medicine and Digital Health* (pp. 277–310). IGI Global Scientific Publishing.

Raz, R., Negev, M., Hauzer, M., Miller, E., Paltiel, O., & Kissinger, M. (2025). Environmental responsibility in the Israeli health system in the era of climate change: A required paradigm shift. *Israel Journal of Health Policy Research*, 14(1), 19.

Ren, L., Cheng, S., Tong, Y., Zhang, Y., Zhu, F., Tian, Y., & Yue, T. (2025). Study on carbon emission accounting method system and its application in the Iron and steel industry. *Sustainability*, 17(9), 3829.

Rizzo, L., Barbetta, E., Ruberti, F., Petz, M., Tornesello, M., Deolmi, M., … & Esposito, S. (2024). The role of telemedicine in children with obstructive sleep apnea syndrome (OSAS): A review of the literature. *Journal of Clinical Medicine*, 13(7), 2108.

Saeed, S., Singhal, M., Kaur, K. N., Shannawaz, M., Koul, A., Arora, K., … & Arora Sr, K. (2024). Acceptability and satisfaction of patients and providers with telemedicine during the COVID-19 pandemic: A systematic review. *Cureus*, 16(3), 1–8.

Saleh, A., Nona, P., Price, E. B., Rickards, J., & Andrikopoulou, E. (2025). Principles of telehealth and telemedicine in cardio-oncology. In S.-A. Brown (Ed.), *Innovations in Cardio-Oncology* (pp. 141–158). Academic Press.

Salemdeeb, M. (2025). AI impact on climate change. In M. Wadi, M. Salemdeeb, & M. Jouda (Eds.), *Innovations and Applications of Artificial Intelligence in Electrical and Electronics Engineering*.

Samal, P., & Samantaray, S. (2024, January). Balancing technology and environmental responsibility: Leveraging telemedicine for sustainable healthcare solutions. In S. Mishra et al. (Eds.), *2024 International Conference on Advancements in Smart, Secure and Intelligent Computing (ASSIC)* (pp. 1–5). IEEE.

Savoldelli, A., Landi, D., & Rizzi, C. (2024). Exploring the environmental impact of telemedicine: A life cycle assessment. In D. Hayn, B. Pfeifer, G. Schreier, & M. Baumgartner (Eds.), *dHealth 2024* (pp. 81–86). IOS Press.

Schmidt Jr, A. F., de Freitas Filho, O., Tsuboi, C. E., Cordeiro, T. A. G., Perondi, M. B. D. M., Utiyama, E. M., & Pego Fernandes, P. M. (2025). Utilizing telemedicine in public health services for the treatment of patients with thoracic surgical conditions. *Telemedicine and e-Health,* 31(4), 556–562.

Sebai, J., Leslie, W., & Lichy, J. (2025). The role of telemedicine during and beyond the COVID-19 pandemic: Shaping our future health organisations and practices. *International Journal of Organizational Analysis*, 33(5), 1236–1259.

Seckam, A., Ordell, R., James, D., & Crone, D. (2025). Experiences and perceptions of using a digital health intervention. *Physiotherapy*, 126 (Supplement 1), 101587.

Şenel Tekin, P., & Bekar, F. (2025). Sustainable development, ecological footprint, carbon footprint, biomimicry, permaculture, and proactive behavior. In F. Özsungur & F. Bekar (Eds.), *Empowering Employee Proactive Behavior: Concepts and Perspectives from Organization and Society* (pp. 239–266). Springer Nature Switzerland.

SHI, Q., CAO, M., & BAI, Y. (2025). Power-aware video transmission in 5G telemedicine: Challenges, solutions, and future directions. *Power*, 16(7), 45–57.

Shinde, S. S., Khandare, N. B., Kale, G. M., & Nalbalwar, S. L. (2025, May). Transforming industries with green business models: Strategic management approaches to sustainable energy and technology. In *2025 International Conference in Advances in Power, Signal, and Information Technology (APSIT)* (pp. 1–6). IEEE, Bhubaneswar, India.

Shokoohi, H., Liteplo, A., Montoya, K., Patnode, C., Hutchinson, A. B., Zalis, M. E., … & Slutzman, J. E. (2025). Climate-smart diagnostic medical imaging: An evidence-based perspective. *The Journal of Emergency Medicine,* 75, 150–157.

Shrivastava, A., & Shrivastava, A. (2024). Modeling telemedicine consumer behavior amid COVID-19 pandemic. *International Journal of Pharmaceutical and Healthcare Marketing*, 18(3), 375–397.

Singh, B., Kaunert, C., & Jermsittiparsert, K. (2025). Advocating medical tourism and healthcare in global health market places: Promoting sustainability and technological advancements. In K. S. Solanki, A. K. Bhoi, & M. K. Mishra (Eds.), *AI Technologies and Advancements for Psychological Well-Being and Healthcare* (pp. 327–350). IGI Global.

Sugawara, Y., Hirakawa, Y., Iwagami, M., Inokuchi, R., Wakimizu, R., & Nangaku, M. (2025). Metrics for evaluating telemedicine in randomized controlled trials: Scoping review. *Journal of Medical Internet Research*, 27, e67929.

Swati, M., Sharma, S., & NishthaThakur, M. (2025). Effectiveness of mobile health apps and telepsychiatry in supporting mental health nursing care: A systematic review. *Journal of Neonatal Surgery*, 14(32s), 840.

Ta, H. D., Van Vu, H., Mai, T. X., Nguyen, H. T. M., Do, T. T. T., & Luu, H. N. (2025). Utilization, demand, and willingness to pay for telehealth services: A study of patients in selected Vietnamese provinces. *Asia Pacific Journal of Health Management*, 20(1), 141–148.

Tseng, M. H., Lian, J. Y., Liu, A. S., & Chen, P. T. (2025). An interpretive structural modeling approach for biomedical innovation strategy models with sustainability. *Sustainability*, 17(15), 6740.

Tshiamala, D., & Tartibu, L. (2025). Telemedicine queuing system study: Integrating queuing theory, Artificial Neural Networks (ANNs) and Particle Swarm Optimization (PSO). *Applied Sciences*, 15(11), 6349.

Umpierre, R. N., Mattiello, R., Schmitz, C. A. A., Falceto de Barros, E., da Silva, R. S., Gonçalves, M. R., & Goldim, J. R. (2025). Greening healthcare and slashing carbon emissions through telemedicine: A cross-sectional study from over 50 thousand remote consults at a leading tertiary hospital. *Frontiers in Digital Health*, 7, 1497770.

van der Zee, C., Chang-Wolf, J., Koopmanschap, M. A., van Leeuwen, R., & Wisse, R. P. (2024). Assessing the carbon footprint of telemedicine: A systematic review. *Health Services Insights*, 17, 11786329241271562.

Van Rhee, N. F., Schoonbeek, R. C., Wegner, I., Vermeulen, K. M., Maat, R. C., de Loos, D. A. D., ... & Plaat, B. E. (2025). Telemedicine follow-up for pre-malignant and malignant glottic lesions: A randomised controlled trial study protocol comparing care close to home versus standard of care. *Acta Oncologica*, 64, 1035–1040.

Vanaria, R. J., Bhupalam, V., Marrero-Perez, A., Chaudry, A., Awad, N., & Nestor, M. (2025). Environmental impact and sustainability associated with the practice of dermatology. *The Journal of Clinical and Aesthetic Dermatology*, 18(2), 50.

Verdonck, P., & Verniers, I. (2025). Environmental sustainability in healthcare: Managerial concerns and solutions. *Best Practice & Research Clinical Anaesthesiology,* 39, 101–113.

Verma, N., Radhakrishnan, D., & Ray, D. (2025). Greening digital healthcare balancing act for sustainable future. In D. K. Sharma, R. Singh, & A. Kumar (Eds.), *Optimization Tools and Techniques for Enhanced Computational Efficiency* (pp. 81–124). IGI Global Scientific Publishing.

Vudathaneni, V. K. P., Lanke, R. B., Mudaliyar, M. C., Movva, K. V., Kalluri, L. M., Boyapati, R., & krishna prasad Vudathaneni, V. (2024). The impact of telemedicine and remote patient monitoring on healthcare delivery: A comprehensive evaluation. *Cureus*, 16(3), e55534.

Weppner, W. G., Jeffreys, A. S., Coffman, C. J., Bosworth, H. B., Edelman, D., & Crowley, M. J. (2025). Decarbonizing health care: Measuring the carbon footprint impact of a national VA telehealth program. *NEJM Catalyst Innovations in Care Delivery*, 6(5), CAT–24.

Wong, Y. L., Aslam, T. M., Chang, D. F., & Erny, B. (2025). Sustaining ophthalmic practices for the future: A high-value care approach to environmental responsibility. *Ophthalmology and Therapy*, 14, 1–20.

Yahia, M. E., Ali, S. B., Aldurra, O. H., & Alagha, A. Y. (2025). Hospital design for rural areas with telemedicine services: Case study in Sudan. *Authorea Preprints*.

Zhang, Y., & Feng, J. (2025). Towards a smart and sustainable future with edge computing-powered internet of things: Fundamentals, applications, challenges, and future research directions. *Journal of The Institution of Engineers (India): Series B*, 106(2), 785–804.

Zhang, Z., Yu, Y., Zheng, H., & Tian, P. (2025). The intersecting impact of aging and affluence on China's household carbon emissions. *Environmental Impact Assessment Review*, 115, 107997.

Zito, A., Prete, D., De Pascalis, A., Ria, P., Elia, G., & Napoli, M. (2025). Sustainable self-assisted home haemodialysis through telemedicine: An economic and environmental perspective. *Measuring Business Excellence,* 29(4), 815–830.

Zurl, H., Qian, Z., Stelzl, D. R., Dagnino, F., Korn, S. M., Labban, M., ... & Cole, A. P. (2025). Carbon emissions from patient travel for health care. *JAMA Network Open*, 8(3), e252513–e252513.

3 Creating Clean, Green, and Smart Learning Spaces in Pharmaceutical Educational Institutes

Somesh Thapliyal, Amit Chaudhary, Aruna Sharma, and Vikas Solanki

1 Introduction

In India, pharmacy education began in 1932, initiated by Professor M.L. Schroff at Banaras Hindu University. The Pharmacy Council of India was formed in 1949 under the Ministry of Health, which governs all statutory regulations of pharmacy education in India, as described in the Pharmacy Act 1948. Neuroplasticity is defined as the brain's "ability to reorganize" itself by forming new neural connections throughout life. Neuroplasticity is especially important in early life. Research has shown evidence that demonstrates experiences and learning can affect brain structure, including how thick the cortex is and how branching dendrites look. It has been found through functional magnetic resonance imaging studies that neuroplasticity can be found even in an adult's brain. The neuroplasticity approach has significant implications for educational psychology and rehabilitation medicine.

Nowadays, the phenomenon of global warming has made environmental sustenance a worldwide concern. Global warming results in unstable weather, too much heat, heavy rain, tornadoes, and intense storms. Various researchers have confirmed through their studies the increased amount of CO_2 in the environment due to increased human activities on a worldwide scale, which include transportation, industries, and domestic practices. The involvement of intellectuals along with the public can aid the solution of environmental problems. This commitment might be observed in several practices or projects concerning various areas of life, including the environment, which covers green marketing strategies, green campuses, green production, green human resource management practices, and sustainable institutes, along with sustainable education.

One of the leading culprits of pollution is the pharma sector; it has to be acknowledged that more than 100,000 tons of medications are used globally each year, of which more than 50% of all pharmaceuticals used globally each year are used only in the United States and then in the European Union. The usage of such a high quantity of pharmaceuticals has a profound impact on the environment that cannot be overlooked; henceforth, it highlights that it is important for pharmaceutical education institutions to adopt a vision that is not only clean and green but also smart (Federation, 2015). All of these are important factors that demand a highly dynamic and responsive approach toward education as a whole; henceforth, it is important to

DOI: 10.4324/9781003640486-3

ensure that the students of tomorrow are prepared to sustain the profound changes that are looming in their fields; it is vital that not only do pharmaceutical industry employees have profound knowledge of science, but it is important that their knowledge of cutting-edge technologies and of working amidst highly controlled and completely efficient working conditions is also extensive.

A sustainable campus refers to an institute that promotes environmentally friendly concepts, social concerns, and economic efficiency measures (Buana et al., 2018). Research about the sustainability of educational institutions revealed that the educational institutions that maintain sustainability provide a high level of comfort in the lives of their citizens rather than those that are not sustainable (Tiyarattanachai and Hollmann, 2016). Offering sustainability can contribute greatly to the formation of a new generation of citizens that can lead a clean and green world.

This chapter's objective is to explore the key elements that contribute to building a clean, green, and smart campus in the context of pharmaceutical education.

2 Concept of Clean, Green, and Smart Campuses

Currently, one of the major issues is that educational institutions are to be clean and smart. The concept of a clean campus is the starting point for sustainability. A green campus is an initiative or a place that brings together environmentally friendly initiatives, sustainable practices, and environmental education. A smart campus is an academic institution that combines technology to achieve sustainability. A modern pharmaceutical institute should prepare students for the complexities of the global pharmaceutical industry by integrating "Clean, Green," and "Smart" principles.

3 Clean Campus

Improved hygiene and sanitation practices in educational institutes play a very important role in preventing contamination and infection, which is paramount for health safety, research, and integrity (Kabir, Roy, Begum, Kabir, & Miah, 2021). Educational institutions, particularly pharmacy institutes, generate a variety of waste owing to their academic, laboratory, and research activities. This waste includes chemicals such as solvents, acids, alkalis, and expired reagents, as well as biomedical waste such as syringes, cotton, and culture media. Additionally, they produce general waste (Elhalwagy, 2024). Various types of waste in pharmaceutical educational institutions include:

- **Biodegradable Waste**: Food scraps, paper, garden waste, human waste, natural polymers, culture media, and so on.
- **Non-biodegradable Waste**: Plastics, metals, glass, etc.
- **Hazardous Waste**: Chemicals and toxins
- **Electronic Waste**: Computers, projectors, printers, etc.
- **Biomedical Waste**: Gloves, syringes, culture plates, etc.

Biodegradable waste is organic matter that can be broken down naturally by microorganisms and other living organisms into simple, non-toxic substances such as carbon dioxide, water, methane, and compost (Katinas, Marčiukaitis, Perednis, & Dzenajavičienė, 2019). In contrast, waste that cannot be decomposed by biological processes is known as non-biodegradable waste (Bharadwaj, Yadav, & Varshney, 2015). Hazardous waste is defined as a material that is discarded because of its inherent properties and poses a potential hazard to human health or the environment (Misra & Pandey, 2005). Biomedical waste is the result of laboratory work, diagnosis, treatment, and associated biomedical research (Hegde, Kulkarni, & Ajantha, 2007). Waste generated by all parts and items of electronic and electrical equipment that are discarded without the intention of being reused is known as electronic waste (Shahabuddin et al., 2023).

3.1 Environmental Hazards of Discarded Pharmaceutical Waste

Water contamination is a major consequence of improper pharmaceutical waste disposal, posing a risk to human health (Rajbongshi, Shah, & Sajib, 2016; MK Vijayalakshmi et al., 2023). Some of the unwanted compounds reached water bodies due to improper waste disposal methods, which adversely affect aquatic systems. These toxic chemicals disrupt the normal behavior and reproductive capabilities of aquatic life. When fish, amphibians, and other water animals absorb these toxic substances, the process of bioaccumulation will occur through the food chain. As a result of improper waste disposal methods, the development of drug-resistant pathogens can occur, which may be transmitted to human, animal, or other environmental media, causing infection that cannot be treated. Degradation of soil quality occurs due to some pharmaceuticals, which leads to an array of negative environmental impacts. Some pharmaceuticals are absorbed into plant parts. Whatever the residual pharmaceutical compound present in the plant parts may be, it enters the human or animal body when it is consumed as food and causes health effects such as allergic reactions, endocrine disruption, or development of antimicrobial resistance.

3.1.2 Effective Strategies for Managing Pharmaceutical Waste

Effective management of pharmaceutical waste involves crucial practices such as source segregation accompanied by the active collaboration of all the concerned stakeholders in the direction of sustainability. The different phases of the management of waste comprise the collection, segregation, transportation, processing, recycling, and ultimate disposal of the waste materials. It is important to inculcate a sense of sustainability in educational institutions along with maintaining a good environment in educational institutions. Educational institutes are adopting zero-waste strategies to promote sustainable development, particularly in developing countries such as Turkey, India, Malaysia, and Indonesia (Kasavan, Yusoff, Ali, & Masarudin, 2021; Trihadiningrum, Anandita, & Nadira, 2023) (Table 3.1).

Table 3.1 Pharmaceutical take-back programs

S. No.	*Program*	*Country*	*Reference*
1	National Prescription Drug Take-Back Day	USA	Fleming et al. (2016)
2	Secure and Responsible Drug Disposal Act (2014)	USA	Barenie, Leav, Johnson III, & Wheeler (2022); Perry, Shinn, & Stanovich (2014)
3	National Return Unused Medicines (NatRUM) program	Australia	Kirkpatrick, Dooley, & Charman, (2013); Wheeler, Kelly, Spinks, & Bettington, (2016)

3.1.3 Importance of Waste Management

- In the prevention of pollution of land, water, and air.
- To reduce infections and diseases.
- To conserve resources.
- Meet the legal and regulatory standards set by environmental authorities.
- To raise awareness among students about adopting sustainable practices.

To achieve a safe academic environment, stakeholders of any institute need regular training in pharmaceutical waste management. One of the most effective ways to deal with expired drugs is through the pharmaceutical take-back program, an initiative for collecting and disposing of expired drugs from households, healthcare centers, and other sources (Mitkidis, Chrysochou, Obolevich, & Mitkidis, 2022). The USA, European countries, Australia, New Zealand, Malaysia, and Brunei have implemented this program (Ariffin & Zakili, 2019; Rogowska & Zimmermann, 2022).

Waste undergoes various treatments to reduce its harmful effects and is then disposed of through methods such as incineration, landfilling, and recycling (M Vijayalakshmi, 2020).

According to the World Health Organization (WHO) guidelines (Frontières & Frontières, 1999), pharmaceutical solid waste, like tablets, capsules, and semisolid waste, such as creams and ointments, can be managed by the processes of incineration, encapsulation, and landfilling. Specially designed incinerators are used in the incineration method to destroy the pharmaceutical waste, minimizing the release of harmful byproducts. In the encapsulation method, pharmaceutical waste is immobilized in a solid block within a drum. Impermeable linings and proper drainage systems are designed in landfill sites to prevent soil and groundwater contamination. Dilution and sewage flushing are two methods to dispose of liquid pharmaceutical waste.

Disintegration, screening, flotation, and sedimentation, with pH and temperature adjustment, are preliminary treatments to remove pharmaceutical waste (Khalidi-Idrissi et al., 2023). Bioprocesses are commonly used methods for treating biodegradable waste. Activated sludge systems, bioreactors, and biofilm reactors are used for biological treatment (Badia-Fabregat et al., 2016). This technique

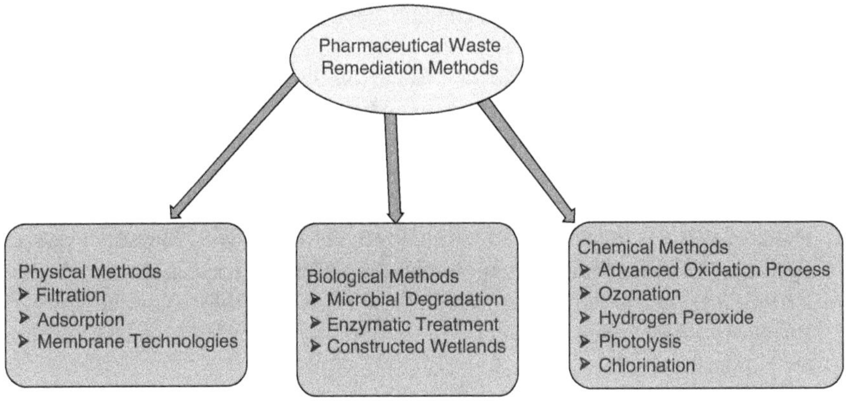

Figure 3.1 Methods of pharmaceutical waste remediation.

is effective for the remediation of pollutants, including β-lactam antibiotics commonly used in medical treatment and halogenated organic compounds often found in industrial processes; however, the application of this technique remains limited. These biological agents exist under various environmental conditions. Further studies are required to optimize these methods and enhance their reliability for wider use in pollution mitigation strategies (Dou et al., 2023).

In the initial stages of wastewater treatment, filtration, sedimentation, and adsorption (including using activated carbon to adsorb trace pharmaceutical residues) are routinely used, followed by mechanical or thermal techniques, such as incineration and ultrafiltration. However, more advanced technologies have produced hybrid systems that combine natural processes, such as constructed wetlands, with controlled microbial degradation in an activated sludge membrane bioreactor for further purification (Aminullah, Khan, Nisar, Arbak, & Ishtiaq, 2025).

Ambient ionization mass spectrometry is a modern method used to identify pharmaceutical pollutants in complex matrices that requires no pre-treatment (Ranjbari et al., 2022).

Oxidation, precipitation, and complex reactions are various methods to neutralize harmful materials, which fall under the chemical method of remediation. Functional materials, such as micro- and nanoparticles, degrade waste by enzymatic hydrolysis and oxidative decomposition of waste (Figure 3.1). Currently, advanced oxidation processes, membrane separation, and bioelectrochemical methods are used for the removal of natural organic matter; however, these technologies require more energy, have limited specificity, and generate secondary waste (Nieminen, Anugwom, Kallioinen, & Mänttäri, 2020).

3.1.4 *Recycling*

Recycling involves the collection, processing, and creation of new products from materials that would otherwise be discarded. It works well for reducing pollution, conserving energy, and protecting natural resources (B. Ma, Li, Jiang, & Jiang, 2019).

Recycling generally involves three main steps:

- **Collection and Sorting**: The first stage of the waste management process involves gathering all waste materials produced within an institute or university from predetermined collection points, either through scheduled curbside pickup programs, drop-off centers where people can bring their waste, or buy-back centers that provide incentives to return recyclable materials. In the next step, gathered waste is transported to a specialized facility called a Material Recovery Facility (MRF) for the sorting and separation of waste for recycling purposes.
- **Processing**: In this step, the sorted material is processed for manufacturing.
- **Purchase of Recycled Products**: In the last step, recycled materials are used for purchase.

3.1.4.1 RECYCLING OF PLASTIC WASTE

Research showed that approximately 66% of the plastic produced each year ends up in the environment, with less than 10% being recycled. Microplastics have been detected in Arctic ice, the deep sea, and even human biological samples, such as blood, breast milk, and placenta (Le, 2025).

Recycling plastic waste is essential to preserve resources and improve the economy. Converting plastic waste into high-value carbon materials may provide a helpful role in achieving sustainability and maintaining the economy. Examples of carbon material include graphene, carbon nanotubes, and activated carbon, which have excellent electrical, thermal, and mechanical properties, due to which these materials are facilitated for use in various waste management applications. Depending on their source, plastics can be classified into three broad groups comprising natural polymers, such as lignin, chitin, and starch; semi-synthetic polymers obtained from natural polymeric materials like chemically modified cellulose; and synthetic polymers obtained from petrochemicals, including styrene, silicone, nylon, and polyethylene.

Three main approaches in the management of plastic wastes are landfilling, mechanical recycling, and incineration. Of these three approaches, landfilling is the most employed method for managing plastic waste; it embraces large amounts of land and often presents various ecological risks. For example, the leachate collected from the landfill can comprise resistant biological matter such as naphthalene, phenanthrene, and chlorinated polycyclic aromatic hydrocarbons.

Mechanical recycling is one common method of recycling plastic materials, and some processes included in mechanical recycling processes for plastic materials are cutting, grinding, washing, flaking, and pelletizing. However, during the recycling process, heat and physical effects can influence the degradation and reduction of thermal, physical, and mechanical properties. On the same note, plastic materials have a lifespan to undergo mechanical recycling processes before the waste is subjected to other recycling processes.

In particular, thermosetting plastics like polyurethanes, which undergo degradation easily when heat treatment is employed, ought to be addressed in terms of incineration. There are also significant environmental impacts when using the incineration techniques. For example, fewer than 6% of plastic wastes can be treated through incineration. Urgent approaches in handling wastes need to be put in place.

When disposed in the environment, they decompose over a long period of time through a series of physical, chemical, and biological changes to ultimately decompose into little fragments called microplastics. Increased temperature can increase the brittleness of plastic polymers to speed up their breakdown, while changes in pH can affect the chemical stability of plastic materials, also contributing to fragmentation by mechanical forces such as abrasion, ultraviolet radiation, wave or wind action, and eventually breaking larger items into particles smaller than 5 mm in diameter. These microplastics are persistent and emerging pollutants because they are not biodegradable and accumulate in ecosystems, where they can be ingested by aquatic organisms and enter the food chain (Liu et al., 2023).

Microfiltration, ultrafiltration, reverse osmosis, and membrane bioreactor (MBRs) technologies are useful for microplastic management (Hanif et al., 2022). Adsorption has been shown to be highly effective for removing microplastics from water sources. One study examined the extraction of polystyrene-based nanoparticles from water using a chromium-based metal-organic framework (Cr-MOF) adsorbent synthesized using the hydrothermal method (Modak, Kasula, & Esfahani, 2023).

Chemical recycling is a method that affects the molecular structure of materials using chemical reactions under certain conditions of temperature, pressure, and catalysts to transform plastics into their original monomers and other products such as hydrogen, oxygen, carbon monoxide, carbon dioxide, and methane (Luo, Tyrrell, Bai, Muazu, & Long, 2024). Some typical methods of this technique include chemolysis, pyrolysis, gasification, bioconversion, and catalysis (J. Chen et al., 2022).

Waste plastic pyrolysis can be achieved through direct thermal or catalytic cracking. In direct thermal cracking, plastic waste is heated to high temperatures, causing the breakdown of large polymers into smaller hydrocarbons, such as gases, oils, and char. Catalytic cracking employs specific catalysts, such as zeolites and metal oxides, causing the breakdown of polymers. This process lowers the operating temperature and increases the yield of desirable products, particularly light hydrocarbons and liquid fuels, while producing a more stable pyrolysis oil with fewer impurities (J. Ma et al., 2023; Park, Jeong, Guzelciftci, & Kim, 2019).

In photolysis, ultraviolet (UV) radiation from sunlight causes radical-mediated reactions in which polymer molecules absorb energy; due to this reaction, the chemical bonds of plastics break down. Polyethylene (PE) and polypropylene (PP) are the polymer molecules that are commonly used in this method (Fueki, Takeuchi, Torikai, & Nagaya, 1986; Gewert, Plassmann, & MacLeod, 2015). Thermal catalysis, catalytic conversion, and hydrocracking are the methods to convert waste plastic into valuable chemicals and fuels (Lee, Jing, Wang, & Yan, 2022).

3.1.4.2 RECYCLING OF FOOD WASTE

Food waste consists of food items along with inedible items discarded in the human food supply chain. This has a considerable influence on the environment, economy, and society as a whole. Food waste happens in different phases of the supply chain, including the production phase, processing phase, distribution phase, and consumption phase.Creating valuable materials or products from food waste in the form of biofertilizer products, animal feed materials, or functional food materials helps in the establishment of a sustainable food system in the circular economy. Traditional methods of food waste recycling comprise composting, anaerobic digestion methods, and upcycling methods.

3.1.5 Sanitation and Hygiene

The promotion of a sound practice of sanitation and hygiene in an educational environment is of critical use in reducing the infection risk while helping in the promotion of a conducive lifestyle (Aiello, Coulborn, Perez, & Larson, 2008). The use of improved access to sanitation, coupled with a sound practice of hygiene, was emphasized by the United Nations as an important dimension of Sustainable Development Goal 6, thus directing itself toward the attainment of a sound practice of sustainable economic development while creating a sound future for the communities at large (Mara & Evans, 2018).

3.1.6 Air and Water Quality

Poor quality of indoor air can have negative effects on human health, including breathing problems like asthma, bronchitis, and tiredness. This usually comes about because of poor ventilation, pollutants, dust mites, or chemicals coming from the construction materials used or the furniture in the buildings. This condition needs attention in the development toward a healthy, better environment for all (Mendell & Heath, 2005).

4 Green Campus

The main objectives of the Green Campus Initiatives (GCIs) are the creation of sustainable infrastructure, reduction of environmental impacts and economic costs, and raising the awareness of the students regarding the principles of sustainable development (Joao Marcelo Pereira Ribeiro et al., 2021).

4.1 Advantages of Green Campus

- It reduces environmental impact and operational costs.
- It creates a healthy and inspiring learning environment.
- It fosters environmental responsibility and awareness among students.
- It encourages innovation and research in green technologies and practices.
- Enhances the institution's reputation and aligns it with global sustainability goals.

4.2 Categories of Green Campus

Education on Sustainable Development: It remains critical in the awareness of issues concerning the environment. Education for Sustainable Development

(ESD) combines sustainability, academics, research, and management practices while at the same time participating in activities related to it among the students, academics, and administration. ESD has a broad scope, including different types of courses such as climate change, green technology, sustainable development, and research, as well as protecting the environment and the use of renewable energy, among others. Furthermore, there are campus organizations that are crucial in participating in the activities, especially concerning sustainable development among the students, a factor that has been essential in raising awareness in society at large regarding issues affecting the environment, as observed in literature.

Clean Energy: The need for renewable energy, energy conservation measures, and the development of sustainable buildings, in addition to measures to respond to and reduce the impacts of climate change, are all essential for a greater future, such as the reduction of greenhouse gases and increased forest-like flora to counter urbanization and natural systems.

Energy Efficiency: Using smart thermostats, motion sensors, Energy Star–rated appliances, lighting, etc., and retrofitting old infrastructure with newer windows, roofs, etc., that allow natural lighting, proper ventilation, the use of non-toxic materials, etc., are beneficial in increasing energy efficiency in schools, which would, in turn, improve the health of the teaching staff as well as the children, freeing them from exposure to toxic materials like those in traditional school infrastructure, as recommended in the literature.

Waste Management: It involves segregation of waste at the source with proper bins provided for paper, plastic, metals, and other wastes placed at strategic positions around the campus. It also involves collecting these wastes for transportation to recycling facilities as well as organizing awareness campaigns among students and employees to promote waste reduction and proper disposal practices. It also involves collecting and handling hazardous wastes like toxic materials as well as e-waste and biomedical waste for proper disposal through composting and vermicomposting organic waste, followed by sorting and dispatching inorganic waste to recycling facilities for proper disposal and recycling. Universities collaborate with vendors to boost efficiency in the process as sewage plants treat both gray and black waters for use in landscaping and flushing toilets instead of fresh water for publication purposes.

4.2.1 Water Efficiency

Water efficiency is the process of making the minimum use of water in the various activities of the pharmaceutical education institutions while maintaining the quality of education and infrastructure.

Water conservation programs can be conducted in these institutes through government or institutional initiatives that advocate the efficient use of water and reduce the wastage of water. Water-saving habits can be brought about among the students by organizing seminars, posters, and events. Water wastage can also be reduced by regular audits on water supply. Water-saving devices should be installed in laboratories and toilets. Water supply pipes in institutes should be regularly maintained to check wastage of water. Treated wastewater can also be used for watering purposes in a medicinal plant garden, cleaning of floors, or flushing.

The rainwater harvesting system is a method for the collection and storage of rainwater collected from rooftops, paved areas, and open grounds. This will lower the water bill and reliance on an outside source, be positive for green cover, support the herbal or botanical garden, and aid sustainability goals and green certification efforts.

In pharmaceutical colleges, where medicinal plant gardens are maintained, the use of harvested rainwater for irrigation is both sustainable and cost-effective. It also serves as a live model for students to understand environmental practices and water management in real life.

Planting resistant plants on campus is recommended, as they require less water. A few examples of these plants are cactus, agave, aloe vera, and lavender, which reduce dependence on groundwater, municipal water, or irrigation. Due to the deep root system in these plants, they improve soil aeration, help to maintain moisture, and help to increase the organic content of soil.

4.3 Sustainable Transportation

The idea of sustainable transport systems can be defined as using a transport system to meet present needs without affecting its utility in the future. Therefore, successfully offering sustainable transport options on campuses addresses not just local mobility but also serves as a high bar for broader changes to be made in society toward sustainability.

5 Smart Campus

The advancement and integration of cutting-edge technology have resulted in a paradigm shift in the overall concept and nature of a smart campus, an environment previously considered an academic campus, shifting toward a modern environment that is inclusive and sustainable, intelligent, and innovative in terms of cutting-edge technology integration and intelligent data systems and analytics. A smart campus is an academic institution, mentioned in literature and considered to have evolved into a contemporary campus through "cutting-edge technology integration, such as Internet of Things Technology, Digital Twin Technology, Cloud Computing Technology, Data Analytics Technology, and Artificial Intelligence Technology, to enhance efficiency, streamline resource management, and enhance the overall learning experience". References to the integration and development of smart campuses have been identified to have emerged during the 2000s, a period considered to have marked a major milestone in the overall evolution and development of campuses and their infrastructure to integrate cutting-edge technology and create a smart campus environment: a "structured effort to integrate digital technology into campus environments" was, for the most part, considered and was initiated (Figure 3.2).

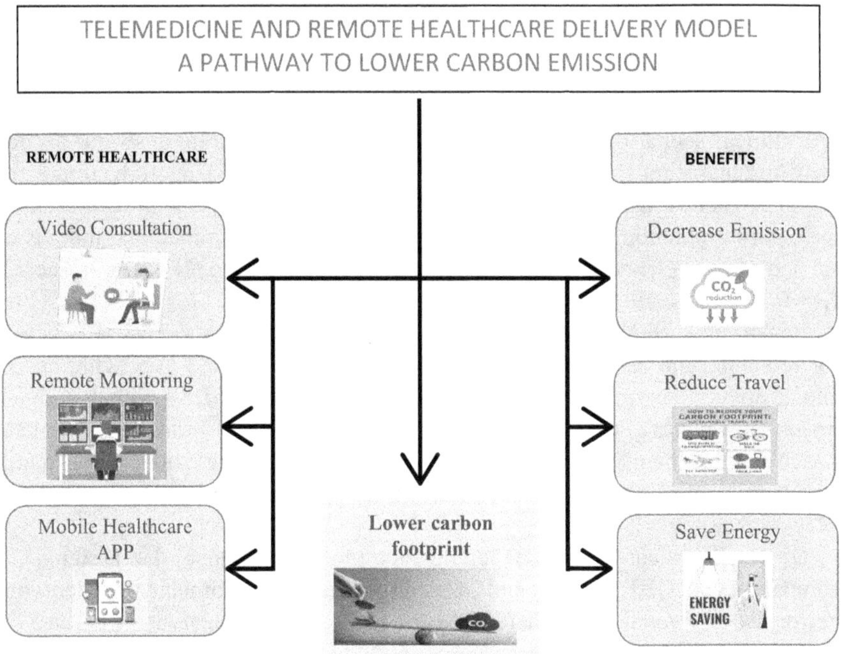

Figure 3.2 Enhancing technologies for the development of a smart campus.

In the economic sector, the top pharmaceutical institutes can encourage entrepreneurial activities by developing innovation centers and research incubation centers. The pharmaceutical institutes can use a blockchain platform to bring transparency in research funding and an AI system to manage resources efficiently. Furthermore, adopting cost-saving strategies, such as energy-efficient buildings, smart grids, and intelligent procurement systems, will not only reduce utility expenses but also ensure the continuity of services (Sciarelli, Landi, Turriziani, & Tani, 2021).

Artificial intelligence is a technology intended to boost productivity in the field in which it is applied. The term artificial intelligence was first used in 1956 (Jessica, Britney, Sarira, Parisa, & Joe, 2025). The use of computers in pharmacy education is thought to have begun in 1980, and the use of AI in pharmacy may have followed (Raza et al., 2022). In the initial phase, machine learning technology plays an important role in increasing computer capabilities and streamlining a range of work in the pharmacy field, such as data collection, dispensing histories, drug storage, clinical research, clinical pharmacy, and pharmacy education (Dasta, 1992; Raza et al., 2022). The use of AI has increased recently, as evidenced by the rise of chatbots for medication management and systems to prioritize potential drug-related issues for clinical pharmacists performing medication reconciliations (Raza et al., 2022). It is a game changer in digital health (Kolluri, Lin, Liu, Zhang, & Zhang, 2022; Raza et al., 2022).

Carou-Senra et al. evaluated the ability of large language models (LLMs), including ChatGPT, Gemini, and Copilot, to support clinical pharmacy students in adjusting drug dosages using pharmacokinetic problems with drugs having narrow therapeutic windows (tacrolimus, vancomycin, and lidocaine) in various clinical scenarios. ChatGPT provided the most accurate answers, particularly for tacrolimus, owing to the simpler calculations. The study found that prompt structure significantly influenced model performance and that these tools have strong potential as educational aids when users are trained and models are refined (Carou-Senra, Delgado-Taboada, Alvarez-Lorenzo, Diaz-Rodriguez, & Goyanes, 2025).

Benjamin J. Shultz and Jeffrey Mucksavage found that GPT-4 was helpful for retaining and revising a significant number of items and improving answer choice quality; however, there was a limitation in aligning GPT-4 with the original intent. However, rejected GPT-4 outputs can provide useful formatting templates, which suggest the need for human review of AI-generated revisions but also indicate the potential use of AI to assist faculty in growth for item writing (Shultz & Mucksavage, 2024).

Do et al. evaluated artificial intelligence tools in pharmacy lab assignments, comparing ChatGPT, Copilot, and Gemini with student performance. Students outperformed AI overall, with ChatGPT scoring 73%, Copilot 72%, and Gemini 54%. Notably, ChatGPT performed on par with students for two in-depth patient case activities (Do et al., 2025).

The social domain is dedicated to enhancing the overall quality of campus life through user-centric and humanized approaches. Intelligent health monitoring, AI-enabled surveillance, the Internet of Things (IoT) for air and water quality monitoring, smart classrooms with virtual labs, AR/VR simulations in pharmacology and anatomy, mobile apps for community engagement, peer collaboration, and stakeholder feedback via cloud-based platforms would contribute toward a safe and healthy learning environment and help bridge the gap between theory and practice. It will also make the institute socially responsible by engaging with communities, stakeholders, peers, and other partners to ensure inclusivity (Meddeb, Maraoui, & Zrigui, 2021; Zhang, Dong, Yip, & Swift, 2020).

A blockchain-enabled secure intelligent health monitoring (BSSHM) system plays an essential role in observing patients' physiological conditions. In this system, healthcare devices are connected to users, such as patients, doctors, nurses, and pharmacists, through a health server. These devices collect data and send them to a server for analysis. With the help of some machine learning models, these data may be beneficial for valuable outputs, such as the prediction of diseases (Li, Weng, Lee, & Wang, 2015; Thapliyal, Singh, Wazid, Singh, & Das, 2023). Reliance on fossil fuels can be greatly decreased from an environmental perspective by including several green energy solutions on intelligent pharmaceutical campuses, such as solar panels for energy generation. Additionally, installing IoT-enabled lighting systems that automatically adjust brightness according to occupancy and natural light levels, or even constructing eco-friendly infrastructure, such as buildings made with energy-efficient materials and green roofs, can reduce operational costs. A crucial aspect of sustainability is holistic waste management, particularly for biomedical and

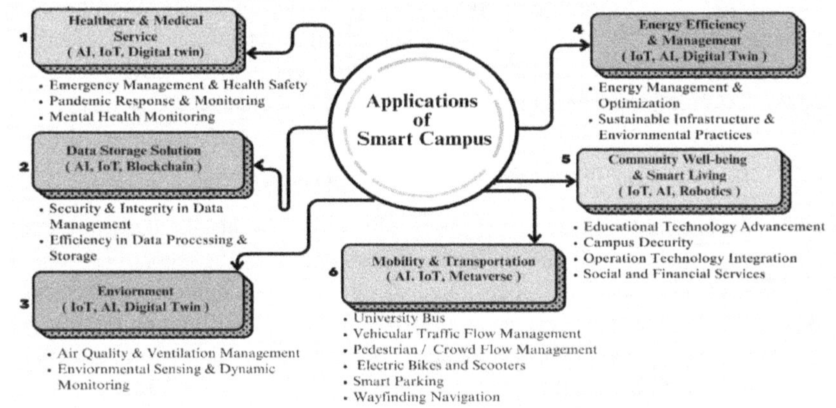

Figure 3.3 Applications of a smart campus.

chemical wastes. Developing a comprehensive waste disposal strategy that adheres to regulatory compliance is essential for protecting public health and the environment of the region (Yigitcanlar, 2009; Yigitcanlar et al., 2017).

5.1 Applications of Smart Campus

The application of a smart campus is depicted in Figure 3.3. The benefits of a smart campus include the following:

- Enhanced student learning outcomes and practical skills are also observed.
- Reduced environmental footprint and operational costs:
- Enhance innovation and industry-academic collaborations.
- This is for the improvement of safety, transparency, and campus management.

6 Designing of Clean, Green, and Smart Space in Pharmaceutical Educational Institutes

6.1 Campus Layout with Green Architecture

Green spaces in pharmaceutical institutes are respected resources for mental health and well-being. Campuses with rich greenery can reduce stress and may be helpful for the mental health of students, faculty, and stakeholders (Cui, He, & Liu, 2025; Dzhambov et al., 2021). Greening refers to initiatives focused on minimizing harmful social and environmental effects (Ribeiro et al., 2016).

6.2 Energy-Efficient Buildings

Advanced architectural designs and technologies of energy efficiency, such as ventilation, air quality, temperature control, and lighting, should be applied to laboratories and classrooms. Energy-efficient buildings not only enhance energy efficiency but also ensure a safe environment for handling chemicals and biological samples (Ribeiro et al., 2016). Solar panels can efficiently generate electricity to power essential laboratory systems, including ventilation systems that ensure proper air circulation and energy-efficient lighting that enhances visibility.

6.3 Establishment of Medicinal Plant/Botanical Gardens

Medicinal plant gardens may be helpful in educating students about the pharmacological importance of such plants. These gardens will be living laboratories with an abundance of plant species needed for research into their chemical characteristics and possible medical applications (G. Chen & Sun, 2018). Kumamoto University is an example of a step that can be taken to develop medicinal plant gardens. On their campus, they launched the "Medicinal Plant Park Initiative" in the year 2015 to promote better utilization of medicinal plants (Devkota & Watanabe, 2020).

6.4 Smart Classrooms and Labs

Students will benefit from smart labs and classrooms that use virtual reality and simulation software to better comprehend the intricacies of the pharmaceutical industry and various courses.

Smartboards are white interactive boards used to display images on a computer monitor with a surface similar to a giant touch screen (Preston & Mowbray,

Table 3.2 Advantages and disadvantages of various learning management systems

S. No.	*Type of LMS*	*Advantages*	*Disadvantages*
1	Proprietary	• They were first developed and widely used. • They are suitable for large institutions with well-developed infrastructure.	• They require a well-developed infrastructure. • Installation on HEO servers and computers are necessary. • Limited external access if the institutional infrastructure is not well developed. • Cost-effective only for large educational institute.
2	Open-source	• Freely available. • Better financial solution. • Does not require well-developed infrastructure.	• Requires more technical expertise to customize and maintain.
3	Cloud-based	• Low-cost solution. • No need to install an LMS platform. • Accessed directly through an internet connection. • No need for costly infrastructure.	• Reliance on internet connectivity. • Potential data security concerns as data is stored on a third-party server.

2008), significantly enhancing interaction between teachers and students by enabling instructors to display vibrant animations of drug mechanisms, intricate molecular structures, and detailed pharmacokinetic processes in real time. Through interactive learning experiences, this technology turns conventional classrooms into dynamic learning spaces that promote greater student participation and engagement.

6.5 Learning Management Systems

Learning Management Systems (LMSs) are platforms used by instructors to share content, track assignments, and provide training online. They can be proprietary, open-source, cloud-based, or hybrid. Proprietary LMSs require licensed use; open-source LMSs are free and customizable, while cloud-based LMSs offer affordable, accessible education anytime and anywhere (Dobre, 2015). Advantages and disadvantages of different types of LMSs are summarized in Table 3.2.

7 Role of Stakeholders in Creating Clean, Green, and Smart Pharmaceutical Educational Institutes

The transformation of pharmaceutical educational institutions into clean, green, and technologically advanced environments requires joint efforts of administration, faculty, and students to promote excellence, sustainability, and innovation.

7.1 Role of Administration

- **Policy Formulation**: Any educational institution, including a pharmacy college, needs a strong policy framework to integrate sustainability, technology, and innovation. Adopting the multidisciplinary and digital approach of NEP 2020, maintaining cleanliness through the Swachh Bharat Mission, and engaging in community health and sustainable practices under the Unnat Bharat Abhiyan, following energy-efficient infrastructure as guided by IGBC, Green Rating for Integrated Habitat Assessment (GRIHA), and ECBC, and digital initiatives as part of National Mission on Education through Information and Communication Technology (NMEICT) along with policies like NISP 2019 and Atal Innovation Mission for green entrepreneurship and start-ups, together with strict compliance to the National Green Policy and EPA for safe waste and chemical management, create healthy and green campuses, which contribute to a better environment and society (Table 3.3).

7.2 Budgeting

Dedicated funding should support sustainability and advanced technologies in pharmaceutical institutes by investing in energy-efficient instruments, adopting VR/AR for drug design, and implementing IoT-based smart building systems to optimize resources, cut costs, and reduce the carbon footprint.

Table 3.3 Policy framework for green and smart pharmaceutical institutes

S. No.	*Policy Name*	*Relevance*	*Application*
1	National Education Policy (NEP 2020)	Emphasizes sustainability, multidisciplinary learning, digital infrastructure, and quality education.	Encourages integration of green and smart technologies in educational institutes, including pharmaceutical colleges.
2	Swachh Bharat Mission (Urban & Rural)	Focus on sanitation, hygiene, and waste management.	Promotes clean campus initiatives and biomedical waste disposal systems in pharma institutes.
3	Unnat Bharat Abhiyan (UBA)	Aims to connect higher education institutions with rural development.	Encourages institutes to develop sustainable practices and engage in eco-friendly community health projects.
4	Energy Conservation Building Code (ECBC) & Green Building Guidelines by GRIHA and IGBC	Promotes energy efficiency in institutional infrastructure.	Adoption of green buildings, solar panels, LED lighting, and smart HVAC systems in pharma colleges.
5	Smart Campus Initiative by Ministry of Education	Supports digital learning and ICT infrastructure.	Encourages installation of smart classrooms, biometric attendance, cloud labs, and Wi-Fi-enabled campuses.
6	National Mission on Education through ICT (NMEICT)	Promotes digital content and e-learning in higher education.	Supports virtual labs, e-learning modules, and digital repositories in pharmaceutical education.
7	National Innovation and Start-up Policy (NISP) 2019	Encourages innovation and sustainability in academic institutions.	Fosters green entrepreneurship and pharma tech-based start-ups in institutes.
8	Atal Innovation Mission (AIM)	Promotes innovation hubs and labs.	Establishment of eco-friendly, tech-driven incubation centers in pharma institutions.
9	National Green Policy & Environment Protection Act (EPA), 1986	Mandates pollution control and environmental safety.	Regulates waste disposal, chemical handling, and emission standards in pharma labs.
10	AICTE Guidelines for Green and Sustainable Campuses	Recommends practices for energy saving, waste management, and clean technologies.	Encourages pharma institutes to adopt green practices and meet sustainable development goals (SDGs).

7.3 Role of Faculty

Faculty members have an important role to play as disseminators of knowledge and must be actively involved to make an impact through education that incorporates the principles of sustainability as well as smart technologies.

7.4 Curriculum Development

Faculties should renew existing courses by including topics such as "green chemistry," "sustainable drug manufacture," "waste management," and "environmental implications of pharmacy," while making increased use of "smart tools," such as "data analysis tools" and "simulation tools," to make the curriculum "personalized" and "adaptive."

7.5 Research Integration

Faculty should engage in research that promotes and aids in the process of developing green pharma and innovative manufacturing techniques employing AI for drug discovery.

7.6 Hands-on Training

Hands-on training should introduce students to greener approaches for laboratory practices, including the careful handling and minimization of solvent use, conducting reactions on a microscale to reduce waste generation, and integrating advanced technologies such as fully automated synthesis systems and robotic screening platforms to enhance efficiency, precision, and sustainability in laboratory workflows.

7.7 Mentorship and Guidance

Academic staff members should mentor pupils in pharmaceutical-related projects on aspects of environmental sustainability.

7.8 Continuous Professional Development

Faculty members need to focus on continuous development through various training activities, seminars, and workshops related to sustainable practices and smart technologies, imparting knowledge with effectiveness.

7.9 Empower Students for Clean, Green, and Smart Campus Development

The areas below represent the major areas where the students can have an impact.

Green Clubs and Initiatives: Students can participate in green clubs and lead green initiatives such as running environmental awareness campaigns, tree plantations, waste segregation drives and recycling, and competitions on energy savings.

Cleanliness Drives: Pharmaceutical institutes ought to arrange regular cleanliness drives, especially in high-risk zones such as laboratories.

Smart Learning Adoption: Online resources, virtual lab environments, simulations, online textbooks, and interactive projects can be used to help students practically understand the course content better.

Innovation and Advocacy: Students should promote environmental responsibility by encouraging peer discussions on sustainability in academic and professional settings.

Feedback and Improvement: Student feedback through surveys, focus groups, and forums helps improve campus programs and align them with learners' needs.

8 Conclusion

In addition to encouraging sustainability and creativity, transforming pharmaceutical schools into clean, green, and smart campuses equips aspiring chemists to ethically address global health issues.

References

Aminullah, A., Khan, W. A., Nisar, A., Arbak, S., & Ishtiaq, M. (2025). Pharmaceutical waste reduction in hospitals: The impact of segregation practices and regulatory compliance. In B. Yingngam, M. S. Aslam, & A. K. Haghi (Eds.), *Sustainable Pharmaceutical Product Development and Optimization Processes: From Eco-Design to Supply Chain Integrity* (pp. 229–245): Springer.

Ariffin, M., & Zakili, T. S. T. (2019). Household pharmaceutical waste disposal in Selangor, Malaysia—policy, public perception, and current practices. *Environmental Management, 64*(4), 509–519.

Badia-Fabregat, M., Lucas, D., Pereira, M. A., Alves, M., Pennanen, T., Fritze, H., … Caminal, G. (2016). Continuous fungal treatment of non-sterile veterinary hospital effluent: Pharmaceuticals removal and microbial community assessment. *Applied Microbiology and Biotechnology, 100*(5), 2401–2415.

Barenie, R. E., Leav, K., Johnson III, W. T. E., & Wheeler, J. S. (2022). Review and assessment of drug disposal state statutes in the United States, 2022. *Journal of the American Pharmacists Association, 62*(6), 1865–1869.

Bharadwaj, A., Yadav, D., & Varshney, S. (2015). Non-biodegradable waste–its impact & safe disposal. *International Journal of Advanced Technology in Engineering and Sciences, 3*(1), 184–191.

Carou-Senra, P., Delgado-Taboada, I., Alvarez-Lorenzo, C., Diaz-Rodriguez, P., & Goyanes, A. (2025). Exploring the role of LLMs like ChatGPT in pharmacy education for supporting students' therapeutic decision-making. *American Journal of Pharmaceutical Education*, 101462, 89(8).

Chen, G., & Sun, W. (2018). The role of botanical gardens in scientific research, conservation, and citizen science. *Plant Diversity, 40*(4), 181–188.

Chen, J., Wu, J., Sherrell, P. C., Chen, J., Wang, H., Zhang, W. x., & Yang, J. (2022). How to build a microplastics-free environment: Strategies for microplastics degradation and plastics recycling. *Advanced Science, 9*(6), 2103764.

Cui, C., He, Q., & Liu, H. (2025). Depression restoration in university students: Data-driven insights across three types of campus greenness. *Data in Brief*, 111831, 61.

Dasta, J. (1992). Application of artificial intelligence to pharmacy and medicine. *Hospital Pharmacy, 27*(4), 312–315, 319.

Devkota, H. P., & Watanabe, M. (2020). Role of medicinal plant gardens in pharmaceutical science education and research: An overview of medicinal plant garden at Kumamoto University, Japan. *Journal of Asian Association of Schools of Pharmacy, 9*, 44–52.

Do, V., Donohoe, K. L., Peddi, A. N., Carr, E., Kim, C., Mele, V., … Crawford, A. N. (2025). Artificial intelligence (AI) performance on pharmacy skills laboratory course assignments. *Currents in Pharmacy Teaching and Learning, 17*(7), 102367.

Dobre, I. (2015). Learning management systems for higher education-an overview of available options for higher education organizations. *Procedia-Social and Behavioral Sciences, 180*, 313–320.

Dou, B., Zhu, Z., Merkurjev, E., Ke, L., Chen, L., Jiang, J., … Wei, G.-W. (2023). Machine learning methods for small data challenges in molecular science. *Chemical Reviews, 123*(13), 8736–8780.

Dzhambov, A. M., Lercher, P., Browning, M. H., Stoyanov, D., Petrova, N., Novakov, S., & Dimitrova, D. D. (2021). Does greenery experienced indoors and outdoors provide an escape and support mental health during the COVID-19 quarantine? *Environmental Research, 196*, 110420.

Elhalwagy, E. N. (2024). Waste management in educational institutes. *Assiut University Bulletin for Environmental Researches, 27*(1), 40–50.

Fleming, E., Proescholdbell, S., Sachdeva, N., Alexandridis, A. A., Margolis, L., & Ransdell, K. (2016). North Carolina's operation medicine drop: Results from one of the nation's largest drug disposal programs. *North Carolina Medical Journal, 77*(1), 59.

Frontières, M. S., & Frontières, P. S. (1999). Guidelines for safe disposal of unwanted pharmaceuticals in and after emergencies. *World Health Organization*, **WHO/EDM/PAR/99.2**, Geneva. pp. 31.

Fueki, K., Takeuchi, A., Torikai, A., & Nagaya, S. (1986). Photodegradation of polyethylene: Effect of crosslinking on the oxygenated products and mechanical properties. *Polymer Photochemistry, 7*, 199–211.

Gewert, B., Plassmann, M. M., & MacLeod, M. (2015). Pathways for degradation of plastic polymers floating in the marine environment. *Environmental Science: Processes & Impacts, 17*(9), 1513–1521.

Hanif, M. A., Ibrahim, N., Dahalan, F. A., Ali, U. F. M., Hasan, M., & Jalil, A. A. (2022). Microplastics and nanoplastics: Recent literature studies and patents on their removal from aqueous environment. *Science of the Total Environment, 810*, 152115.

Hegde, V., Kulkarni, R. D., & Ajantha, G. (2007). Biomedical waste management. *Journal of Oral and Maxillofacial Pathology, 11*(1), 5–9.

Jessica, H., Britney, R., Sarira, E.-D., Parisa, A., & Joe, Z. (2025). Applications of artificial intelligence in current pharmacy practice: A scoping review. *Research in Social and Administrative Pharmacy, 21*(3), 134–141.

Kabir, A., Roy, S., Begum, K., Kabir, A. H., & Miah, M. S. (2021). Factors influencing sanitation and hygiene practices among students in a public university in Bangladesh. *PLoS One, 16*(9), e0257663.

Kasavan, S., Yusoff, S., Ali, N. I. M., & Masarudin, N. A. (2021). Reducing food waste at school canteens: The behaviour of school communities. *Geografia, 17*(2), 52–64.

Katinas, V., Marčiukaitis, M., Perednis, E., & Dzenajavičienė, E. F. (2019). Analysis of biodegradable waste use for energy generation in Lithuania. *Renewable and Sustainable Energy Reviews, 101*, 559–567.

Khalidi-Idrissi, A., Madinzi, A., Anouzla, A., Pala, A., Mouhir, L., Kadmi, Y., & Souabi, S. (2023). Recent advances in the biological treatment of wastewater rich in emerging pollutants produced by pharmaceutical industrial discharges. *International Journal of Environmental Science and Technology, 20*(10), 11719–11740.

Kirkpatrick, C. M., Dooley, M. J., Charman, B. E., Bergen, P. J., Kong, D. C. M., George, J., Hussainy, S. Y., & Stehlik, P. (2013). The National Return and Disposal of Unwanted Medicines (NatRUM) Project Audit: Final report. Monash University, Faculty of Pharmacy and Pharmaceutical Sciences.

Kolluri, S., Lin, J., Liu, R., Zhang, Y., & Zhang, W. (2022). Machine learning and artificial intelligence in pharmaceutical research and development: A review. *The AAPS Journal, 24*(1), 19.

Le, P.-A. (2025). A review of commercial plastic waste recycling into graphene materials. *RSC Advances, 15*(25), 20239–20267.

Lee, K., Jing, Y., Wang, Y., & Yan, N. (2022). A unified view on catalytic conversion of biomass and waste plastics. *Nature Reviews Chemistry, 6*(9), 635–652.

Li, C.-T., Weng, C.-Y., Lee, C.-C., & Wang, C.-C. (2015). A hash based remote user authentication and authenticated key agreement scheme for the integrated EPR information system. *Journal of Medical Systems, 39*(11), 144.

Liu, Z., Sokratian, A., Duda, A. M., Xu, E., Stanhope, C., Fu, A., … Bobay, B. G. (2023). Anionic nanoplastic contaminants promote Parkinson's disease–associated α-synuclein aggregation. *Science Advances, 9*(46), eadi8716.

Luo, H., Tyrrell, H., Bai, J., Muazu, R. I., & Long, X. (2024). Fundamental, technical and environmental overviews of plastic chemical recycling. *Green Chemistry, 26*(23), 11444–11467.

Ma, B., Li, X., Jiang, Z., & Jiang, J. (2019). Recycle more, waste more? When recycling efforts increase resource consumption. *Journal of Cleaner Production, 206*, 870–877.

Ma, J., Tominac, P. A., Aguirre-Villegas, H. A., Olafasakin, O. O., Wright, M. M., Benson, C. H., … Zavala, V. M. (2023). Economic evaluation of infrastructures for thermochemical upcycling of post-consumer plastic waste. *Green Chemistry, 25*(3), 1032–1044.

Meddeb, O., Maraoui, M., & Zrigui, M. (2021). Personalized smart learning recommendation system for Arabic users in smart campus. *International Journal of Web-Based Learning and Teaching Technologies (IJWLTT), 16*(6), 1–21.

Misra, V., & Pandey, S. (2005). Hazardous waste, impact on health and environment for development of better waste management strategies in future in India. *Environment International, 31*(3), 417–431.

Mitkidis, P., Chrysochou, P., Obolevich, V., & Mitkidis, K. (2022). Effectiveness of environmental health and loss framing on household pharmaceutical take-back schemes. *Waste Management, 143*, 61–68.

Modak, S., Kasula, M., & Esfahani, M. R. (2023). Nanoplastics removal from water using metal–organic framework: Investigation of adsorption mechanisms, kinetics, and effective environmental parameters. *ACS Applied Engineering Materials, 1*(2), 744–755.

Nieminen, J., Anugwom, I., Kallioinen, M., & Mänttäri, M. (2020). Green solvents in recovery of aluminium and plastic from waste pharmaceutical blister packaging. *Waste Management, 107*, 20–27.

Park, K.-B., Jeong, Y.-S., Guzelciftci, B., & Kim, J.-S. (2019). Characteristics of a new type continuous two-stage pyrolysis of waste polyethylene. *Energy, 166*, 343–351.

Perry, L. A., Shinn, B. W., & Stanovich, J. (2014). Quantification of an ongoing community-based medication take-back program. *Journal of the American Pharmacists Association, 54*(3), 275–279.

Preston, C., & Mowbray, L. (2008). Use of'SMART' Boards for teaching, learning and assessment in kindergarten science. *Teaching Science, 54*(2), 50–53.

Rajbongshi, S., Shah, Y. D., & Sajib, A. U. (2016). Pharmaceutical waste management: A review. *European Journal of Biomedical and Pharmaceutical Sciences, 3*(12), 192–206.

Ranjbari, M., Esfandabadi, Z. S., Shevchenko, T., Chassagnon-Haned, N., Peng, W., Tabatabaei, M., & Aghbashlo, M. (2022). Mapping healthcare waste management research: Past evolution, current challenges, and future perspectives towards a circular economy transition. *Journal of Hazardous Materials, 422*, 126724.

Raza, M. A., Aziz, S., Noreen, M., Saeed, A., Anjum, I., Ahmed, M., & Raza, S. M. (2022). Artificial Intelligence (AI) in pharmacy: An overview of innovations. *Innovations in pharmacy, 13*(2), 10.24926/iip.v13i2.4839..

Ribeiro, J. M. P., Barbosa, S. B., Casagrande, J. L., Sehnem, S., Berchin, I. I., da Silva, C. G., … de Andrade Guerra, J. B. S. O. (2016). Promotion of sustainable development at universities: The adoption of green campus strategies at the University of Southern Santa Catarina, Brazil. In L. F. Walter, Brandli, L., Castro, P., & Newman, J. (Eds.), *Handbook of Theory and Practice of Sustainable Development in Higher Education: Volume 1* (pp. 471–486): Springer International Publishing AG, Cham.

Rogowska, J., & Zimmermann, A. (2022). Household pharmaceutical waste disposal as a global problem—a review. *International Journal of Environmental Research and Public Health, 19*(23), 15798.

Sciarelli, M., Landi, G. C., Turriziani, L., & Tani, M. (2021). Academic entrepreneurship: Founding and governance determinants in university spin-off ventures. *The Journal of Technology Transfer, 46*(4), 1083–1107.

Shahabuddin, M., Uddin, M. N., Chowdhury, J., Ahmed, S., Uddin, M., Mofijur, M., & Uddin, M. (2023). A review of the recent development, challenges, and opportunities of electronic waste (e-waste). *International Journal of Environmental Science and Technology, 20*(4), 4513–4520.

Shultz, B. J., & Mucksavage, J. (2024). Exploring the role of ChatGPT in enhancing multiple-choice questions for pharmacy education. *American Journal of Pharmaceutical Education, 88*(9).

Thapliyal, S., Singh, S., Wazid, M., Singh, D. P., & Das, A. K. (2023). Design of blockchain-enabled secure smart health monitoring system and its testbed implementation. *Cyber Security and Applications, 1*, 100020.

Trihadiningrum, Y., Anandita, F. D., & Nadira, A. (2023). Electronic waste management in schools: A case of Surabaya City, Indonesia. *Journal of Material Cycles and Waste Management, 25*(1), 597–611.

Vijayalakshmi, M. (2020). Modern waste management techniques—a critical review. *IOC, Innovation Sustainability Through E-STEM-14th 15th October*, 2020 (IOC-2020 Proceedings), 64–72.

Vijayalakshmi, M., Showbharnikhaa, S., Snega, K., Nadhiya, J., Akshaya, T., & Muthu Kaviya, M. (2023). Pharmaceutical waste management. *Journal of Pharma Insights and Research, 1*(2), 166–173.

Wheeler, A. J., Kelly, F., Spinks, J., & Bettington, E. (2016). National Return and Disposal of Unwanted Medicines (RUM) Project Audit 2016. Return Unwanted Medicines (RUM) Project, The Pharmacy Guild of Australia, Melbourne, Australia.

Yigitcanlar, T. (2009). Planning for smart urban ecosystems: Information technology applications for capacity building in environmental decision making. *Theoretical and Empirical Researches in Urban Management, 4*(3 (12), 5–21.

Yigitcanlar, T., Edvardsson, I. R., Johannesson, H., Kamruzzaman, M., Ioppolo, G., & Pancholi, S. (2017). Knowledge-based development dynamics in less favoured regions: Insights from Australian and Icelandic university towns. *European Planning Studies, 25*(12), 2272–2292.

Zhang, Y., Dong, Z. Y., Yip, C., & Swift, S. (2020). Smart campus: A user case study in Hong Kong. *IET Smart Cities, 2*(3), 146–154.

4 Green Technology for Creating a Sustainable Future in the Pharmaceutical Sector

Progress and Barriers

Kapil Kumar Goel, Shalini Juglan, Suraj Tyagi, Ritu Vishnoi, Neha Kanojia, and Peeush Singhal

1 Introduction

Green synthesis will also aim at ensuring that consumption is optimal so that the energy which is generated is wasted to a minimum as well as providing the power with renewable energy sources. The other reasons that have led to the carbon footprint were that it was also one of the primary causes of the carbon footprint that generated about 1.9 Mt CO_2 even though the pharmaceutical companies are the biggest earners in the world economy with a total revenue amounting to 1.27 trillion U.S. dollars (Agrawal et al., 2024). The seeds of the concept of the environment protection implementation were sown ten years ago, and the majority of them were not fulfilled, as the industries did not cooperate. The industrial nations have constantly been seeking a mode of regulating production and selecting the process that would cause the least impact on the environment, yet neither of the former ideas passed the test (Al-Emran & Griffy-Brown, 2023). The vision of any pharma company has never been otherwise, as it has always been guaranteed that it introduces groundbreaking drugs to improve the quality of life in the world. To achieve this in a friendly manner, the companies are supposed to come up with an alternative to the traditional synthetic process of the traditional type to a modern, advanced process (Ali et al., 2024). Chemical manufacturers generate a huge amount of byproducts and pollutants, e.g., used-up reagents, air pollutants, and contaminated solvents. All these are enormous contributors to the pharmaceutical industry (Amin & Oláh, 2024). Gaps and efforts must be sought to develop tailored education and training content that will enable the adoption of green and sustainable practices that are required in the bioprocess units, such as in the pharmaceutical industries, that will reduce their environmental impact. Green chemistry is currently at the high command of the situation (Amin et al., 2024; Andreani et al., 2019). The pharmaceutical industries in recent decades have developed in a different direction, i.e., the way of solving the problem of pollution and limited use of the environmental resources, as well as renewable, sustainable sources. In that way, the implementation of the green chemistry concept might be considered another obstacle (Ayanle et al., 2022). The population is increasingly conscious of environmental pollution and has more advanced testing procedures, and the pharmaceutical

DOI: 10.4324/9781003640486-4

industry is being pressured not only to be more efficient in its production but also to have products with a lesser effect. This is also explained by the fact that capital investment cannot be used to commercialize a green technology (Bauer et al., 2015). Green is not always cost-effective, and vice versa is justified in a holistic way (Bejgam et al., 2021).

1.1 Conceptual Framework of Green Technology in Pharmaceuticals

The building has four blocks of the holistic framework, which include (1) life cycle processes and stages, (2) data inventory, (3) impact categories, and (4) sustainability pillars. The final objective ought to be the measurement of the three pillars of sustainability (building block four) (Bieker, 2021). It is, thus, very essential to examine the first blocks carefully and then go on to the last ones (Table 4.1). Figure 4.1 reflects the major advantages of implementing sustainability in the pharmaceutical industry.

Figure 4.1 illustrates four major advantages gained by the pharmaceutical industry through the implementation of sustainable approaches: (i) enhanced regulatory compliance through adherence to emerging environmental standards; (ii) improved reputation and market advantage driven by greater trust among eco-conscious consumers and stakeholders; (iii) cost-effectiveness achieved via resource efficiency and reduced waste; and (iv) strengthened, resilient supply chains with lowered operational risks through stable and responsible sourcing.

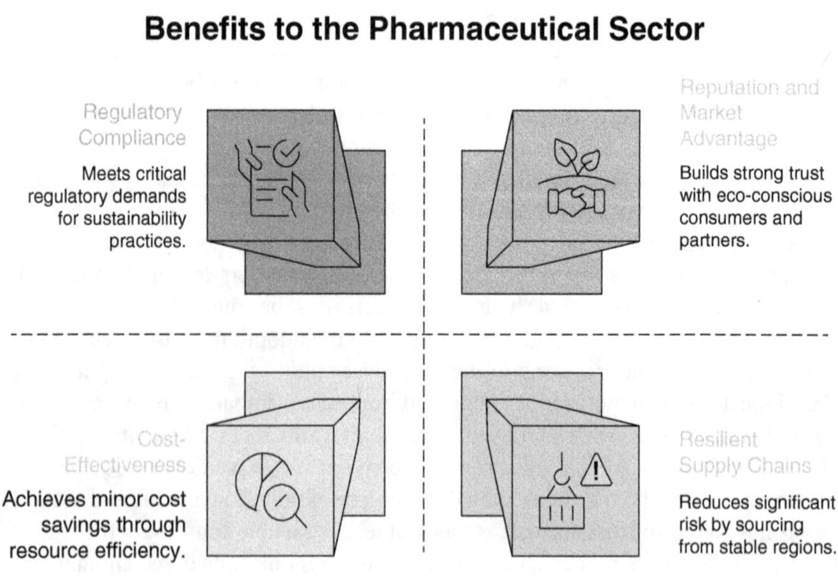

Figure 4.1 Summary of the key benefits of adopting sustainability practices in the pharmaceutical sector.

Table 4.1 Overview of building blocks used in pharmaceutical sustainability assessment

Building Block	*Key Components*	*Description*	*Examples*
1 Life cycle stages and processes	Eight cradle-to-grave stages (raw material extraction → production → distribution → use → disposal). Technosphere processes	Covers the full pharmaceutical life cycle, including all material/energy inputs and environmental/social/economic outputs. Used to identify sustainability hotspots	• API synthesis, formulation, packaging • Distribution logistics • Waste generation and emission points • End-of-life treatment
2 Data inventory	Physical flows; non-physical flows; primary and secondary data sources	Systematic collection of input–output data required to quantify impacts across life cycle stages. Data may be generic or site-specific, depending on user and geographical context	**Physical data:** raw material use, energy consumption, transport distances, waste volumes, and emissions to air/water/soil. **Non-physical data:** labor hours, employment, costs, revenues, health/well-being metrics
3 Impact categories	Environmental impacts, social impacts, economic impacts, and pharma-specific impacts (e.g., AMR, residues)	Links data inventory to specific sustainability outcomes. Lack of harmonized categories creates variability across studies; impacts may intersect across pillars, risking double counting	**Environmental:** CO_2 footprint, toxicity, biodiversity loss **Social:** DALY, QALY, WELLBY **Economic:** cost of illness avoided, treatment affordability **Pharma-specific:** AMR pathways, persistence of residues
4 Sustainability pillars	• Environmental • Social • Economic	Final evaluation of beneficial or adverse effects of pharmaceutical processes/products across the three pillars of sustainability	**Environmental:** greener APIs, solvent reduction, waste treatment **Social:** workplace safety, access to medicines, patient well-being. **Economic:** R&D expenditure, labor productivity, market affordability

1.1.1 Life Cycle Stages

A pharmaceutical life cycle in general is normally a complicated process with a huge range of environmental/social/economic demands (BloombergNEF, 2022). Several sub-processes are present in eight sequential stages (Bonou et al., 2016). The technosphere, alternatively referred to as the human-made environment, represents the different processes in the areas of stage one to eight. Every process has an input that gets into the system and output.

1.1.2 Data Inventory

The information about inputs and outputs of every process in the pharmaceutical life cycle should be gathered in order to measure the contribution of every stage of the life cycle (Bošnjaković et al., 2023). Preferably, data can be gathered to take into account the entire life cycle and category of impacts in the sustainability analysis to balance out with the integrated assessment. Also, the data inventory depends on the focus of the one who uses the assessment system, as well as their geographical location. The information may thus be generic and/or site based, quantitative and/or qualitative, and be both primary and secondary (Chowdhury et al., 2024).

Material and energy flows are related to the physical ones. Among the examples of the data that will be gathered to define the physical flows quantitatively are the number of raw material inputs (e.g., solvent, catalysts), the amount of energy used, the distance of transportation of a product, the amount and the nature of waste (solid/liquid), air/soil/water emissions, etc. (Fu et al., 2022). The non-physical flows in their turn indicate socio-economic data about activities or events in the pharmaceutical life cycle such as labor hours, total employment, health and well-being data, costs, and revenues (Gaustad et al., 2018).

1.1.3 Impact Categories

Each and every input or output obtained in the data inventory is then tied to categories of impact. At present, the question of the correct categories of impact to be used in assessing the overall sustainability of the pharmaceutical sector remains unresolved. Current pharmaceutical life cycle analysis (LCA) literature uses divergent impact categories (between 5 and 16 impact categories), and no literature took social and/or economic impacts and pharma-related impacts on the environment (i.e., the presence of residues in the environment, such as antibiotics) into account (Gazi et al., 2024). The category of some impacts is located in the overlaps of sustainability pillars; it may result in a greater risk of counting the same impact twice.

As an example, antimicrobial resistance has two categories of impact, but they deal with a similar impact. Nevertheless, antimicrobial resistance genes that persist in the environment and present a health concern to humans follow other cause-and-effect patterns of ecological impact of the antimicrobial resistance genes (Gong et al., 2024; Hasan et al., 2023). This means that the various types of impact, and therefore, their evaluation strategies, are necessary.

Once the last category of impact is determined, the most relevant indicators should be found. There are varying indicators that can be used to measure impacts (e.g., CO_2 releases, possibly lost percentage of species, DALY) (Hossain et al., 2023; Hepburn et al., 2020). Nonetheless, other categories of effects are hard to measure, like access to healthcare, social conditions of the workers, or how a patent protection would contribute to future prosperity.

1.1.4 Sustainability Pillars

The whole movement of the pharmaceutical life cycle causes positive/negative effects on the three pillars of sustainability:

1.1.4.1 ENVIRONMENTAL SUSTAINABILITY

The environment pillar deals with the effects of pharmaceutical processes on the environment and biodiversity (Islam et al., 2024). Increased focus is on environmental sustainability concerns associated with pharmaceutical manufacturing, greener APIs (Jabessa et al., 2023), less solvents through microfluidics (Jafarizadeh et al., 2024), pharmaceutical waste disposal, and pharmaceutical contaminant treatment.

1.1.4.2 SOCIAL SUSTAINABILITY

The social pillar will enhance the social conditions across the life cycle (Jafrin et al., 2024). It includes workplace safety, human rights, equality, and the well-being of workers, patients, and communities (Jelle, 2011). However, social impacts strongly depend on local context, and compliance varies across regions (Kaffine et al., 2013).

Studies highlight employee conditions, access to medicines for developing countries, and consumer behavior toward drug advertisement (Kaldellis & Apostolou, 2017; Karakaya & Sriwannawit, 2015).

1.1.4.3 ECONOMIC SUSTAINABILITY

The economic pillar describes impacts on economic systems and includes costs, revenues, productivity, R&D expenditure, and healthcare affordability (Karim et al., 2023). Economic sustainability issues often relate to patents (Khalid, 2024), technology adoption, labor productivity, and organizational capital (Kim et al., 2021; Laskowicz, 2022).

2 Challenges in the Implementation of Green Chemistry

2.1 Economic and Financial Barrier

A green chemistry product must be economical and environmentally friendly, as it is reported (Mukherjee et al., 2023). A product must be aimed at making profits by doing good to the environment and health. As stated by Plageras et al. (2018), the measurement of success in business is based mainly on economic stability instead of social and economic stability. Such insignificant reductions in the price of waste, adoption of operations less damaging to health, and slight increases in efficiency cannot compensate for the cost of great investments when the value of the saving is uncertain or immeasurable.

The green chemistry process can be introduced only in case it can cover the investment in a matter of a few years to interest the investors (Qing et al., 2023). Mark the presence of basic economic and financial obstacles: the excessive cost of capital, the impossibility of future benefits, and the unwillingness to denounce sunken capital (Rabbi & Amin, 2024). Companies cannot afford to rid themselves of the old technology, which is capital intensive, and invest in new green technology (Randau et al., 2020). The comparison between old unsustainable approaches and the current green approaches is created to inform on the economic and environmental advantages of the green approaches (Saif et al., 2021). It is found that in certain instances, government scientists were using copyrighted techniques extensively without understanding the consequences of green practices (Mondal & Palit, 2022).

2.2 Regulatory Barriers

Regulatory risk remains one of the most significant challenges for the adoption and implementation of green chemistry and green technologies in both generic and API-manufacturing pharmaceutical industries. Over the years, environmental regulations have become increasingly stringent, directly influencing industrial practices, operational costs, and compliance responsibilities. For example, in 2005, chemical industries in the United States spent more on pollution control and environmental compliance than any other industrial sector (Schnieders et al., 2015), reflecting the scale of regulatory burden on manufacturers.

When a pharmaceutical firm needs to alter an already established process, whether it is converting to a more eco-friendly synthetic process, substituting solvents, or switching to a biocatalytic process, the company goes through lengthy and time-consuming and expensive regulatory steps (Shakeel, 2021). Such legal and documentation processes are not the same in all countries and can take months and sometimes years to be approved, which becomes a significant obstacle in terms of innovation and sustainability transitions (Sharif et al., 2022). Internal compliance departments, external law firms, and regulatory authorities like the FDA also subject the administrative procedures to regulatory reviews and deter companies from abandoning their traditional process (Sun, 2024).

Writing off assets, depreciation of infrastructure, and accounting of process redesigns are also other complexities to the financial regulations. Lack of expedited approval procedures to green drug products or environmentally friendly manufacturing systems also demoralizes adoption. Furthermore, insufficient investment in green chemistry R&D works is also a contributor to regulatory inertia (U.S. DOE, 2023).

2.3 Leadership and Management Challenges

Transformational leadership is a critical factor that can facilitate organizational change to green chemistry and green technology. A top-down response: the top management in most instances will fail to involve or prioritize the green initiatives so that they are pushed aside for short-term financial or operational objectives. These are aggravated by the misalignment of organizational goals, internal power, and lack of strategic clarity (Vollmer et al., 2020).

Lack of a clear vision and mission clearly stated in support of sustainability does not lead to adoption on a company-wide basis. The management is also in charge of fostering capacity building—like training, workshops, and technical skills building—that is required to implement the green processes effectively. The lack of cultural and structural support led by leaders makes the attempts to incorporate green chemistry disjointed and unsuccessful (Wicki & Hansen, 2019).

2.4 Lack of Expertise

Green chemistry is a collection of specialized fields, and this aspect of it can tend to be an obstacle toward its application in industries. Numerous chemists and engineers do not have sufficient knowledge and exposure to the principles of green engineering, sustainable process design, and environmentally friendly synthetic strategies (Yamaguchi et al., 2018). This knowledge difference in the API industry is even more acute due to the requirement of great precision in reaction control, scalability, and regulatory compliance.

The branches of green chemistry, such as catalysis, biomass conversion, solvent engineering, molecular design, and nanotechnology, demand different skills. A specialist in a specific field might lack the feasible knowledge in another vital field, which results in a discontinuous provision of efforts (Yigitcanlar et al., 2019). The nanotechnology-based pharmaceutical inventions are also limited to expertise. Chemists must not only devise effective processes but also get rid of environmentally dangerous intermediates and byproducts of drug syntheses (Yusoh et al., 2024). This barrier is further enhanced by the fact that the technical proficiency of the personnel who are in direct contact with the customers and stakeholders is lacking (Ahuja & Morris Lampert, 2001).

2.5 Lack of Standardization in Definitions and Metrics

Although the character of green chemistry is usually informed by the principles of green chemistry (The Twelve Principles of Green Chemistry), it remains controversial how the principles can be interpreted and quantified. Overall, there is a conceptual overlap and confusion because many stakeholders consider green chemistry the same concept as sustainable development or overall environmental responsibility (Ardabili et al., 2020).

There is as yet no generally accepted certification, metric system, or generally accepted framework to define a process or product as green. This absence of standardized assessment criteria, as well as homogeneity in definition, complicates the task of industries to benchmark performance or confirm claims (Barbieri et al., 2020). This ambiguity in definition, as noted by Bianchini et al. (2023), is a key obstacle to popularization.

2.6 Lack of Awareness and Knowledge among Stakeholders

Although significant progress has been made with regard to green chemistry in the past few years, consciousness and knowledge among most major stakeholder groups have been lacking. Numerous chemists, managers, consumers, and industry experts continue to have a poor understanding of green chemistry and frequently think that it is more expensive, less effective, or a marketing-related initiative of greenwashing (Bloom et al., 2019). The scarcity of knowledge in green chemistry tools, techniques, and measurement metrics also plays a role in this knowledge gap (Bollobás, 2001).

Other departments of a company like marketing, supply chain, and operations do not often know about the strategic and economic advantages of using green technology. Market acceptance as well is influenced by limited consumer awareness since the common population might view the green products as inferior or expensive (Brevini, 2023). To address these gaps, green chemistry should be integrated into university curricula, advanced training programs, and industrial capacity-building initiatives. Practical knowledge and hands-on expertise should be imparted to chemists, engineers, and decision-makers to enable sustainable technological adoption across all levels of the pharmaceutical value chain (Cattani et al., 2023).

3 Green Manufacturing Practices

Although the nature of green chemistry is usually guided by the principles of green chemistry (The Twelve Principles of Green Chemistry), much is still debated on how the principles should be implemented and quantified (Crespi et al., 2015). All this is based on the reality that therapeutic activity and the safety of patients have to be ensured. The interdependence of human health and the environment has become a familiar phenomenon, which is confirmed by the One Health approach. However, the current level of communication between environmental scientists and drug discovery and development specialists regarding these issues is not significant (Damioli et al., 2024). Nevertheless, only the cross-sectoral approach, which will involve the healthcare sector in collaboration with the environmental experts, regulators, and drug design and development experts sharing their experiences and views on the available opportunities and challenges and collaborating toward the potential solution, will be effective in reducing the effect of pharmaceuticals on the environment (De Jesus & Mendonca, 2018). The corresponding phases of the current drug discovery and development procedures should be provided with the knowledge of environmental concerns, the vision of sustainable pharmacy, and green chemistry regulations (Dechezleprêtre et al., 2013). The discovery and development of APIs and other drug constituents with a low environmental burden

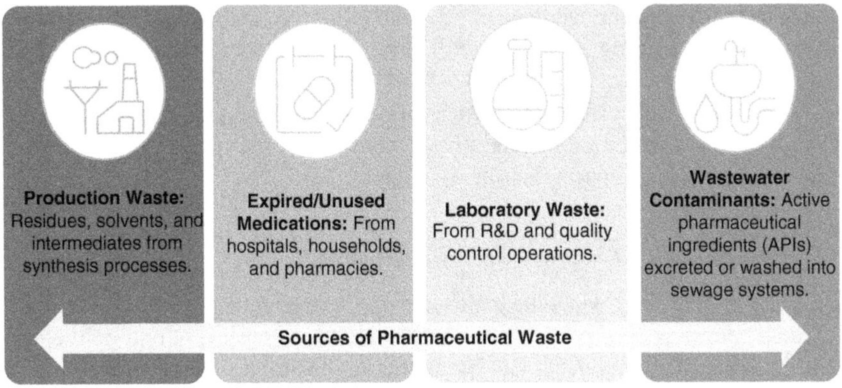

Figure 4.2 General description of the pharmaceutical waste sources and their connection to the green practice.

after use can be integrated with innovations in the product design, drug delivery, clinical diagnosis, and treatment (Diodato et al., 2023). Taking both the natural environment and the patient into consideration, the suggested GREENER concept is benign by design (Fazio et al., 2024; Fusillo et al., 2024). Figure 4.2 provides the summary of the key sources of pharmaceutical waste and their applicability to green practices.

3.1 *G: Good Practice for Patients*

The fear that the environmental factor may be used to underestimate the availability of or access to medicines by patients is one of the factors that may impede the communication and interaction across sectors (Fusillo, 2023). The overall aim in drug development and discovery is to end up with a clinically effective API with few side effects to the patients. Before any drug is subjected to human usage, all drugs must have a good benefit/risk ratio in regard to their efficacy and safety to the patient. The idea of GREENER, which is rooted in being benign by design, is the way in which human and environmental health can be assisted in the case of specific conditions in which the decision-making process of drug discovery and development is carried out. The overall principle of good practice to patients is that patient health must not be compromised in favor of environmental health (Ghisetti & Quatraro, 2017). The close interconnection between environmental and human health makes it urgent to emphasize that the aspect of the environment should be represented in growing numbers in this general principle (Griliches, 1990).

3.2 *R: Reduced Off-Target Effects and High Specificity*

Design of drugs should be facilitated with high specificity as well as efficacy on specific biological targets that relate to the disease being treated. Most of these drug targets are somehow conserved in environmental species (Hall et al., 2001), where they can also have pharmacological effects comparable to their actions in humans. These changes in drug specificity will lower the unwanted off-target effects on wildlife or on patients.

Drug targets and off-target conservation in environmental species should be identified and assessed by comparative genomics to predict and prevent undesirable environmental impacts (Haščič & Migotto, 2015).

3.3 E: Exposure Reduction via Less Emissions

Ecosystems are at risk when the exposures of the environment reach critical levels to cause an adverse effect (Higham et al., 2021). Exposure is one of the ways that the risks can be reduced, i.e., by having less pharmaceuticals in the environment. The reduction of the exposure can be done through the minimization of API emissions.

It entails new drug forms, which can be given in low doses, or drug delivery processes, which are more precise in their delivery modes like individualized medicine, antibody drug conjugates, and nanodrug delivery systems (Howell, 2017). Strategies of directed delivery are used to assist in making sure that the APIs are delivered into the target organ in an efficient manner, which implies that less of the API is needed to be effective and thus less of the API is discharged into the environment. However, the procedures may also introduce additional ambiguity in environmental risk and carbon footprint (IEA, 2021).

3.4 E: Environmental (Bio)Degradability

Exposure can be decreased by avoiding the development of persistent APIs. Persistent and hydrophilic APIs may find their way into drinking water sources. APIs need to be stable in production, distribution, and the body of the patient (IPCC, 2018) but optimally dissolve into nonpersistent metabolites in sewage treatment systems (Iori et al., 2022). Examples of APIs that are fully biodegradable in the environment are summarized elsewhere (Juo & Wang, 2022). Medium-throughput assays are required to screen environmental degradability at an early drug discovery stage (Iori et al., 2022).

3.5 N: No PBT (Persistent, Bioaccumulative, and Toxic) Properties

PBT substances could be deposited in food webs and present long-term hazards in the food webs at low concentrations (Kamilaris et al., 2017). In the majority of EU regulatory authorities, authorization is limited by meeting PBT requirements (Kogan et al., 2017).

Because most oral APIs are water soluble, bioaccumulation is reduced (Laurent, 2008). However, some metabolites may be highly mobile in aquatic environments, which is undesirable (Lerner, 1994).

3.5.1 E: Effect Reduction

Some APIs contain structural moieties (e.g., fluorinated groups) that are persistent and toxic to organisms (Li et al., 2023). These should be avoided when possible without compromising efficacy or stability (Martinelli et al., 2021).

Example: cytarabine is more biodegradable than gemcitabine and 5-fluorouracil because it contains no fluorine (Montresor & Vezzani, 2023).

3.5.2 R: Risk and Hazard Mitigation

If risks cannot be avoided, targeted environmental monitoring can validate predictions (Popp, 2019). Risk mitigation options include:

- Limited advertising
- Controlled availability
- Specific waste-collection systems (e.g., urine bags for contrast media) (Reichstein et al., 2019)

However, such mitigation can increase ecological footprint.

Improved prescription practices, optimized dosing, collection schemes, and advanced sewage treatment can be part of broader mitigation (Robinson et al., 2020).

Advanced treatment is effective but costly, energy-intensive, and may generate unknown byproducts (Rolnick et al., 2022).

3.6 Implementation of the GREENER Concept

The pharmaceutical firms, academic partners, and regulators are defining how and whether the existing drug discovery and development can be changed to embrace the idea of GREENER (Santoalha et al., 2021). One of the methods of ensuring sustainable healthcare is the production of greener APIs (Santoleri et al., 2022; Sloczyński & Wooldridge, 2018).

4 Early Drug Discovery

Environmental criteria may be integrated using:

- In silico tools (Soleimanpouromran & Ahmadimoghadam, 2021; Squicciarini et al., 2013)
- Biodegradation models (Steinmueller, 2010; Sun et al., 2023)

4.1 Later Development

During formulation and dosage optimization, environmental refinements are possible. But once clinical studies begin, options for change are limited (Swiatek,

2024). Figure 4.2 overviews the major sources of pharmaceutical waste and their relevance to green practices.

This number identifies four major sources of pharmaceutical waste, namely production residues, unused or expired pharmaceuticals, laboratory wastes, and wastes in water with active pharmaceutical ingredients (APIs). Identifying these waste streams is vital in carrying out green pharmaceutical practices that will reduce the environmental emissions, enhance waste management, reduce toxicity burdens, and integrate sustainable manufacturing and disposal plans throughout the pharmaceutical life cycle.

5 Digitalization and Industry 4.0 for Green Pharma

Modern pharmaceutical production is undergoing changes through digitalization and Industry 4.0 that allow for making smarter, predictive, and resource-efficient production systems. These technological innovations are important facilitators of green chemistry and sustainable production, with less energy used, less waste generated, better control of the process, and the promotion of the model of the circular operation. Cyber-physical systems, automation, AI, Internet of Things (IoT), and data analytics are finding applications to enable pharmaceutical companies to shift to a more responsive, cleaner, and greener manufacturing platform based on batch manufacturing (Bloom et al., 2019; Cattani et al., 2023).

5.1 Artificial Intelligence and Machine Learning for Process Optimization

AI and ML promise considerable possibilities to maximize chemical synthesis, formulation processes, and API manufacturing. With big data, AI can be used to anticipate the outcomes of reactions, find greener reaction conditions, and minimize the necessity of the solvent-intensive trial and error of reaction experimentation (Cockburn et al., 2018).

The machine learning-based models are able to predict the behavior of the equipment, predict the energy requirements, and optimize the flow of materials, resulting in decreased carbon footprints and less chemical waste. Moreover, AI-based predictive maintenance lowers unexpected downtime, losing materials, and increasing the life of the equipment, which also leads to sustainability (Cowls et al., 2023).

5.2 Digital Twins and Energy Forecasting Models

Digital twins—virtual replicas of physical manufacturing systems—play a transformative role in sustainable pharmaceutical production. By simulating process changes, scaling scenarios, and environmental effects, digital twins allow industries to evaluate greener alternatives without interrupting existing operations (Crespi et al., 2015). They enable real-time optimization of:

- Energy consumption
- Solvent flow

- Resource allocation and supporting sustainable decision-making.

Digital twins also support LCA by providing continuous data on environmental impacts, enabling comparisons between conventional and green process routes (Damioli et al., 2024).

5.3 IoT-Enabled Waste, Emission, and Resource Monitoring (Saif et al., 2022)

The IoT enhances transparency across the pharmaceutical supply chain by enabling real-time monitoring of:

- Waste generation
- Emission levels
- Water use
- Energy flows

  Smart sensors and automated data acquisition systems detect inefficiencies early, allowing corrective actions before environmental harm occurs (De Jesus & Mendonça, 2018).

  IoT platforms integrate with environmental dashboards to visualize resource consumption patterns and support ISO-aligned sustainability compliance (Dechezleprêtre et al., 2013).

  IoT-enabled systems can also track:

- API residues in effluents
- chemical pollutant leakage
- wastewater toxicity

  which is essential for green manufacturing (Diodato et al., 2023).

5.4 Automation and Smart Manufacturing for Resource Efficiency

Automation under Industry 4.0 reduces human error, enhances precision, and ensures consistent quality—critical for both sustainability and regulatory compliance (Fazio et al., 2024).

Smart robotic systems, automated reactors, and continuous manufacturing platforms significantly improve process efficiency compared to traditional batch processes. Continuous manufacturing:

- reduces solvent use
- minimizes waste
- increases safety
- reduces cycle time
- lowers energy consumption

Automated quality-control systems further reduce material loss by enabling real-time defect detection and process corrections (Fusillo et al., 2024).

5.5 Integration with Circular Economy and Sustainable Supply Chains

Digitalization supports circular economy principles by enabling:

- Optimized resource recovery
- Advanced recycling strategies
- Reverse logistics
- Transparent material tracking: Blockchain systems strengthen accountability by providing immutable records of:
- Raw material sourcing (Mouloudi et al., 2022)
- Carbon footprints
- Eco-compliance

Supply chain analytics improve demand forecasting, reducing overproduction, expired stock, and pharmaceutical wastage (Fusillo, 2023).

Smart distribution networks further minimize logistical emissions through:

- Predictive routing
- Optimized cold-chain transport
- Dynamic fleet management (Ghisetti & Quatraro, 2017)
- Digitalization therefore becomes a key enabler of sustainable, circular, and efficient pharmaceutical supply systems (Griliches, 1990).

6 Greening the Pharma Industry: The Avenues and Exemplary Endeavors

The pharmaceutical sector is at a critical crossroads, where it is encouraged to substitute the fossil-based organic chemical raw materials and plastics in packaging and manufacturing with the aim of reducing the emission massively (Hall et al., 2001). This change does not only revolve around the sourcing of renewable feedstocks/non-fossil carbon but also requires renewable energy sources in production strategies. This will be possible by ensuring supply chain transparency by making detailed material declarations, which will also lessen dependence on unstable oil markets. Although just replacing fossil chemicals is a step in the right direction, a long-term measure will be to design the processes considering green chemistry and de-fossilization since the beginning. To their credit, other firms are changing starting materials and substitutes to greener ones and encourage sustainable pharmaceutical production (Haščič & Migotto, 2015).

There is an attempt to utilize biobased feedstocks within the pharma industry. Cashew nut shell liquid (CNSL), which is a type of agro-waste but contains rich bioactive compounds including anacardic acid, cardol, cardanol, and 2-methylcardol, was transformed into pharmaceuticals through a green metathesis strategy (Higham et al., 2021). It was found that the compounds exhibit strong antiparasitic activities against Trypanosoma cruzi, the causative agent of Chagas disease, and two of them are much more selective than the existing drug, benznidazole. Valorization of such biobased wastes in Asian and African countries (leaders in CNSL production) might

a catalyze the establishment of local pharma industries
b augment job creation and economic progress
c lessen dependence on pharmaceutical imports
d reduce carbon emissions linked to long-distance freight (Howell, 2017)

Synthesis of drugs is usually a multi-step reaction. To this end, the key strategies to increase the sustainability of the economies and environment are the maximization of atom economy, reduction of solvent use and solvent waste, the use of alternative reaction media, and process intensification (IEA, 2021). Similarly, microwave and sonochemical methods are reportedly used in more research articles and patents (IPCC, 2018), but the problem of scalability cannot be ignored. However, in liquid–liquid reactions, biphasic catalysis and sonochemical activation are promising scalable, mild reactions (Iori et al., 2022).

Conversely, untreated and improperly disposed of antibiotic-containing pharmaceutical wastewater containing resistance genes poses a serious risk to the ecosystem and human health (Juo & Wang, 2022). It requires prompt, intersectoral, and interdisciplinary responses, a One Health approach to setting universal standards on effluent antibiotic residues, creating treatment technologies, and enhancing antimicrobial resistance (AMR) action plans to uphold the health of the population and the environment (Kamilaris et al., 2017).

The model was able to predict PBT-relevant substructures in drug molecules by grouping the data to be considered fairly. It is hoped that these findings will serve as a kind of structural flag to drug designers, allowing them to design drug candidates that are more environmentally friendly at the first stages of the discovery process without compromising therapeutic efficacy (Kogan et al., 2017).

The introduction of carbon emission reduction should also be the issue of concern and should be discussed simultaneously with the renewable energy sources and water efficiency and waste management use (Lerner, 1994). Despite the fact that the concept of green chemistry has long been a welcome one within the context of the scientific community, the technical green chemistry development is one of the matters that can only be given the required attention and effort as a consequence of the impact of education and awareness (Li et al., 2023). It takes radical change in order to transform the traditional chemical companies into a sustainable one. Nevertheless, it needs to be supported by the basis of cooperation between education, politics, economics, interdisciplinary commitment, equity, metrics, regulation, and awareness (Martinelli et al., 2021). Yes, green chemistry had long been beckoning the direction of many research establishments and universities and is now slowly starting to toy with at least some realities in the industry. However, we still have much to do not only to carry out research, but also to change the way to go about chemistry and synthesis, what it can bring to our life in terms of wellness and technological and social achievements (Montresor & Vezzani, 2023; Popp, 2019).

7 Conclusion and Future Prospects

Green chemistry is now a significant dimension in the global arena. It also makes quality products whose residues of toxic substances are minimal in numbers, besides solving most of the environmental issues. Analyzing the overall state of the pharmaceutical sector and the issues related to it like the ecological challenges, high prices of medicines, and many other issues of this kind, it might be assumed that green chemistry is a novel approach to make life better and decrease the number of environmental issues (Reichstein et al., 2019). This will allow keeping the carbon and water footprint to a minimum; the hazardous chemicals and solvents can be reduced and replaced with renewable and green solvents and feedstocks. The future opportunities are that green chemistry has the capability of transforming the pharmaceutical industry and drug production. It is both environmental and cost-effective. It will result in the transformation of the traditional pharmaceutical industries into green ones and the sustainability of the environment (Robinson et al., 2020). In the future, the concept of integrating GREENER into drug discovery and development is likely to be a key to sustainable pharmaceutical innovation. The current trends in computational toxicology, AI-based drug design, high-throughput screening of environmental fate and ecotoxicology, and predictive biodegradation modeling will allow researchers to evaluate environmental fate and ecotoxicological risks in the discovery pipeline at earlier stages (Rolnick et al., 2022). As the regulatory bodies begin to incorporate the environmental sustainability requirements in their approval systems, the trend toward pharmaceutical companies achieving benign-by-design approaches as a competitive and compliance advantage will increase.

The cross-sectoral collaboration that includes drug designers, environmental scientists, clinicians, and policymakers will help to develop APIs with therapeutic effects and the smallest environmental impact (Santoalha et al., 2021). With the emergence of new technologies like precision dosing, nanodelivery systems, microfluidic production, and circular waste-management structures, the emissions and environmental exposure will be reduced further.

Over time, sustainable education in pharmacy, One Health efforts on a global scale, and harmonized international guidelines will help turn the GREENER principles from a novelty into a conventional practice and create a pharmaceutical environment that ensures the health of patients and the health of the planet (Santoleri et al., 2022; Słoczyński & Wooldridge, 2018; Soleimanpouromran & Ahmadimoghadam, 2021; Squicciarini et al., 2013; Steinmueller, 2010).

Bibliography

Agrawal, R., Agrawal, S., Samadhiya, A., Kumar, A., Luthra, S., & Jain, V. (2024). Adoption of green finance and green innovation for achieving circularity: An exploratory review and future directions. *Geoscience Frontiers, 15*(4), 101669.

Ahuja, G., & Morris Lampert, C. (2001). Entrepreneurship in the large corporation: A longitudinal study of how established firms create breakthrough inventions. *Strategic Management Journal, 22*(6–7), 521–543.

Al-Emran, M., & Griffy-Brown, C. (2023). The role of technology adoption in sustainable development: Overview, opportunities, challenges, and future research agendas. *Technology in Society, 73*, 102240.

Ali, S. M., Norhashim, M., & Jaffar, N. (2024). Tax avoidance and earnings management in Malaysian firms: Impact of tax incentives. *Bangladesh Journal of Multidisciplinary Scientific Research, 9*(2), 30–44. https://doi.org/10.46281/bjmsr.v9i2.2223

Amin, M. B., & Oláh, J. (2024). Effects of green HRM practices on circular economy-based performance of banking organizations in an emerging nation. *Banks and Bank Systems, 19*(2), 75–87. https://doi.org/10.21511/bbs.19(2).2024.06

Amin, M. B., Asaduzzaman, M., Debnath, G. C., Rahaman, M. A., & Oláh, J. (2024). Effects of circular economy practices on sustainable firm performance of green garments. *Oeconomia Copernicana, 15*(2), 637–682. https://www.ceeol.com/search/article-detail?id=1265145

Andreani, L. C., Bozzola, A., Kowalczewski, P., Liscidini, M., & Redorici, L. (2019). Silicon solar cells: Toward the efficiency limits. *Advances in Physics: X, 4*(1), 1548305.

Ardabili, S., Mosavi, A., Dehghani, M., et al. (2020). Deep learning and machine learning in hydrological processes, climate change and Earth systems: A systematic review. In *Engineering for sustainable future: Selected papers of the 18th International Conference on Global Research and Education Inter-Academia 2019* (Vol. 18, pp. 52–62). Springer.

AL-Maamari, O. A., Aljonaid, N., & Alrefaei, N. (2025). Impact of microcredit on the performance of micro and small enterprises (MSEs) in Yemen. *Cogent Economics & Finance, 13(1)*. https://doi.org/10.1080/23322039.2025.2460083

Barbieri, N., Marzucchi, A., & Rizzo, U. (2020). Knowledge sources and impacts on subsequent inventions: Do green technologies differ from non-green ones? *Research Policy, 49*(2), 103901.

Bauer, C., Hofer, J., Althaus, H. J., Del Duce, A., & Simons, A. (2015). The environmental performance of current and future passenger vehicles: Life cycle assessment based on a novel scenario analysis framework. *Applied Energy, 157*, 871–883.

Bejgam, R., Sunkari, S., Keshipeddi, S. B., Rangaraju, M. R., & Dunde, V. (2021, September). A brief study on hybrid electric vehicles. In *2021 Third International Conference on Inventive Research in Computing Applications (ICIRCA)* (pp. 54–59). IEEE.

Bianchini, S., Damioli, G., & Ghisetti, C. (2023). The environmental effects of the "twin" green and digital transition in European regions. *Environmental and Resource Economics, 84*(4), 877–918.

Bieker, G. (2021). *A global comparison of the life-cycle greenhouse gas emissions of combustion engine and electric passenger cars*. International Council on Clean Transportation. https://theicct.org/publication/a-global-comparison-of-the-life-cycle-greenhouse-gas-emissions-of-combustion-engine-and-electric-passenger-cars

Bieńkowska A, Koszela A, Sałamacha A, Tworek K. COVID-19 oriented HRM strategies influence on job and organizational performance through job-related attitudes. PLoS One. 2022 Apr 13;17(4):e0266364. doi: 10.1371/journal.pone.0266364. PMID: 35417468; PMCID: PMC9007351.

Bloom, N., Van Reenen, J., & Williams, H. (2019). A toolkit of policies to promote innovation. *Journal of Economic Perspectives, 33*(3), 163–184.

Bloomberg NEF. (2022). *Electric vehicle outlook 2022*. https://about.bnef.com/electric-vehicle-outlook

Bollobás, B. (2001). *Random graphs*. Cambridge University Press.

Bonou, A., Laurent, A., & Olsen, S. I. (2016). Life cycle assessment of onshore and offshore wind energy—from theory to application. *Applied Energy, 180*, 327–337.

Bošnjaković, M., Santa, R., Crnac, Z., & Bošnjaković, T. (2023). Environmental impact of PV power systems. *Sustainability, 15*(15), 11888.

Brevini, B. (2023). Myths, techno-solutionism and artificial intelligence: Reclaiming AI materiality and its massive environmental costs. In S. Lindgren (Ed.), *Handbook of critical studies of artificial intelligence* (pp. 869–877). Edward Elgar Publishing.

Cattani, L., Montresor, S., & Vezzani, A. (2023). Firms' eco-innovation and Industry 4.0 technologies in urban and rural areas. *Regional Studies*. https://doi.org/10.1080/00343404.2023.2243984

Chowdhury, R. S., Islam, M. A., Yuauf, D. H. B. M., Amin, M. B., Hassan, M. S., Barua, S., & Abdullah, M. (2024). Implications of artificial intelligence (AI) and machine learning-based fintech for financial assets related traditional investment theories. *Journal of Infrastructure, Policy and Development, 8*(12), 7415. https://doi.org/10.24294/jipd.v8i12.7415

Cockburn, I. M., Henderson, R., & Stern, S. (2018). The impact of artificial intelligence on innovation: An exploratory analysis. In A. Agrawal, J. Gans, & A. Goldfarb (Eds.), *The economics of artificial intelligence: An agenda* (pp. 115–146). University of Chicago Press.

Cowls, J., Tsamados, A., Taddeo, M., et al. (2023). The AI gambit: Leveraging artificial intelligence to combat climate change—Opportunities, challenges, and recommendations. *AI & Society, 38*, 283–307.

Crespi, F., Ghisetti, C., & Quatraro, F. (2015). Environmental and innovation policies for the evolution of green technologies: A survey and a test. *Eurasian Business Review, 5*, 343–370.

Czarnitzki, D., Ebersberger, B., & Fier, A. (2007). The relationship between R&D collaboration, subsidies and R&D performance: Empirical evidence from Finland and Germany. *Journal of Applied Econometrics, 22*(7), 1347–1366.

Damioli, G., Bianchini, S., & Ghisetti, C. (2024). The emergence of a "twin transition" scientific knowledge base in the European regions. *Regional Studies*. https://doi.org/10.1080/00343404.2024.2355998

De Jesus, A., & Mendonça, S. (2018). Lost in transition? Drivers and barriers in the eco-innovation road to the circular economy. *Ecological Economics, 145*, 75–89.

Dechezleprêtre, A., Martin, R., & Mohnen, M. (2013). *Knowledge spillovers from clean and dirty technologies: A patent citation analysis*. Grantham Research Institute on Climate Change and the Environment.

Diodato, D., Huergo, E., Moncada-Paternò-Castello, P., et al. (2023). Introduction to the special issue on "The twin (digital and green) transition: Handling the economic and social challenges." *Industry and Innovation, 30*(7), 755–765.

Fazio, G., Maioli, S., & Rujimora, N. (2024). The twin innovation transitions of European regions. *Regional Studies*. https://doi.org/10.1080/00343404.2024.2309176

Fu, F., Li, J., Yang, T. C. J., Liang, H., Faes, A., Jeangros, Q., …& Hou, Y. (2022). Monolithic perovskite–silicon tandem solar cells: From the lab to fab? *Advanced Materials, 34*(24), 2106540.

Fusillo, F. (2023). Green technologies and diversity in the knowledge search and output phases: Evidence from European patents. *Research Policy, 52*(4), 104727.

Fusillo, F., Quatraro, F., & Santhià, C. (2024). Leveraging circular economy technologies for recombinant dynamics: Do localised knowledge and digital complementarities matter? *Regional Studies*. https://doi.org/10.1080/00343404.2024.2329255

Gaustad, G., Krystofik, M., Bustamante, M., & Badami, K. (2018). Circular economy strategies for mitigating critical material supply issues. *Resources, Conservation and Recycling, 135*, 24–33.

Gazi, M. A. I., Rahman, M. K. H., Masud, A. A., Amin, M. B., Chaity, N. S., Senathirajah, A. R. B. S., & Abdullah, M. (2024). AI capability and sustainable performance: Mediating effects of organizational creativity and green innovation with knowledge-sharing culture as a moderator. *Sustainability, 16*(17), 7466. https://doi.org/10.3390/su16177466

Ghisetti, C., & Quatraro, F. (2017). Green technologies and environmental productivity: A cross-sectoral analysis of direct and indirect effects in Italian regions. *Ecological Economics, 132*, 1–13.

Gong, X., Yee, C. L., Lee, S. Y., Cao, E. Y., & Saif, A. N. M. (2024). Knowledge mapping of impulsive buying behavior research: A visual analysis using CiteSpace. *Humanities and Social Sciences Communications, 11*(1), 1–18.

Griliches, Z. (1990). *Patent statistics as economic indicators: A survey, part II*. National Bureau of Economic Research.

Hall, B. H., Jaffe, A. B., & Trajtenberg, M. (2001). *The NBER patent citation data file: Lessons, insights and methodological tools* (NBER Working Paper No. 8498).

Hasan, M., Abedin, M. Z., Amin, M. B., Nekmahmud, M., & Oláh, J. (2023). Sustainable biofuel economy: A mapping through bibliometric research. *Journal of Environmental Management, 336*, 117644. https://doi.org/10.1016/j.jenvman.2023.117644

Haščič, I., & Migotto, M. (2015). *Measuring environmental innovation using patent data* [Technical report].

Hepburn, C., O'Callaghan, B., Stern, N., Stiglitz, J., & Zenghelis, D. (2020). Will COVID-19 fiscal recovery packages accelerate or retard progress on climate change? *Oxford Review of Economic Policy, 36*(Suppl 1), S359–S381.

Higham, K., de Rassenfosse, G., & Jaffe, A. B. (2021). Patent quality: Towards a systematic framework for analysis and measurement. *Research Policy, 50*(4), 104215.

Hossain, M. M., Khan, M. Y. A., Halim, M. A., Elme, N. S., & Hussain, M. N. (2023). A review on stability challenges and probable solutions of perovskite–silicon tandem solar cells. *Signal and Image Processing Letters, 5*(1), 62–71.

Howell, S. T. (2017). Financing innovation: Evidence from R&D grants. *American Economic Review, 107*(4), 1136–1164.

Intergovernmental Panel on Climate Change. (2018). *Global warming of 1.5°C* (IPCC Special Report). https://www.ipcc.ch/sr15/

International Energy Agency. (2021). *Net zero by 2050: A roadmap for the global energy sector*. https://www.iea.org/reports/net-zero-by-2050

International Energy Agency. (2023). *Global EV outlook 2023*. IEA.

Iori, M., Martinelli, A., & Mina, A., et al. (2022). The direction of technical change in AI and the trajectory effects of government funding. *LEM Working Paper* (Vol. 2021).

Islam, M. S., Rubel, M. R. B., Rimi, N. N., Amin, M. B., & Quadir, P. (2024). Attaining sustainable excellence: Impact of sustainable SCM and circular economy on the green garment industry in Bangladesh. *Sustainable Futures*, 100234. https://doi.org/10.1016/j.sftr.2024.100234

Jabessa, T., Tesfaye, G., & Bekele, K. (2023). Evaluation of genotypes with environmental interactions of lablab (Purpureus L.) and its dry matter yield stability in the midland of Guji Zone, Southern Oromia, Ethiopia. *Bangladesh Journal of Multidisciplinary Scientific Research, 8*(1), 34–43. https://doi.org/10.46281/bjmsr.v8i1.2169

Jafarizadeh, H., Yamini, E., Zolfaghari, S. M., Esmaeilion, F., Assad, M. E. H., & Soltani, M. (2024). Navigating challenges in large-scale renewable energy storage: Barriers, solutions, and innovations. *Energy Reports, 12*, 2179–2192.

Jafrin, N., Saif, A. N. M., Masud, M. M., Ghosh, D., & Nesa, M. (2024). Nexus between demographic dividend and economic growth: A systematic review with bibliometric exploration. *Multidisciplinary Reviews, 7*(8), 2024182.

Jelle, B. P. (2011). Traditional, state-of-the-art and future thermal building insulation materials and solutions: Properties, requirements, and possibilities. *Energy and Buildings, 43*(10), 2549–2563.

Juo, W. J., & Wang, C. H. (2022). Does green innovation mediate the relationship between green relational view and competitive advantage? *Business Strategy and the Environment, 31*(5), 2456–2468.

Kaffine, D. T., McBee, B. J., & Lieskovsky, J. (2013). Emissions savings from wind power generation in Texas. *The Energy Journal, 34*(1), 155–176.

Kaldellis, J. K., & Apostolou, D. (2017). Life cycle energy and carbon footprint of offshore wind energy: Comparison with onshore counterpart. *Renewable Energy, 108*, 72–84.

Kamilaris, A., Kartakoullis, A., & Prenafeta-Boldú, F. X. (2017). A review on the practice of big data analysis in agriculture. *Computers and Electronics in Agriculture, 143*, 23–37.

Karakaya, E., & Sriwannawit, P. (2015). Barriers to the adoption of photovoltaic systems: The state of the art. *Renewable and Sustainable Energy Reviews, 49*, 60–66.

Karim, M. R., Nordin, N., Yusof, M. F., Amin, M. B., Islam, M. A., & Hassan, M. S. (2023). ERP implementation as a mediator between knowledge management and perceived organizational performance in the healthcare sector. *Cogent Business & Management, 10*(3), 2275869. https://doi.org/10.1080/23311975.2023.2275869

Khalid, M. (2024). Smart grids and renewable energy systems: Perspectives and grid integration challenges. *Energy Strategy Reviews, 51*, 101299.

Kim, H., Choi, H., Kang, H., An, J., Yeom, S., & Hong, T. (2021). A systematic review of the smart energy conservation system: From smart homes to sustainable smart cities. *Renewable and Sustainable Energy Reviews, 140*, 110755.

Kogan, L., Papanikolaou, D., Seru, A., et al. (2017). Technological innovation, resource allocation, and growth. *The Quarterly Journal of Economics, 132*(2), 665–712.

Laskowicz, T. (2022). Offshore wind energy potential in Europe: A forecast of installed capacities and costs. *Europa XXI, 42*, 129–148.

Laurent, W. (2008). Green intelligence. *Information Management, 18*(12), 35.

Lerner, J. (1994). The importance of patent scope: An empirical analysis. *The RAND Journal of Economics, 25*(2), 319–333.

Li, W., Xu, X., Huang, S., et al. (2023). Assessment of green technology innovation on energy–environmental efficiency in China under the influence of environmental regulation considering spatial effects. *Scientific Reports, 13*(1), 20789.

Liu, Z., Li, H., Chu, Z., Xia, R., Wen, J., Mo, Y., …& Tan, H. (2024). Reducing perovskite/C60 interface losses via sequential interface engineering for efficient perovskite/silicon tandem solar cells. *Advanced Materials, 36*(8), 2308370.

Martinelli, A., Mina, A., & Moggi, M. (2021). The enabling technologies of Industry 4.0: Examining the seeds of the fourth industrial revolution. *Industrial and Corporate Change, 30*(1), 161–188.

Metawa, N., Dogan, E., & Taskin, D. (2022). Analyzing the nexus of green economy, clean and financial technology. *Economic Analysis and Policy, 76*, 385–396.

Moher, D., Liberati, A., Tetzlaff, J., Altman, D. G., & PRISMA Group. (2009). Preferred reporting items for systematic reviews and meta-analyses: The PRISMA statement. *Annals of Internal Medicine, 151*(4), 264–269.

Mollah, M. A., Pal, D., Amin, M. B., Rahaman, M. A., & Abdullah, M. (2024). Effect of technological culture and knowledge sharing on organizational performance: Digital innovation as mediator and self-efficacy as moderator. *Journal of Infrastructure, Policy and Development, 8*(12), 7594. https://doi.org/10.24294/jipd.v8i12.7594

Mondal, S., & Palit, D. (2022). Challenges in natural resource management for ecological sustainability. In S. Mondal & D. Palit (Eds.), *Natural resources conservation and advances for sustainability* (pp. 29–59). Elsevier.

Montresor, S., & Vezzani, A. (2023). Digital technologies and eco-innovation: Evidence of the twin transition from Italian firms. *Industry and Innovation, 30*(7), 1–35.

Mouloudi, L., & Evrard Samuel, K. (2022). Critical materials assessment: A key factor for supply chain risk management. *Supply Chain Forum: An International Journal, 23*(1), 53–67.

Mukherjee, A., Bruijnincx, P., & Junginger, M. (2023). Techno-economic competitiveness of renewable fuel alternatives in the marine sector. *Renewable and Sustainable Energy Reviews, 174*, 113127.

Plageras, A. P., Psannis, K. E., Stergiou, C., Wang, H., & Gupta, B. B. (2018). Efficient IoT-based sensor big data collection, processing and analysis in smart buildings. *Future Generation Computer Systems, 82*, 349–357.

Popp, D. (2019). *Environmental policy and innovation: A decade of research.* National Bureau of Economic Research.

Qing, W., Amin, M. B., Gazi, M. A. I., Khan, W., Al Masud, A., & Alam, M. N. (2023). Mediation effect of technology adaptation capabilities between service quality attributes and customer satisfaction: Evidence from young e-commerce customers in China. *IEEE Access, 11*, 123904–123923. https://doi.org/10.1109/ACCESS.2023.3328775

Rabbi, M. F., & Amin, M. B. (2024). Circular economy and sustainable practices in the food industry: A comprehensive bibliometric analysis. *Cleaner and Responsible Consumption*, 100206. https://doi.org/10.1016/j.clrc.2024.100206

Randau, S., Weber, D. A., Kötz, O., Koerver, R., Braun, P., Weber, A., … & Janek, J. (2020). Benchmarking the performance of all-solid-state lithium batteries. *Nature Energy, 5*(3), 259–270.

Reichstein, M., Camps-Valls, G., Stevens, B., et al. (2019). Deep learning and process understanding for data-driven Earth system science. *Nature, 566*(7743), 195–204.

Robinson, C., Dilkina, B., & Moreno-Cruz, J. (2020). Modeling migration patterns in the USA under sea level rise. *PLOS ONE, 15*(1), e0227436.

Rolnick, D., Donti, P. L., Kaack, L. H., et al. (2022). Tackling climate change with machine learning. *ACM Computing Surveys, 55*(2), 1–96.

Saif, A. N. M., Islam, K. A., Haque, A., Akhter, H., Rahman, S. M., Jafrin, N., … & Mostafa, R. (2022). Blockchain implementation challenges in developing countries: An evidence-based systematic review and bibliometric analysis. *Technology Innovation Management Review, 12*(1–2), 1–20.

Saif, A. N. M., Rahman, A. A., & Mostafa, R. (2021). Post-implementation challenges of ERP adoption in the apparel industry of a developing country. *LogForum, 17*(4), 519–529.

Santoalha, A., Consoli, D., & Castellacci, F. (2021). Digital skills, relatedness and green diversification: A study of European regions. *Research Policy, 50*(9), 104340.

Santoleri, P., Mina, A., Di Minin, A., et al. (2022). The causal effects of R&D grants: Evidence from a regression discontinuity. *The Review of Economics and Statistics*. https://doi.org/10.1162/rest_a_01233

Schnieders, J., Feist, W., & Rongen, L. (2015). Passive houses for different climate zones. *Energy and Buildings, 105*, 71–87.

Shakeel, S. R. (2021). Cleantech: Prospects and challenges. *Journal of Innovation Management, 9*(2), viii–xvii.

Słoczyński, T., & Wooldridge, J. M. (2018). A general double robustness result for estimating average treatment effects. *Econometric Theory, 34*(1), 112–133.

Soleimanpouromran, M., & Ahmadimoghadam, A. (2021). The study of green intelligence on environmental experiences and environmental citizenship behavior. *Central Asian Journal of Environmental Science and Technology Innovation, 2*(2), 79–90.

Squicciarini, M., Dernis, H., & Criscuolo, C. (2013). *Measuring patent quality: Indicators of technological and economic value* [Technical report]. Organisation for Economic Co-operation and Development.

Steinmueller, W. E. (2010). Economics of technology policy. In B. H. Hall & N. Rosenberg (Eds.), *Handbook of the economics of innovation* (Vol. 2, pp. 1181–1218). Elsevier.

Sun, D. (2024). The role of green technology and green utility performance in advancing energy utilities' commitment to sustainability. *Economic Change and Restructuring, 57*(2), 53.

Sun, Y., Gao, P., Tian, W., et al. (2023). Green innovation for resource efficiency and sustainability: Empirical analysis and policy. *Resources Policy, 81*, 103369.

Swiatek, L. (2024). Strengthening the sustainability of artificial intelligence: Fostering green intelligence for a more ethical future. In T. Walker, S. Wendt, S. Goubran, & T. Schwartz (Eds.), *Artificial intelligence for sustainability: Innovations in business and financial services* (pp. 83–103). Springer.

U.S. Department of Energy. (2023). *Hydrogen and fuel cell technologies office accomplishments and progress*. https://www.energy.gov/eere/fuelcells/hydrogen-and-fuel-cell-technologies-office-accomplishments-and-progress

Vollmer, I., Jenks, M. J., Roelands, M. C., White, R. J., Van Harmelen, T., De Wild, P., … & Weckhuysen, B. M. (2020). Beyond mechanical recycling: Giving new life to plastic waste. *Angewandte Chemie International Edition, 59*(36), 15402–15423.

Wicki, S., & Hansen, E. G. (2019). Green technology innovation: Anatomy of exploration processes from a learning perspective. *Business Strategy and the Environment, 28*(6), 970–988.

Yamaguchi, S., Yamamoto, C., Ohdaira, K., & Masuda, A. (2018). Comprehensive study of potential-induced degradation in silicon heterojunction photovoltaic cell modules. *Progress in Photovoltaics: Research and Applications, 26*(9), 697–708.

Yigitcanlar, T., Kamruzzaman, M., Foth, M., Sabatini-Marques, J., Da Costa, E., & Ioppolo, G. (2019). Can cities become smart without being sustainable? A systematic review. *Sustainable Cities and Society, 45*, 348–365.

Yusoh, N. N. A. M., Mat, T. Z. T., & Abdullah, A. (2024). Impacts of environmental management accounting system (EMAS) adoption phases on sustainability performance: A social issue life cycle theory approach. *Bangladesh Journal of Multidisciplinary Scientific Research, 9*(4), 25–38. https://doi.org/10.46281/bjmsr.v9i4.2245

5 Strategies for Sustainable Development in Drug Discovery and Development

Devika Rana and Dhriti Verma

1 Introduction

The world's population continues to grow, and the importance of pharmaceuticals in maintaining public health is increasing. It has been observed that as the diseases are progressing among individuals, there will be more than double the demand for medications in the coming years. This increased demand and use of pharmaceuticals has led to increased exposure of these pharmaceutical drugs and crude substances to the environment, which not only disrupts ecosystems but also potentially harms human health if exposed for a longer duration. This type of exposure results in problems like antibiotic resistance and reproductive health issues (Steffen, 2015; Raworth, 2018; Block, 2019). Sustainability can be defined in different ways depending on the situation. Sustainable development meets the needs of the current population without any harmful effect on the environment and does not compromise with future needs by preserving the renewable stock. In view of sustainable drug discovery and development, there are various principles like environmental impact, meeting the medical needs, focusing on green synthesis, and many more that are considered to achieve this goal (Rittel, 1973; Puhlmann, 2021).

In drug designing and development, one must keep in mind the risk–benefit assessment for the environment, as the environmental impact of drugs on both humans and animals has become an increasing concern as these substances accumulate in nature. Active pharmaceutical ingredients (APIs), their metabolites, and breakdown products are increasingly found in the environment, which leads to hazardous conditions. For example, the diclofenac breakdown products and residues have led to the deaths of animals and birds feeding on contaminated cattle, and another is naproxen, which, when exposed to light, degrades itself into its byproducts that are more toxic to aquatic organisms than the original drug itself. After a drug is taken and excreted, many drugs and their metabolites, along with other waste products, are passed through a wastewater treatment plant (Puhlmann, 2021). These sewerage plants are not usually equipped to treat or filter out pharmaceutical waste (drug metabolites). If sustainability principles are not implemented at the earliest stages of drug discovery, these environmental burdens will ultimately fall to future generations, which will affect the health and environment (Smale, 2021; Belew, 2021; European Centre for Disease Prevention and Control (ECDC), 2021).

DOI: 10.4324/9781003640486-5

These issues require a fundamental transformation in the approach to drug discovery and development, with sustainability as the major guiding principle. Sustainable drug development (SDD) focuses on minimizing environmental harm and maintaining therapeutic efficacy and safety. SDD involves following eco-friendly practices at every stage, from initial compound design through to manufacturing and post-market surveillance (Peake, 2015). Green chemistry has a major role in SDD; it prioritizes synthetic routes that use fewer hazardous reagents, produces less waste or eco-friendly waste, and requires lower energy for the completion of reactions. Innovations in developing solvent-free syntheses, catalytic processes, and use of biocatalysts and renewable feedstocks help to achieve SDD. Researchers are placing more emphasis on designing drugs that are not only effective in treating diseases but also biodegradable, eco-friendly, and safer to decompose (Peake, 2015; van der Gronde, 2018).

Industrial research and development (R&D) teams are exploring innovative technologies and methodologies to accelerate the discovery process from other scientific fields. Despite the number of efforts and experiments to discover or develop a promising chemical compound from the initial active hit stage to lead and then finally to a potential drug candidate, it is a major challenge not only for the pharmaceutical industry but also for scientists involved in drug discovery. These challenges are most affected by the increasing expectations for drug sustainability, its efficiency, and safety in the development stage. As the growing environmental hazards, which have led to strict regulations and public awareness on ecological impacts, are growing, pharmaceutical companies are also asked and compelled to rethink the traditional practices of drug development. Many large organizations are now implementing green chemistry and sustainable methodologies in their drug development methodologies. They are implementing this practice not only to build their standards but also to future-proof their operations and reputation. They are also doing partnerships with academic institutions, technology firms, and regulatory agencies; pharmaceutical R&D teams can access novel insights and tools that drive sustainable innovation. Ultimately, the path towards drug discovery requires a holistic thinking and approach that has the entire life cycle of a medicine, i.e. from the concept of design to post-market surveillance. Implementing sustainability is not just an ethical approach/technique but a strategic advantage that leads to safer therapies, reduces environmental harm, and ensures the long-term survival of the pharmaceutical industry (Berdigaliyev, 2020; Dhasmana, 2018; Bandichhor, 2018).

The path from initial drug discovery to regulatory approval is a challenging and expensive process. Generally, bringing a new medicine to market or starting from scratch takes more than a decade along with a huge investment of approximately $1 billion or more. These investment figures, however, can fluctuate significantly depending on the complexity of the drug candidate and the targeted disease. Treatments for rare diseases or particularly challenging medical conditions eventually have longer, more demanding timelines and even higher costs due to limited patient populations or the challenges involved in validating therapeutic efficacy and safety. This lengthy process rotates around numerous stages of drug

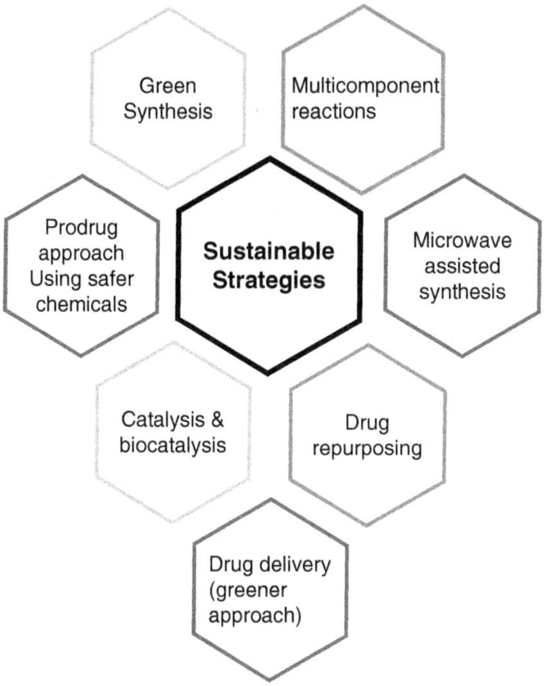
Green Synthesis
Multicomponent reactions
Prodrug approach Using safer chemicals
Sustainable Strategies
Microwave assisted synthesis
Catalysis & biocatalysis
Drug repurposing
Drug delivery (greener approach)

Figure 5.1 Sustainable pathway in drug design, discovery, and development.

development, especially ranging from early compound identification and preclinical testing to multi-phase clinical trials and rigorous regulatory review. In drug discovery, risk and decision-making models are important for SDD. Drug discovery constitutes identifying a hit or ligand for a particular disease acting through a specific mechanism. The understanding on how these ligands modulate cellular networks is a greater challenge in itself. Figure 5.1 shows the strategies in drug discovery, which are environmentally friendly, cost-effective, fast, efficient, and value-creating with optimal experimental designs (Dhasmana, 2018; Berdigaliyev, 2020; Wynendaele, 2021).

2 Strategies for Sustainable Development in Drug Discovery and Development

2.1 *Green Chemistry/Synthesis*

This strategy is dedicated to developing techniques and analytical methods that will reduce waste and decrease the factors driving climate change. It will optimize resource consumption, cut down on energy waste, and incorporate renewable energy sources into production. The pharmaceutical companies have a major role in the global economy for generating a total revenue of $1.27 trillion, along with a significant world carbon production of about 1.9 million tonnes of CO_2.

Therefore, as the demand for drug discovery and development grows, there is also concern about the environmental impact; it becomes important to wisely choose sustainable approaches in drug synthesis. Different strategies to lower solvent usage include adopting flow chemistry and conducting reactions in water, inspired by biological systems. To encourage environmentally friendly synthesis producing less waste, use green solvents and safer chemicals whose degradation and decomposition can be easily done. A green chemistry strategy is based on various principles. We can harness the principle towards sustainable drug discovery and development (Mishra, 2021; Moermond, 2022; Martinengo, 2024).

In "Greener chemical synthesis", the chemical synthetic methodologies for drug development usually generate toxic, harmful chemicals not only for humans but also for the environment. Whenever a chemical process/synthesis is designed, it should be monitored to ensure that it is greener and safe and uses less toxic chemicals. For example, the antibacterial and antiprotozoal agent metronidazole followed the traditional synthetic approach and uses toxic methylating agents such as dimethyl sulphate and methyl iodide. To overcome this drawback, a green chemistry route was developed with methanol (a green solvent) as a methylating reagent (Martinengo, 2024; Erythropel, 2018). Another key aspect of green chemistry is "reducing derivatization" in chemical synthesis. Each step in the synthesis of compounds comes with a burden of increased resources and increased waste. The streamlining of synthetic routes by using solvent-free, one-pot, and multicomponent methods can improve the overall efficiency of synthesis (Martinengo, 2024; Kavthe, 2022).

In earlier times, traditional chemical synthesis methods often led to unwanted waste products which caused environmental pollution. Therefore, a green chemist designs a chemical process in such a way that it becomes more important to prevent waste than to treat or clean up waste after it has been created and hence reduces the burden on the ecosystem. "E-factor" is the first green metric dealing with waste prevention. The E-factor is calculated by dividing a particular kg of waste by a particular kg of product. The waste was defined as the byproducts which are not the desired product. Tafenoquine succinate, an antiparasitic drug synthesized by GlaxoSmithKline with E-factor = 69. Lipshutz's team successfully developed a green and economic method for the same drug with E-factor = 17, resulting in a 3-fold decrease in waste products (Erythropel, 2018; Martinengo, 2024).

Most of the chemical synthesis require "**solvents**". The solvents used earlier, such as aniline, benzene, and many more, are more toxic and less environmentally friendly. They often pose significant risks to both the environment and human health. Green chemistry supports the use of safer options, such as water or bio-based solvents, which are less toxic and less hazardous to both humans and the environment. Water, the most economical solvent, has numerous advantages, such as being non-flammable, non-hazardous, nontoxic, redox-stable, inexpensive, and mostly unlimited. Therefore, there is increasing interest in developing chemical reactions that use water as the primary medium for the reaction. However, attention must be paid to potential water scarcity (Erythropel, 2018; Martinengo, 2024; Prat, 2014).

The raw materials to be used for drug development should be "renewable" and not depleting. Annually, a large amount of biowaste and residues are generated worldwide. This concern highlights the need for recovering these materials. The green chemistry goal is to create sustainable chemical building blocks by suitable utilization of renewable sources which are practically economic. Although sustainable practices for generating energy and the chemicals generated from biomass are common, their use for pharmaceutical production is still a challenge. The renewable bioactive sources from agricultural and food waste have tremendous potential to be used in drug development. Since these byproducts are an abundant source of high-value molecules. For example, cashew nutshell liquid (CNSL) biomass is converted to an active bioactive compound. It is chemically composed of phenol compounds which have a high degree of unsaturation. CNSL is not a potent drug compound, but it is linked with a quinone scaffold to develop antiparasitic applications (Erythropel, 2018; Cerone, 2019).

The use of plants as folk herbal medicines to treat various disorders has been used since ancient times. The different natural products have inspired the design, discovery, and development of new drugs. With the discovery and identification of recent molecular targets based on proteins, there is a growing need for fresh chemical diversification in screening. The drug discovery from medicinal plants plays an important role in the development of novel therapeutic leads, which mainly includes identifying and executing suitable high-throughput screening bioassays. The increasing supply of bioactive molecules has increased the momentum of drug discovery from natural plants. The development from these natural sources has led to various multidisciplinary fields joining together and leading to the generation of potential lead compounds (Chaachouay, 2024).

Metal nanoparticles (NPs) possess unique properties that continue to captivate researchers, prompting investigations into their potential applications. Among the various noble metal NPs, silver and gold nanoparticles have gained significant attention. But because of its toxic chemicals and risks involved for humans and the environment, there is an urgent need for the development of environmentally friendly methods in the emergence of green synthesis techniques. The plant-derived biological molecules, particularly in the form of extracts, serve as the foundation for plant-mediated NP production, which offers advantages over traditional chemical methods. Also, plant-based metallic NPs exhibit well-documented biological properties, including anti-tumour, antioxidant, antibacterial, and wound healing activities. The significant advantages associated with this eco-friendly approach have paved the way for exciting innovations in NP synthesis (Nadaf, 2022).

Nanomaterials (NMs) have drawn curiosity in agrochemical scientists due to possessing unique properties, particularly nanoparticle size, surface designs, elevated solubility, and flexible chemical compositions. Such characteristics make nanotechnology quite unique in reducing various disadvantages of traditional agrochemical compounds: reducing bioavailability, the high photodegradation tendency, and environmental contamination caused by organic solvents. The modern research defines NMs as effective supplements to traditional pesticides and fertilizers, representing two major groups of nanotechnological applications in the agricultural field. Similar studies also indicated its potential in the new fields, including biopesticides, nucleic acid-derived pesticides, plant growth regulators, and pheromone-based systems. Such aspects are used to expand the sphere of nanomaterials into the contemporary area of agrochemistry (An, 2022).

The resultant new category of nano-delivery systems has been shown to increase the stability of ingredients, increase dispersion, allow clear targeting, and reduce residue contamination. Such performance benefits are similar to sustainable development goals, in particular, the use of resources, smaller ecological footprints, and facilitation of long-term food security. In that respect, nanotechnology draws a parallel with pharmaceutical drug development and delivery, where similar techniques enjoy a quality of increased therapeutic action, reduced side effects, and guaranteed controlled release at the biological target. Despite a great promise, mass application of nano-agrochemicals is still limited by multiple barriers: standardized testing, scalable production procedures, complete regulatory protection, and improved social acceptance. However, as protracted and interdisciplinary research and favourable policy frameworks evolve, it is not improbable that nanotechnology will revolutionize the agricultural industry with regard to the profile of agrochemical efficacy, exactitude, and sustainability (An, 2022; Arabi, 2021; Shahiwala, 2025).

2.2 Multicomponent Reactions (MCRs)

The synthetic process should be designed to focus on ensuring that most of the starting materials ends up in the final product. MCRs are atom-economic reactions, as most reactants are there in the product. Atom economy (AE) calculates and measures the efficiency of a reaction. The way to calculate AE is the division of molecular weight of the final product by the combined molecular weights of all substances produced in the reaction. Chemical reactions such as isomerization, molecular rearrangements, and cycloadditions have high AE because all the starting reagents are contained in the product. Similarly, the multicomponent reactions (MCRs) are also efficient, as they also retain most reactant atoms in the product. Moreover, these reactions often occur in a single vessel, which saves organic solvents and chromatographic materials, further reducing waste and supporting sustainability. Medicinal chemists faced the dual challenge of developing safer, more effective drugs while also making the process greener and more sustainable. This is especially urgent for treating diseases that disproportionately affect low-income populations, like certain parasitic diseases linked to poverty. Making medicines both accessible and affordable is a vital public health goal. The popular MCR reaction is the Ugi four-component reaction (U-4CR); it is a type of condensation reaction. The reaction occurs among an amine, an oxo compound, isocyanide, and carboxylic acid. It is a type of one-pot synthesis; the drug praziquantel is synthesized by this approach (Martinengo, 2024; Cioc, 2014; Domling, 2012; Trost, 1991).

2.3 Prodrugs Approach

Another strategy for sustainable development is "designing synthetic process for degradation". As discussed earlier, the waste developed in the reaction should be minimal. The drug developed has the potential to become waste; therefore, its breakdown into harmless substances is important. Green chemistry encourages the development of those products whose degradation is harmless to the environment. This aspect is very similar to the use and design of "safer chemical". The metabolites of various pharmaceuticals have influence on microbial ecological processes and affect the environment. Since drugs are essentially chemical substances, they can sometimes be toxic to humans, leading to serious side effects. The developed drugs at a particular dose should have nontoxic absorption, distribution, metabolism, and excretion. The prime focus is on the development of these compounds or their metabolites into biodegradable derivatives (Fortuin, 2020).

The use of safer chemicals improves the drug development process and helps to have the most promising candidates. Usually, drugs enter the environment as unmetabolized compounds or their metabolites, primarily through wastewater, hospital discharge, households, and pharmaceutical manufacturing. Wastewater treatment plants process these substances, but the breakdown of drug compounds varies greatly (Cioc, 2014).

The approach to enhance safety is the use of prodrug strategies. Prodrugs are the chemically modified, inactive or less active forms of drugs that are converted to their active state inside the body by some enzymatic reaction at the time of degradation. This method reduces potential toxicity for patients and environmental hazard concerns. It designs drugs to be more biodegradable and have a reduced ecological impact and maintains effective pharmacokinetics. The artemether and lumefantrine combination is the recommended drug combination for malaria by the World Health Organization. Later, to achieve more stability and solve the uptake issue of this combination drug, a biodegradable and highly effective polymeric prodrug (PVP–PVL/VEBCPs) is developed (Chung, 2008; Fortuin, 2020). Another example is naltrexone; it is a narcotic antagonist whose biodegradable polymeric prodrug improves the patient compliance in the treatment of opiate addiction (Bennett, 1991).

2.4 Microwave-Assisted Synthesis

Energy efficiency is considered while designing a chemical synthesis. The process should use fewer energy sources and should be conducted at ambient temperature and pressure. Chemical manufacturing processes in pharmaceutical industries that consume large amounts of energy significantly impact the environment. A green synthetic approach aims to address the situation by promoting energy-saving methods and the combination of renewable energy sources for chemical production. Ideally, chemical reactions should be restructured and modified to consume minimal energy input. The most promising method is microwave-assisted synthesis, and it is closely linked to the energy efficiency principles of green chemistry. It has a number of advantages over traditional synthesis. Microwave synthesis follows the dielectric heating method and maintains its energy efficacy. The advantage of using this synthesis is that it directly heats the reaction mixture without heating the apparatus or reaction vessels having the reactants. It is less time- and energy-consuming; it employs the use of safer solvents or no solvents and generally attains a high selectivity and yields. Microwave-assisted continuous flow organic synthesis (MACOS) has been successfully investigated for organic reactions such as heterocycle synthesis and metal-catalysed chemistry and for semi-industrial preparation of aromatic compounds. This approach can often operate without solvents; due to this direct nature of microwave heating, it typically reduces reaction times compared to conventional heating methods, ultimately improving overall energy efficiency (Martina, 2021; Moseley, 2011). Triazole, a nitrogen-containing five-membered heterocycle, has widespread importance in drug design and the development of pharmaceutical and medicinal drugs. Several synthetic methods for its synthesis were explored; most were affected by harsh reaction conditions, high temperatures, low AE, and long reaction times. The triazole derivatives are synthesized using MW synthesis, which is much safer, energy-efficient, and higher scalability (Swami, 2025). Microwave synthesis is effective not only for medicine manufacturing but also for the degradation of pharmaceutical products. Mn-based catalysts with oxygen are used for degrading contaminants in the air using oxidation processes such as catalytic ozonation (Stefanache, 2025).

2.5 Catalysis and Biocatalysis

Nowadays, synthetic methods such as metathesis, biocatalysis, and photocatalysis are used for drug development. These methods represent innovative, efficient, and environmentally friendly approaches. Catalysis is an important principle of green chemistry, as it allows reactions to occur under milder conditions. It uses less energy and increases selectivity. Earlier traditional reagents were used which were ineffective compared to catalysts that are more sustainable and play a key role in synthesizing active pharmaceutical ingredients and bioactive compounds. Synthetic reactions such as transition metal-catalysed cross-coupling reactions are used in drug production in the pharmaceutical industry. Nickel, copper, and iron are selected for low cost, less toxicity, less reactivity, and environmental sustainability (Erythropel, 2018; Xiang, 2014; Lungu, 2024; Rabiee, 2020; Turan, 2019). Grubbs' ruthenium catalysts are used in olefin metathesis, which is very similar to the Wittig reaction. This catalyst avoids the production of a larger amount of waste and therefore has a large number of applications in the pharmaceutical industry (Abera Tsedalu, 2021).

"Biocatalysis", also known as enzymatic catalysis, has become prominent in SDD techniques. It is defined as enzymes derived from natural, biological sources to accelerate the chemical reaction. They use green solvents for the reaction, such as water, which have higher selectivity, and no product contamination occurs. This technique has been used in pharmaceutical industries to manufacture various active pharmaceutical ingredients (API). Drugs such as sitagliptin (Januvia), atorvastatin (Lipitor), rosuvastatin (Crestor), and montelukast (Singulair) are chiral medicines, which are manufactured through biocatalysis. In a recent study, keto reductases, a biocatalyst, were used in the synthesis of an Akt inhibitor (Stefanache, 2025; Paul, 2019; France, 2023).

The green chemistry approach and its aim are to focus on the use of safer solvents and chemicals. Therefore, it minimizes accidental risks with the adoption of chemical processes and technologies that are fundamentally safer, reducing both the likelihood and impact of potential accidents. This principle increases the chances for the development of a safer and more robust chemical industry.

2.6 Drug Repurposing Strategy

The drug development is lengthy, highly expensive, and has significant risk of late-stage failure. The repurposing or repositioning of the already reported drugs is an attractive and cost-efficient alternative. Drug repurposing works by identifying new therapeutic applications for already approved drugs. Therefore, the drug development timeline shortens, and the cost associated with it is reduced. Traditional drug discovery methods use extensive biological testing; they have financial and resource limitations, whereas repurposing offers lower costs and fewer hurdles. It focuses on discovering new applications from marketed drugs rather than starting from scratch with novel compounds. Drug repurposing is finding new therapeutic uses for approved drugs. This strategy is designed to address certain challenges associated with traditional drug discovery. It has one notable challenge that it has limited intellectual property protection. There are strict regulatory requirements regarding safety, efficacy, and quality in both animal and clinical testing. New drug development usually takes around approx. 12–17 years, but drug repositioning can significantly shorten the timeline, allowing research to bring an existing drug to a new therapeutic use (Pushpakom, 2019; Xue, 2018; Oprea, 2015; Gns, 2019).

The aim of drug repositioning is to explore other uses for existing medications apart from their original indication. The criteria for the selection of drugs for drug repurposing can be the following:

(i) Marketed drugs, (ii) drugs that lacked specific indications or faced safety concerns during clinical trials, and (iii) drugs whose development was halted for reasons such as budget constraints. Unlike traditional drug development, repurposing can sometimes allow these compounds to bypass early clinical phases, moving directly to Phase II, which helps shorten the time to market and lower development costs. Furthermore, since clinical data are typically available from the outset, the risks associated with advancing these drugs are significantly minimized. The complete understanding of pharmacology or the clinical efficacy followed by elaborate analysis of original indications increases the success rate in drug repurposing. The intellectual property rights are usually weak in this strategy and reduce companies' return on investments. Most of its applications are based on clinical observations or in vivo efficacy (Kaitin, 2010; Tobinick, 2009; Sleigh, 2010; Novac, 2013).

Drug repurposing in "Neurological diseases" is a challenge. Drug repurposing is a cost-effective and time-efficient process. This approach has been successfully implemented in Alzheimer's disease (AD). AD causes dementia: loss of memory and other mental disabilities that affect a patient's daily life. The brain tissue of the persons with AD led to dementia. The pathology of disease displays two types of lesions in the brain, senile plaque (SP) and neurofibrillary tangles (NFTs), the major cause of AD [49–52]. There are a number of drugs from different indications, which are repurposed for AD, as in Table 5.1.

Table 5.1 Drug repurposing examples with their drug class and repurposed indication in neurological diseases

Sno	*Drug*	*Drug Class*	*Repurposed Indication*
1	Carmustine	Anti-cancer	Alzheimer's disease
2	Bexarotene	Anti-cancer	Alzheimer's disease
3	Tamibarotene	Synthetic retinoid	Alzheimer's disease
4	Imatinib	Anti-cancer	Alzheimer's disease
5	Valsartan	Anti-hypertensive	Alzheimer's disease
6	Nitrendipine	Anti-hypertensive	Alzheimer's disease
7	Liraglutide	Type II diabetes	Alzheimer's disease
8	Acitretin	Severe psoriasis and dyskeratosis	Alzheimer's disease
9	Minocycline	Broad-spectrum antibiotics	Alzheimer's disease

Oncological diseases are the most widespread of all. They are one of the leading causes of death worldwide. The significant work has been done to search for novel methods for the treatment of cancer. The methods for drug development in cancer mainly consist of de novo drug design. A drug repurposing strategy is also used in various types of cancer. "Colorectal cancer", the second leading cause of death worldwide, is caused by mutations in the TP53 gene (Hua, 2022). The drugs of different classes repurposed for colorectal cancer with proposed mechanisms are shown in Table 5.2. Many drugs are also repurposed for "ovarian cancer". The occurrence of ovarian malignant tumours ranks third in gynaecological tumours. The nuclear hormone receptor family has ligand-activated receptors called peroxisome proliferator-activated receptors (PPARs). They can be categorized as PPARα, PPAR β/δ, and PPARγ. It was seen in studies that drugs that activate PPARγ can be used to inhibit ovarian cancer (Adachi et al., 2015; Nicol et al., 2004). Therefore, the repurposed drugs for ovarian cancer are also displayed in Table 5.2 (Kumar, 2003; Yokoyama and Ramakrishnan, 2007).

The current development in the class has decreased from the past decade. The reason is the development of antimicrobial resistance. The de novo discovery in antibiotics is a very long and time-consuming process. Therefore, drug repositioning has progressed in the field of antibiotics and become one of the major strategies for drug development. Recent studies on the drug bithionol, a drug for treating parasitic infections in horses, are being reused against methicillin-resistant *Staphylococcus aureus* (MRSA). This is a successful example of drug repurposing. The challenge is mainly the chances of relapse and drug resistance (Tande, 2014; Payne, 2007; Jackson, 2018). Table 5.3 displays the drugs repurposed as antimicrobial agents (Ayerbe-Algaba, 2018; Mazumdar, 2010; Foye, 2008; Silva, 2017; Alem, 2024)

Virus infections, such as influenza, due to their infectivity, have become a serious worldwide health problem. Researchers have successfully developed a number of antiviral drugs against viral proteins. Another infection is Zika virus (ZIKV) infection, which currently has no effective treatment. It is studied that ZIKV infection leads to increased caspase-3 activation, which eventually causes cell death.

Table 5.2 Drug repurposing examples with their drug class and repurposed indication in oncological diseases

Sno	*Drug*	*Drug Class*	*Repurposed Indication*
1	Chlorpromazine (CPZ)	Antipsychotic agent	Colorectal cancer (CRC)
2	Dehydroepiandrosterone (DHEA)	Over-the-counter dietary supplements	Colorectal cancer (CRC)
3	Orlistat	Treat obesity	Colorectal cancer (CRC)
4	Pantoprazole	Gastric protection	Colorectal cancer (CRC)
5	Dichloroacetate (DCA)	Treat brain cancer	Colorectal cancer (CRC)
6	Raloxifene	Decrease the risk of breast cancer	Colorectal cancer (CRC)
7	Itraconazole	Histoplasmosis; Blastomycosis; *Cryptococcal meningitis*	Colorectal cancer (CRC)
8	Tanshinone IIA	Treatment of coronary heart disease; angina and myocardial infarction	Colorectal cancer (CRC)
9	Fluspirilene	Chronic schizophrenia	Colorectal cancer (CRC)
10	Ciglitazone	Never used as a medication	Ovarian cancer
11	Clofibric acid	Regulate blood lipids	Ovarian cancer
12	Ritonavir	HIV infection	Ovarian cancer
13	Alendronate	Anti-osteoporotic drugs	Ovarian cancer
14	Lovastatin	Antidyslipidemic drugs	Ovarian cancer
15	Ivermectin	Antiparasitic agent	Ovarian cancer
16	Metformin	Diabetes	Ovarian cancer

Table 5.3 Drug repurposing examples and their repurposed indication

Sno	*Drug*	*Drug Class*	*Repurposed Indication*
1	Amlodipine	Cardiovascular	Antibacterial
2	Pentamidine	Antiprotozoal	Antibacterial
3	Sertraline	Antidepressant	Antifungal
4	Aspirin	NSAIDs	Methicillin-resistant *Staphylococcus aureus* (MRSA)
5	Flupentixol	Antipsychotics	Antibacterial
6	Thioridazine	Antipsychotics	Methicillin-resistant *Staphylococcus (S.) aureus*
7	Rapamycin (TOR)	Potent immunosuppressant	Antifungal; antineoplastic
8	Prochlorperazine	Antipsychotics	Antibacterial
9	Lacidipine	Cardiovascular drug	Gram-positive and Gram-negative
10	Nifedipine	Cardiovascular drug	Gram-positive and Gram-negative
11	Zidovudine	Antiretroviral drug	Synergistic effects with polymyxin
12	Tamoxifen	Breast cancer	Antifungal
13	Clioquinol	Antiseptic	Antifungal

Most of the active antiviral drugs were screened again against the ZIKV strain, and with the help of a drug repurposing strategy, many drugs were identified against the infection, e.g. Emricasan, the first caspase inhibitor, is used for protecting liver cells from excessive apoptosis in humans. Emricasan acts by reducing neuronal cell death and inhibiting the activity of caspase 3 and exerts its antiviral action. ZIKV has a similar set of action. The repurposing strategy uses the similar target, but repurposing for different diseases results in Emricasan for ZIKV (Phougat, 2017; Huang, 2014; Sanphui, 2015).

Another viral infection is the coronavirus SARS-CoV-2, a causative pathogen of COVID-19. It is a serious respiratory disease. There are no drugs to treat this viral infection. Therefore, drug repurposing is an effective approach for drug development against this infection. Remdesivir, a prodrug, is a nucleoside analogue and has antiviral activity and is responsible for inhibiting viral RNA polymerase. Other drugs are raltegravir, paritaprevir, bictegravir, and dolutegravir, which are repurposed for COVID-19 (Agostini, 2018; Indu, 2020).

2.7 Pharmaceutical Cocrystals and Nanoparticles for Drug Development

Cocrystals have gained importance in sustainable and green research due to their ability to improve drug delivery systems, mostly solubility and bioavailability. The production of these crystals requires renewable raw materials and greener solvents. The APIs have promising pharmacological properties, but their scope for improvement in physiological properties can be modified to cocrystals. Some compounds are weakly soluble, which can be overcome by formation of cocrystals (Chettri, 2024; Gadade, 2016). Pterostilbene: piperazine is a cocrystal whose solubility is modified, as piperazine has higher solubility properties. Other examples are theophylline: oxalic acid for stability; baicalein: nicotinamide for bioavailability; and hydrochlorothiazide: four aminobenzoic acids for permeability (Phougat, 2017; Trask, 2006; Daisy, 2012; Sanphui, 2015).

Green chemistry principles are emerging as a suitable tool for developing "nanoparticle". They have an increased surface area due to decreased particle size. Most of the particles are open to their environment and freely available for reactions; at the nanoscale, they have different physical and chemical properties. The most commercialized metal for nanoparticles is silver. They can be synthesized by chemically, physically, biologically and by using microorganisms. Silver nanoparticle synthesis using plant extracts is a green synthetic approach for SDD. Plant families such as Euphorbiaceae, Rutaceae, Poaceae, Myrtaceae, Solanaceae, and Asteraceae have an ability to synthesize silver nanoparticles. Euphorbiaceae family nanoparticles have promising antibacterial and insecticidal activities. Plant extract-based silver nanoparticles have a well-known antimicrobial activity (Duan, 2015; Phougat, 2017). The nanoparticle of aloe vera can be made by using metal, either silver or gold, Datura metal, Nelumbo nucifera (lotus) nanoparticle, uses silver. There are many examples of plants which have developed nanoparticles (Nadaf, 2022; Mittal, 2012; Shahiwala, 2025).

3 Conclusion

The path to sustainable drug discovery and development constitutes not only a scientific challenge but also an equal responsibility for protecting both human health and the environment. The pharmaceutical demand for drugs and drug development grows due to the growing global population. The ecological impact of drug synthesis, its use and disposal cannot be ignored. Therefore, we need to change the drug development strategies from traditional synthetic approaches to more innovative, eco-friendly approaches. These strategies led to prolonged safety and efficacy along with a sustainable environment. Sustainable approaches such as green synthesis, multicomponent reactions focusing on AE, drug repurposing, microwave-assisted synthesis, catalysis, biocatalysis, cocrystal engineering, and the use of nanoparticles have displayed promising results in reducing hazardous waste, optimizing renewable sources and minimizing energy consumption. Majorly, green chemistry and its approach towards sustainable development have led to more effective drug manufacturing and have reduced the environmental burden. Another strategy of drug repurposing has accelerated the drug discovery process but also has solved challenges faced by many diseases. The greener approaches for development of cocrystals and nanoparticles are opening new frontiers in drug formulation and delivery systems along with following the principle of sustainability.

These strategies are necessary for the pharmaceutical industry today and determine its future aspects of development and growth. By following these strategies, industry can deliver effective therapies that safeguard public health and reduce environmental burden.

Bibliography

Abera Tsedalu, A. (2021). A review on olefin metathesis reactions as a green method for the synthesis of organic compounds. *Journal of Chemistry*, 2021(1), 3590613.

Adachi, M., Banno, K., Yanokura, M., Iida, M., Nakamura, K., Nogami, Y., ... & Aoki, D. (2015). Risk-reducing surgery in hereditary gynecological cancer: Clinical applications in Lynch syndrome and hereditary breast and ovarian cancer. *Molecular and Clinical Oncology*, 3(2), 267–273.

Agostini, M. L. (2018). Coronavirus susceptibility to the antiviral remdesivir (GS-5734) is mediated by the viral polymerase and the proofreading exoribonuclease. *MBio*, 9(2), 10–1128.

Alem, M. A. (2024). Effects of aspirin and other nonsteroidal anti-inflammatory drugs on biofilms and planktonic cells of Candida albicans. *Antimicrobial Agents and Chemotherapy*, 48(1), 41–47.

An, C. S. (2022). Nanomaterials and nanotechnology for the delivery of agrochemicals: Strategies towards sustainable agriculture. *Journal of Nanobiotechnology*, 20(1), 11.

Arabi, M. O. (2021). Molecular imprinting: Green perspectives and strategies. *Advanced Materials*, 33(30), 2100543.

Ayerbe-Algaba, (2018). Synergistic activity of niclosamide in combination with colistin against colistin-susceptible and colistin-resistant Acinetobacter baumannii and Klebsiella pneumoniae. *Frontiers in Cellular and Infection Microbiology*, 8, 348.

Bandichhor, R. (2018). *Hazardous reagent substitution: A pharmaceutical perspective*. Green Chemistry Series, Vol. 52. Royal Society of Chemistry. London, United Kingdom.

Barrows, N. J.-L.-A.-B. (2016). A screen of FDA-approved drugs for inhibitors of Zika virus infection. *Cell Host & Microbe,* 20(2), 259–270.

Belew, S. S. (2021). Environmental risk assessment of the anthelmintic albendazole in Eastern Africa, based on a systematic review. *Environmental Pollution*, 269, 116106.

Bennett, D. B. (1991). Biodegradable polymeric prodrugs of naltrexone. *Journal of Controlled Release*, 16(1–2), 43–52.

Berdigaliyev, N. (2020). An overview of drug discovery and development. *Future Medicinal Chemistry*, 12(10), 939–947.

Bethune, S. J. (2011). Improving the poor aqueous solubility of nutraceutical compound pterostilbene through cocrystal formation. *Crystal Growth & Design*, 11(7), 2817–2823.

Block, T. (2019). Four misunderstandings about sustainability and transitions. In: K. Van Poeck, L. Östman, & J. Öhman (Eds.), *Sustainable Development Teaching: Ethical and Political Challenges* (pp. 15–27). Routledge, United Kingdom.

Cerone, M. U. (2019). Discovery of sustainable drugs for neglected tropical diseases: Cashew Nut Shell Liquid (CNSL)-based hybrids target mitochondrial function and ATP production in Trypanosoma brucei. *ChemMedChem*, 14(6), 621–635.

Chaachouay, N. (2024). Plant-derived natural products: A source for drug discovery and development. *Drugs and Drug Candidates*, 3(1), 184–207.

Chen, Y. W. (2020). Prediction of the SARS-CoV-2 (2019-nCoV) 3C-like protease (3CL pro) structure: Virtual screening reveals velpatasvir, ledipasvir, and other drug repurposing candidates. *F1000Research*, 9, 129.

Chettri, A. S. (2024). Pharmaceutical co-crystals: A green way to enhance drug stability and solubility for improved therapeutic efficacy. *Journal of Pharmacy and Pharmacology*, 76(1), 1–12.

Chung, M. C. (2008). Prodrugs for the treatment of neglected diseases. *Molecules*, 13(3), 616–677.

Cioc, R. C. (2014). Multicomponent reactions: Advanced tools for sustainable organic synthesis. *Green Chemistry*, 16(6), 2958–2975.

Daisy, P. (2012). Biochemical analysis of *Cassia fistula* aqueous extract and phytochemically synthesized gold nanoparticles as hypoglycemic treatment for diabetes mellitus. *International Journal of Nanomedicine*, **7**, 1189–1202.

Dhasmana, A. U. (2018). Scope of nanoparticles in environmental toxicant remediation. In: R. C. Sobti, N. K. Arora, & R. Kothari (Eds.), *Environmental Biotechnology: For Sustainable Future* (pp. 31–44). Springer Singapore, Singapore.

Domling, A. W. (2012). Chemistry and biology of multicomponent reactions. *Chemical Reviews*, 112(6), 3083–3135.

Drouin, E. (2017). The first report of Alzheimer's disease. *The Lancet Neurology*, 16(9), 687.

Duan, H. W. (2015). Green chemistry for nanoparticle synthesis. *Chemical Society Reviews*, 44(16), 5778–5792.

Erythropel, H. C. (2018). The Green ChemisTREE: 20 years after taking root with the 12 principles. *Green Chemistry*, 20(9), 1929–1961.

European Centre for Disease Prevention and Control (ECDC), E. F. (2021). Third joint interagency report on integrated analysis of consumption of antimicrobial agents and occurrence of antimicrobial resistance in bacteria from humans and food-producing animals in the EU/EEA: JIACRA III 2016-2018. *EFSA Journal*, 19(6), e06712.

Farha, M. A. (2019). Drug repurposing for antimicrobial discovery. *Nature Microbiology*, 4(4), 565–577.

Fortuin, L. L. (2020). Facile route to targeted, biodegradable polymeric prodrugs for the delivery of combination therapy for malaria. *ACS Biomaterials Science & Engineering*, 6(11), 6217–6227.

Foye, W. O. (2008). *Foye's Principles of Medicinal Chemistry*. Lippincott Williams & Wilkins, Philadelphia, PA.

France, S. P. (2023). The evolving nature of biocatalysis in pharmaceutical research and development. *ACS Au*, 3(3), 715–735.

Gadade, D. D. (2016). Pharmaceutical cocrystals: Regulatory and strategic aspects, design and development. *Advanced Pharmaceutical Bulletin*, 6(4), 479.

Gns, H. S. (2019). An update on drug repurposing: Re-written saga of the drug's fate. *Biomedicine & Pharmacotherapy*, 110, 700–716.

Hua, Y. D. (2022). Drug repositioning: Progress and challenges in drug discovery for various diseases. *European Journal of Medicinal Chemistry*, 234, 114239.

Huang, Y. Z. (2014). Baicalein–nicotinamide cocrystal with enhanced solubility, dissolution, and oral bioavailability. *Journal of Pharmaceutical Sciences*, 103(8), 2330–2337.

Indu, P. R.-D. (2020). Raltegravir, Indinavir, Tipranavir, Dolutegravir, and Etravirine against main protease and RNA-dependent RNA polymerase of SARS-CoV-2: A molecular docking and drug repurposing approach. *Journal of Infection and Public Health*, 13(12), 1856–1861.

Ippolito, M. (2021). *Selective activation of G Protein signaling through the β2AR via novel and redefined small molecule ligands*. Thomas Jefferson University, Philadelphia, PA.

Jackson, N. C. (2018). Discovery and development of new antibacterial drugs: Learning from experience? *Journal of Antimicrobial Chemotherapy*, 73(6), 1452–1459.

Kaitin, K. I. (2010). Deconstructing the drug development process: The new face of innovation. *Clinical Pharmacology & Therapeutics*, 87(3), 356–361.

Kavthe, R. D. (2022). An efficient and sustainable synthesis of the antimalarial drug tafenoquine. *ACS Sustainable Chemistry & Engineering*, 10(50), 16896–16902.

Kumar, K. A. (2003). Amlodipine: A cardiovascular drug with powerful antimicrobial property. *Acta Microbiologica Polonica*, 52(3), 285–292.

Lee, H. J. (2011). Biological synthesis of copper nanoparticles using plant extract. *Nanotechnology*, 1(1), 371–374.

Lungu, I. I. (2024). Insights into Catechin–copper complex structure and biologic activity modulation. *Molecules*, 29(20), 4969.

Martina, K. C. (2021). Impact of microwaves on organic synthesis and strategies toward flow processes and scaling up. *The Journal of Organic Chemistry*, 86(20), 13857–13872.

Martinengo, B. D. (2024). Harnessing the 12 green chemistry principles for sustainable antiparasitic drugs: Toward the One Health approach. *ACS Infectious Diseases*, 10(6), 1856–1870.

Mazumdar, K. K. (2010). Potential role of the cardiovascular non-antibiotic (helper compound) amlodipine in the treatment of microbial infections: Scope and hope for the future. *International Journal of Antimicrobial Agents*, 36(4), 295–302.

Mishra, M. S. (2021). Green synthesis interventions of pharmaceutical industries for sustainable development. *Current Research in Green and Sustainable Chemistry*, 4, 100174.

Mittal, A. K. (2012). Free radical scavenging and antioxidant activity of silver nanoparticles synthesized from flower extract of Rhododendron dauricum. *Nano Biomedicine & Engineering*, 4(3), 118–124.

Moermond, C. T. (2022). GREENER pharmaceuticals for more sustainable healthcare. *Environmental Science & Technology Letters*, 9(9), 699–705.

Moseley, J. D. (2011). A critical assessment of the greenness and energy efficiency of microwave-assisted organic synthesis. *Green Chemistry*, 13(4), 794–806.

Nadaf, S. J. (2022). Green synthesis of gold and silver nanoparticles: Updates on research, patents, and future prospects. *OpenNano*, 8, 100076.

Nicol, C. J., Yoon, M., Ward, J. M., Yamashita, M., Fukamachi, K., Peters, J. M., & Gonzalez, F. J. (2004). PPARγ influences susceptibility to DMBA-induced mammary, ovarian and skin carcinogenesis. *Carcinogenesis*, 25(9), 1747–1755.

Nosengo, N. (2016). Can you teach old drugs new tricks? *Nature*, 534, 314–316.

Novac, N. (2013). Challenges and opportunities of drug repositioning. *Trends in Pharmacological Sciences*, 34(5), 267–272.

Oprea, T. I. (2015). Computational and practical aspects of drug repositioning. *Drug Repurposing, Rescue, and Repositioning*, 1(1), 28–35.

Paul, P. E. (2019). Emerging trends in the industrial production of chemical products by microorganisms. *Recent Developments in Applied Microbiology and Biochemistry*, 1, 107–125.

Payne, D. J. (2007). Drugs for bad bugs: Confronting the challenges of antibacterial discovery. *Nature Reviews Drug Discovery*, 6(1), 29–40.

Peake, B. M. (2015). *The Life-Cycle of Pharmaceuticals in the Environment*. Elsevier, Amsterdam.

Phougat, N. K. (2017). Green chemistry approach towards nanoparticle synthesis. *Metabolic Engineering for Bioactive Compounds: Strategies and Processes,* 1, 249–268.

Prat, D. H. (2014). A survey of solvent selection guides. *Green Chemistry*, 16(10), 4546–4551.

Prince, M. W. (2015). *World Alzheimer report 2015. The global impact of dementia: an analysis of prevalence, incidence, cost and trends* (Doctoral dissertation, Alzheimer's Disease International).

Puhlmann, N. M. (2021). Towards the design of active pharmaceutical ingredients mineralizing readily in the environment. *Green Chemistry*, 23(14), 5006–5023.

Pushpakom, S. I. (2019). Drug repurposing: Progress, challenges and recommendations. *Nature Reviews Drug Discovery*, 18(1), 41–58.

Rabiee, N. B. (2020). Biosynthesis of copper oxide nanoparticles with potential biomedical applications. *International Journal of Nanomedicine*, 15, 3983–3999.

Raworth, K. (2018). *Doughnut economics: Seven ways to think like a 21st century economist.* Chelsea Green Publishing, White River Junction, VT.

Reilly, J. G. (2000). QTc-interval abnormalities and psychotropic drug therapy in psychiatric patients. *The Lancet*, 355(9209), 1048–1052.

Rittel, H. W. (1973). Dilemmas in a general theory of planning. *Policy Sciences*, 4(2), 155–169.

Sanphui, P. D. (2015). Cocrystals of hydrochlorothiazide: Solubility and diffusion/permeability enhancements through drug–coformer interactions. *Molecular Pharmaceutics*, 12(5), 1615–1622.

Sedlacek, M. G. (2007). Aspirin treatment is associated with a significantly decreased risk of Staphylococcus aureus bacteremia in hemodialysis patients with tunneled catheters. *American Journal of Kidney Diseases*, 49(3), 401–408.

Shahiwala, A. (2025). Advancing drug delivery research: Sustainable strategies for innovation and translation. *Drug Delivery and Translational Research*, 15(5), 1513–1524.

Sharma, S. D. (2020). A glimpse into green chemistry practices in the pharmaceutical industry. *ChemSusChem*, 13(11), 2859–2875.

Silva, R. A. (2017). In vitro anti-Candida activity of selective serotonin reuptake inhibitors against fluconazole-resistant strains and their activity against biofilm-forming isolates. *Microbial Pathogenesis*, 107, 341–348.

Sleigh, S. H. (2010). Repurposing strategies for therapeutics. *Pharmaceutical Medicine*, 24(3), 151–159.

Smale, E. M. (2021). Waste-minimising measures to achieve sustainable supply and use of medication. *Sustainable Chemistry and Pharmacy*, 20, 100400.

Stefanache, A. M. (2025). Green chemistry approaches in pharmaceutical synthesis: Sustainable methods for drug development. *AppliedChem*, 5(2), 13.

Steffen, W. R. (2015). Planetary boundaries: Guiding human development on a changing planet. *Science*, 347(6223), 1259855.

Swami, S. S. (2025). Recent advances in microwave-assisted synthesis of triazoles and their derivatives: A green approach toward sustainable development methods. *RSC Advances*, 15(4), 2361–2415.

Tande, A. J.-Q. (2014). Clinical characteristics and outcomes of prosthetic joint infection caused by small colony variant staphylococci. *MBio*, 10–1128.

Tang, H. H. (2016). Zika virus infects human cortical neural progenitors and attenuates their growth. *Cell Stem Cell*, 18(5), 587–590.

Thanacoody, H. K. (2007). Thioridazine: Resurrection as an antimicrobial agent? *British Journal of Clinical Pharmacology*, 64(5), 566–574.

Tobinick, E. L. (2009). The value of drug repositioning in the current pharmaceutical market. *Drug News & Perspectives*, 22(2), 119–125.

Trask, A. V. (2006). Physical stability enhancement of theophylline via cocrystallization. *International Journal of Pharmaceutics*, 320(1–2), 114–123.

Trost, B. M. (1991). The atom economy—A search for synthetic efficiency. *Science*, 254(5037), 1471–1477.

Turan, N. B. (2019). Preparation and spectroscopic studies of Fe (II), Ru (II), Pd (II) and Zn (II) complexes of Schiff base containing terephthalaldehyde and their transfer hydrogenation and Suzuki-Miyaura coupling reaction. *Open Chemistry*, 17(1), 571–580.

Van der Gronde, T. (2018). Assessing pharmaceutical research and development costs. *AMA Internal Medicine*, 178(4), 587–588.

Wynendaele, E. F. (2021). Sustainability in drug discovery. *Medicine in Drug Discovery*, 12, 100107.

Xiang, J. L. (2014). Bimetallic Pd-Ni core-shell nanoparticles as effective catalysts for the Suzuki reaction. *Nano Research*, 7(9), 1337–1343.

Xue, H. L. (2018). Review of drug repositioning approaches and resources. *International Journal of Biological Sciences*, 14(10), 1232.

Yokoyama, Y., & Ramakrishnan, S. (2007). Binding of endostatin to human ovarian cancer cells inhibits cell attachment. *International Journal of Cancer*, 121(11), 2402–2409.

Zhai, B. W. (2012). The antidepressant sertraline provides a promising therapeutic option for neurotropic cryptococcal infections. *Antimicrobial Agents and Chemotherapy*, 56(7), 3758–3766.

6 Innovations Driving Sustainable Development in Pharmaceutical Research for Educational Purposes

Hurmat and Akriti Singh

1 Introduction

In order to eradicate poverty and inequality, achieve world peace and prosperity, and make the planet a safer place for all living things by 2030, the United Nations adopted the concept of sustainable development objectives, or SDGs, in 2015 (Agrawal et al., 2024). Legislators, consumers, and communities have been drawing more and more awareness to the pharmaceutical industry's sustainability in progressive years. Consciousness on this topic has risen due to concerns about combining principles of sustainability into the formation of novel delivery systems, products that are environmentally friendly, greener manufacturing techniques, recycling of waste, water conservation, and packaging that is reused. The necessity to keep costs under control and preserve social, economic, and environmental sustainability has made management in the pharmaceutical industry more difficult. This has led to the development of an economic logic for managing sustainability challenges (Milanesi et al., 2020).

1.1 Importance of Innovation in Achieving Sustainability

Creative research is an elementary examination of change processes, advancement of knowledge, and knowledge emancipation for the intent of creating new combinations. Every innovative idea illustrates conventional knowledge, merged in new ways. In general, innovation should be viewed as an ongoing, progressive process rather than as a singular occurrence. Sustainability and innovation go hand in hand since innovation is a fundamental skill for sustainable businesses (Shin et al., 2018). The therapeutic effect of pharmaceuticals is crucial when it pertains to health and well-being. Under Corporate Social Responsibility (CSR), a number of healthcare companies are leading the fight for sustainability while documenting their sustainability efforts in relation to the 17 Sustainable Development Goals (SDGs). Concerned about the anticipated implications of possible negative influence on the environment, both on land and in water, the pharmaceutical sector is putting more emphasis on sustainability due to legal mandates and ecological responsibility. The goal of sustainable pharma is to operate the pharmaceutical sector in a way that strikes a balance between conservation of the environment,

DOI: 10.4324/9781003640486-6

social consciousness, and economic expansion. A multifaceted strategy incorporating environmental, social, and economic elements is fundamentally needed to establish flexible, ethical, and environmentally responsible pharmaceutical companies. The current approach is admirable, and the need for sustainable pharma is real. The industry may lessen its negative effects on the environment and promote equitable treatment and global wellness by using environmentally friendly procedures. Although the path to sustainable pharmaceuticals is difficult and calls for cooperation along the whole value chain, the advantages for the industry, society, and environment are significant and wide-ranging (Agrawal et al., 2024).

1.2 Background

1.2.1 The Triple Bottom Line: People, Planet, Profit

In order to solve the sustainability issue, triple bottom line (TBL) was provided by researchers that consists of the planet, people, and profits. Following the European Union's release of the Electronic Equipment Declaration and Waste Electrical and the Restriction of Hazardous Substances Directive in 2003, there was a minor increase in the quantity of articles published on this topic. However, because the idea was still in its beginning stages, the TBL's components were not sufficiently explicit to address sustainability, even with increasing numbers of articles. A fundamentally dynamic and multifaceted idea is involved in optimizing the TBL toward sustainability (Tseng et al., 2020). The real-life execution of TBL in the medical industry acknowledges a more comprehensive set of obligations than simply generating money for stakeholders. The introduction of TBL in healthcare, which is frequently encouraged by governments, relies on the significance of shifting toward a more sustainable approach for medical care delivery, one that raises the degree of interdependence between these three triple bottom line pillars. Every proposal highlights the so-called triple-win structure, which holds that national and international socioeconomic objectives can only be achieved when they balance those linked to environmental sustainability. Because health services function at the junction of social well-being, financial stability, and ecological impact, the TBL is essential to current healthcare and has risen in popularity (Alim and Sulley, 2024).

1.2.2 Global Sustainable Development Goals and Their Relevance

The United Nations (UN) High-Level Political Forum for Sustainable Development (HLPF) devised a series of 17 interconnected goals named the SDGs, or Global Goals, in 2015 with the intention of achieving a world that is prosperous and secure both today and in the future (Sharma et al., 2024). As a roadmap for prosperity, the environment, and people, the 2030 Agenda for Sustainable Development was adopted by all UN member states in 2015. The 17 SDGs that make up this ambitious agenda collaboratively tackle important global issues, from eliminating hunger and poverty to advancing environmental sustainability, health, and education (Martinengo et al., 2025).

1.2.3 Principles of Green Chemistry

The application of a set of guidelines that lessen the production of chemical hazards throughout the design, production, and usage of chemical substances is known as the "green chemistry approach." This approach improves the atomic economy and energy usage of the synthetic process while also drastically reducing environmental contamination through the use of safe solvents, catalysts, and suitable reaction conditions (Banik et al., 2021). A fresh chapter in the long tradition of chemistry is now in progress with the rise of "green" chemistry, a freshly integrated scientific route. To generate "green" chemistry, synthetic organic chemistry is combined with toxicology, analytical chemistry, physical chemistry, microbiology, biotechnology, and engineering. The goal of "green" chemistry is to develop methods for more efficient chemical processes. "Green" chemistry encompasses all forms and aspects of chemical processes and aims to minimize pollution from the initial stages of their design and execution in order to lessen environmental concerns. There are two main types of problems that are covered by "green" chemistry. The first is about the use and handling of chemical industry byproducts and trash that poses a risk to the environment. The creation of innovative industrial methods to lower or eradicate the production and utilization of hazardous items is the second and more promising. "Green" chemistry makes it possible to acquire the required material in the most secure manner. Along with emphasizing environmentally friendly industrial processes and holding scientists and manufacturers accountable for the final products, it also provides raw material and process scheme selection that generally avoids the use of dangerous chemicals and other contaminants (Srivastav et al., 2023). In their 1998 book "Green Chemistry: Theory and Practice," Paul Anastas and John Warner developed 12 "green" chemistry concepts. They advise government representatives, entrepreneurs, and scientists to focus their efforts on minimizing or getting rid of the usage of lethal substances and materials. Because of their versatility, precision, and significance, these 12 principles have greatly aided in the development and growth of an innovative philosophy. The guiding principles are as follows: the design of safe chemicals and goods (chemicals that are effective but non-toxic); the creation of less hazardous chemical syntheses (producing and using compounds with little or zero toxicity); the use of safe solvents and reactions (use the safest solvents and additional chemicals if needed and minimize or avoid using them); the maximum growth of components like "atom economy" (synthesis design that optimizes the raw materials ratio in the final product with little or no amount of waste); avoidance of waste (chemical synthesis design that mitigates waste rather than disposal or exploitation); and the identification and reduction of the adverse consequences of energy utilization in chemical synthesis in order to boost energy efficiency. Utilizing sustainable raw materials derived from agricultural waste or products; refraining from chemical derivatives (if at all possible, lowering or doing away with the use of blocking or safeguarding groups or any short-term changes); initiating chemical reactions at room temperature and pressure, if at all possible; using non-stoichiometric catalysts (which reduce waste by using catalytic reactions and relatively small quantities of effective catalysts to

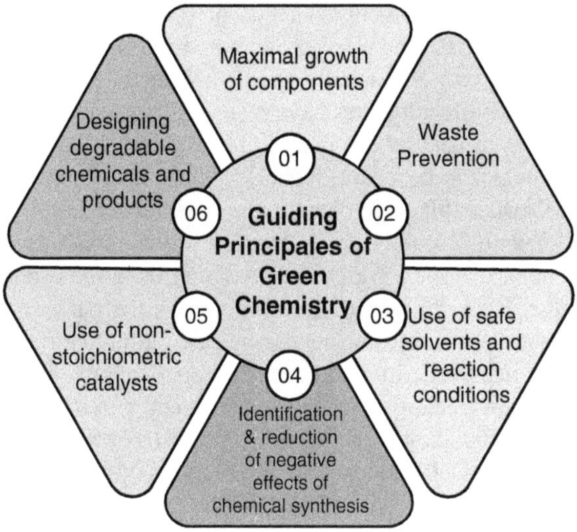

Figure 6.1 Guiding principles of green chemistry.

promote the reaction repeatedly); creating non-persistent chemicals and products (which break down into safe substances); monitoring pollution in real time (by eliminating or limiting byproducts by interfering with the synthesis process); and lowering the risk of accidents (like releases, explosions, and fires) by creating safer chemicals and their physical forms (liquid, solid, or gaseous) (Soltys et al., 2021). These guiding principles are represented in Figure 6.1.

1.2.4 Biocatalysis and Enzyme-Based Synthesis

Over millions of years, enzymes—often recognized as the vital catalysts of life—have developed the ability to precisely coordinate chemical reactions inside living things. Enzymes are excellent candidates for therapeutic uses due to their innate specificity and affinity for mild reaction conditions. In addition to improving reaction selectivity, using enzymes in drug research and synthesis helps pharmaceutical processes adhere to green chemistry principles and reduce their environmental impact. Pharmaceutical enzyme biocatalysis is no longer just a theoretical concept; it has developed into a useful, advantageous reality with apparent advantages. The catalytic power of enzymes has been used by scientists worldwide to carry out a wide variety of transformations, including the manufacture of sophisticated biological therapies and small-molecule drugs.

Enzymes like lipases and hydrolases, for instance, have been essential in maximizing the manufacturing of enantiopure chiral intermediates, a difficult task that is regularly faced in pharmaceutical chemistry. This development emphasizes how important enzyme biocatalysis is to contemporary pharmaceutical research and production. Enzyme biocatalysis, the most cutting-edge field that could drastically change our comprehension of chemical reactions and synthetic processes, is situated at the nexus of biology and chemistry. Fundamentally, this revolutionary subject uses the amazing catalytic capabilities of enzymes, which are biological macromolecules that have been refined over millions of years by evolution to serve as molecular machinery in living things. Enzyme biocatalysis is a reliable and ecologically conscious technology that easily conforms to the values and standards of sustainable development and green chemistry. In the pharmaceutical industry, enzyme biocatalysis has become a game-changer due to its many extremely beneficial qualities, which are revolutionizing the production and drug discovery process. Researchers can greatly improve the purity and effectiveness of medications and therapeutic substances by fine-tuning their synthesis with the help of enzyme biocatalysis. In pharmaceutical applications, enzyme biocatalysis has special benefits, especially in terms of efficiency and affordability. Enzymes exhibit remarkable efficiency and quick catalytic activity while using less energy than conventional chemical catalysts. In addition to saving energy, their ability to trigger reactions at low temperatures improves safety by reducing the possibility of high-temperature reactions. In the pharmaceutical production industry, this quick and energy-efficient feature results in significant cost reductions, confirming the enzyme biocatalysis's economic feasibility. Complex processes can be catalyzed by enzymes in just one stage, which minimizes the need for extra reagents and the number of reaction stages. Enzyme biocatalysis is a financially feasible option for pharmaceutical manufacture because of its efficiency, which results in shorter production periods and lower prices. In conclusion, a number of beneficial characteristics of enzyme biocatalysis in medicines have made it a leader in medication development and manufacturing (Kim et al., 2024).

1.3 Solvent Reduction and Waste Minimization Techniques

Given their vast bulk, complexity, and dangerous nature, pharmaceutical wastes are extremely difficult to dispose effectively. Pharmaceutical wastes include volatile organic compounds (VOCs), which pose a risk to the biosphere and pharmaceutically active compounds (PhACs), such as surfactants, antibiotics, hormones, drug residues, and toxic substances, with higher chemical oxygen demand (COD) and biological oxygen demand (BOD). Hence, the scientific community faces a significant difficulty in effectively managing and disposing of these wastes, particularly due to the existence of chemical residues in the discharge of traditional wastewater treatment facilities. The phrase "pharmaceutical wastewater" primarily describes the wastes and effluents produced during the production of medications. Nonetheless, there is a startling prevalence of improper disposal of unwanted medications in homes and institutions. The fact that pharmaceutical wastewater is constantly changing due to the vast differences in raw material composition between product classes is a major issue that arises often. To get around the strict pollution control standards, many pharmaceutical corporations pretend that their composition is private. As a result, they keep releasing pharmaceutical wastes into the environment without fully disclosing the extent and type of the hazardous materials. The issue is exacerbated by the frequently irrational mixing of hospital waste, home sewage, and industrial effluents in public wastewater treatment facilities. Mixing pharmaceutical wastewater with sewage water or even waste streams released from various unit operations is another improper method of treating pharmaceutical wastewater. Such a combination produces extremely complicated wastewater that is challenging to properly administer and treat. Attempts to separate the recovery-related components result in a significant rise in the overall treatment cost. Individual treatment approaches become unsuccessful, but they also bring with them new wastewater kinds and unidentified issues whose treatment and disposal methods remain mainly unaddressed. In light of this perplexing circumstance, it is imperative to review current treatment technologies and common pharmaceutical wastewater handling procedures in order to provide specific recommendations for formulating the best plans and guiding research to create sustainable technologies. The utilization of microorganisms to break down pharmaceutical waste and transform it into either safe or useful forms has been the subject of a significant portion of research. Composting, aerobic and anaerobic techniques, vermicomposting, and their combination are among the recommended processes; some of these produced useful byproducts. Such hybrid waste mixtures can be handled by biological methods such as built wastelands or activated sludge operations. In order to assess the removal effectiveness of the created wasteland of the particular recovered PhACs, pharmaceuticals found in household wastewater were separated using an activated sludge configuration and then processed separately in a horizontally subsurface flow bed. The zero-discharge method is always the best course of action when it comes to trash management. The idea is to make the procedure environmentally friendly in order to avoid producing any waste. Even though it is very difficult to achieve zero discharge in practice, manufacturing procedures can be made as environmentally friendly as possible, which will result in negligible waste formation.

The green chemistry approach, often known as the green pharmacy approach. This idea involves keeping an eye on a product's whole life cycle and making it as safe as feasible. The production methods have been selected in a way that allows for a relatively short process time, minimal energy and material consumption, minimal production of unwanted byproducts, and even easy biodegradation of the byproducts. Every step of the manufacturing process is ecologically beneficial thanks to this technique. Many studies on the treatment of pharmaceutical waste have been conducted over the years, but the majority of them have concentrated on lab-scale processes employing artificial solutions, just escalating the lack of scale-up confidence in techno-economic feasibility assessments. A revolutionary change in this waste control strategy is required because the issue continues and is made worse by growing populations, rising pharmaceutical production, and the corresponding release of hazardous waste from manufacturing facilities. The most environmentally friendly solution seems to be the utilization of green chemistry in pharmaceutical manufacturing and the biological conversion of waste pharmaceutical materials into innocuous products. The optimal choice of technology will be determined by its efficiency, social acceptance, long-term environmental desirability, and economic feasibility. There is no doubt that research efforts to create new treatment plans will continue (Pal, 2018). Solvents and solutions are used in many aspects of daily life, from painting to applying a soluble painkiller for a headache, from making coffee (and putting sweetener and then rinsing the cup) to cleaning one's hair while taking a shower, from applying and removing nail polish to cleaning an apple under the faucet before eating it. However, what is the answer? What are a solute and a solvent? What distinguishes a suspension, gel, slurry, dispersion, and solution from one another? The necessity to balance solvents' utility with minimizing their negative effects is underscored by the environmental and other repercussions that result from their widespread use. Avoidance (establishing "solvent-free" processes or totally removing the source of a solvent release), reduction (using solvent reduction, reuse, recovery, and recycling), and secure disposal (converting to less toxic substances or annihilating completely (with recuperating energy, if appropriate)) are the three main goals of implementing the waste reduction order for the use of solvents (and additional byproducts) in the manufacturing process of chemicals. Research is still being done on each of these topics. However, it should be noted that products using solvents typically release volatile ingredients either during or after usage. Many of these products, especially those intended for home use, are widely used, making containment or recovery extremely challenging, if not impossible. Mitigation strategies are thus not the same as those applied in the manufacture of chemicals; they are rather more dependent on the replacement of solvents or reduction of their usage. Minimization of the effects of the solvents may be achieved through the prevention of emissions and through the substitution of problematic solvents. Absolute prohibition, either of emissions or solvents, generally needs radical re adaptations in reaction engineering and process technology. Substitutes for the solvents that are currently in use may be realized by (i) repurposing available materials or (ii) the identification of some entirely novel materials. Industry tends to make routes, (i) but academia and industry are both at work developing methods that make efficient and effective the exploration process in seeking alternatives to industrial solvents. Route (ii) is not universally but generally the one followed in the academic area, and it is often funded by industry or done with industry collaboration. The need to reduce the emissions of detrimental or potentially detrimental chemicals should at present be augmented by the demands of sustainability. The result of this is that a significant effort has become established within the industry and academia to look to the potential new solvents available that involve more renewable feedstock, in some cases the use of biomass, and the process technology that can be used in making such new solvents. The fact that solvents are subject to a wide variety of tasks is to be considered when selecting a solvent in a given set of conditions; in most cases this decision is rather complicated. The selection of solvent is never a compromise that is dictated by the peculiarities of its use. Technical, relevant physicochemical, cost, availability on scale, regulatory, sustainability, and safety should be optimized and balanced. Green chemistry is now preoccupied with solvents since the late 1990s. Besides the research on so-called solvent-free processes, with green chemistry emerged the concept of the green solvent, which is mainly used to conduct chemical reactions or chemical processing. A large body of literature emerged about the revelation and application of alleged green solvents. This is more likely to be preferable now to speak in respect of a sustainable solvent as opposed to a new or green solvent, i.e., one to which or in which an evaluation, ideally by life cycle evaluation methodology, has been made of the consequences (economic, toxicological, resource depletion, environmental, and ecotoxicological) of the production chain of that drug (right down its primary feedstock), not to mention formulation and use and disposal or ultimate fate (Winterton, 2021).

2 Sustainable Drug Discovery and Development

Sustainable development can be defined as progress that aims at satisfying the needs of the current generation without interfering with the powers of succeeding generations to satisfy their needs as well. Comparing SDGs and the One Health approach are similar initiatives. Different novel approaches toward ensuring that drug discovery becomes sustainable include in silico screening, pathway matching, and molecular docking, signature mapping, retrospective analysis of clinical data, genetic association, high-throughput screening, drug repurposing, and so forth. Among the many alternatives that may be adopted in drug repositioning, injecting sustainability in drug discovery and development, or using its substitute nomenclature of drug repurposing, drug re-profiling, or drug re-tasking, is the approach of choice since the benefits are much more than ever perceived in trying to sell a drug in a new medical indication, which, in all other cases, is totally different from the drug's originally intended use (Bhar, 2023).

2.1 AI and Machine Learning in Efficient Molecule Screening

Pharmaceutical companies and chemical scientists have an interest in such a research area as drug designing and development. Indeed, off-target delivery, low efficacy, high cost, and time cost come as a challenge as well as a hurdle, and this affects the drug design and drug discovery. Machine learning technology and artificial intelligence have a vital role in drug discovery and drug development. That is, the deep learning algorithms and artificial neural networks have updated the field. Examples of usage of deep learning algorithms and machine learning in various processes of drug discovery include ligand-based virtual screening, quantitative structure–activity relationships, structure-based virtual screening, peptide synthesis, drug monitoring and release, pharmacophore modeling, and toxicity prediction. The fact that it can be proved based on the former results enhances the use of artificial intelligence and deep learning in this sphere. Labor-intensive and hopeless efforts in the drug discovery and drug development process involve the process of searching for pertinent and bioactive drug molecules that exist in the chemical space so large that it consists of 1,060 molecules. Moreover, drug discovery and drug development are said to be a tedious process taking time and money. The worst of all is the fact that in most of the cases, nine of every ten drug molecules do not clear the stage two clinical trials and further regulatory acceptance tests. The mentioned constraints of drug discovery and drug development can be prevented through adopting AI-based methodologies as well as technologies. AI has been used in every stage of the drug development process, including designing small molecules, determining the dosage and effectiveness of drugs, predicting bioactive agents, protein–protein interactions, identifying protein folding and misfolding, and using structure- and ligand-based virtual screening (VS), modeling quantitative structure–activity relationships (QSARs), repurposing drugs, predicting toxicity and bioactive properties, and determining the mode of action of drug compounds, all of which are described below. With recent developments, the biggest issue that the pharmaceutical industry faces in making a new drug is the high cost and low efficiency of the drug. Nonetheless, machine learning methodologies and the new advances in the field of DL have the fantastic potential to decrease this expenditure, embark on a more productive agenda, and rescue time in the drug discovery and development process. With recent developments, the biggest issue that the pharmaceutical industry faces in making a new drug is the development of a high-cost, lower-efficiency drug. Nevertheless, ML methods and recent advances in DL are associated with enormous potential to lower this expense and hike efficiency and time savings in the drug discovery and drug development process (Gupta et al., 2021).

2.2 In Silico Modeling and Virtual Trials

Depending on the activities that are under management in the wet lab, chemistry may be carried out on the computer and at the wet lab. There are three broad experiment categories, namely in vitro, in vivo, and in silico experiments. The in silico studies refer to the studies carried out on a computer or on computer simulations. These studies regard past tried results of activities so as to predict some activity by using a computer. Experimentation on a computer is dubbed in silico. Over and above 20 years in the scientific community, in silico studies are being practiced (Tessema et al., 2025).

2.3 Repurposing Existing Drugs for New Indications

Drug repositioning/reprofiling/redirecting, also known as drug repurposing, is the investigation of the drug molecules regardless of their clinically approved indication to obtain the therapeutic potential in other diseases/conditions than which the drug is meant to treat. Drug repurposing is built out of two other conceptions of polypharmacology, i.e., the potential of a drug molecule to hit more than one target and produce both desired and undesired effects, and the presence of shared or related molecular routes/genetic factors in various illnesses. Through drug repurposing, the bottleneck impediments experienced in the case of conventional de novo drug development procedures can be constructively evaded in terms of timing, expenses, and resources used. Nonetheless, the achievement of drug repurposing programs is not too encouraging. By carefully analyzing a few of the unsuccessful cases of repurposing, we wanted to determine the major influential elements that result in a high attrition rate in such research consultations. Our four foundational pillars consist of: a thorough understanding of the pharmacological characteristics of the repurposed drug (pillar 1: drug pharmacology), considerations for formulating the drug for new uses (pillar 2: drug formulation), evaluation in relevant biological assays with translational potential (pillar 3: assessment in biological assays), and strong clinical trial methodologies, including a biomarker-driven approach, to provide definitive evidence of the drug's efficacy in new indications (pillar 4: clinical evaluation). These pillars are rooted in essential elements of knowledge and assessment. Drug repositioning offers several advantages over a fresh drug development and drug discovery process, specifically a cost-effective drug development process that reduces development risks because the compound's safety, a key factor contributing to high destruction rates in the process of drug development, is already well objectified (Mittal and Mittal, 2021).

3 Role of AI-Based Tools to Ensure Sustainable Development in Pharmaceutical Research

The pharma field is rapidly growing by using a number of smart techniques and different AI-based tools to enhance the efficiency of the pharmaceutical research field. Moreover, these tools are helpful to maintain sustainable education by making education extra interactive, aligned with environmental demands, data-driven, and usable for real-world applications. Different innovative tools, including GraphPad Prism, BioRender, DOE, WinPharm, and molecular docking, are playing a crucial role in making pharmaceutical studies more innovative. These tools are valuable and acknowledged owing to a plethora of significance or applications, as shown in Figure 6.2. To be more precise about the innovative features of BioRender, it is

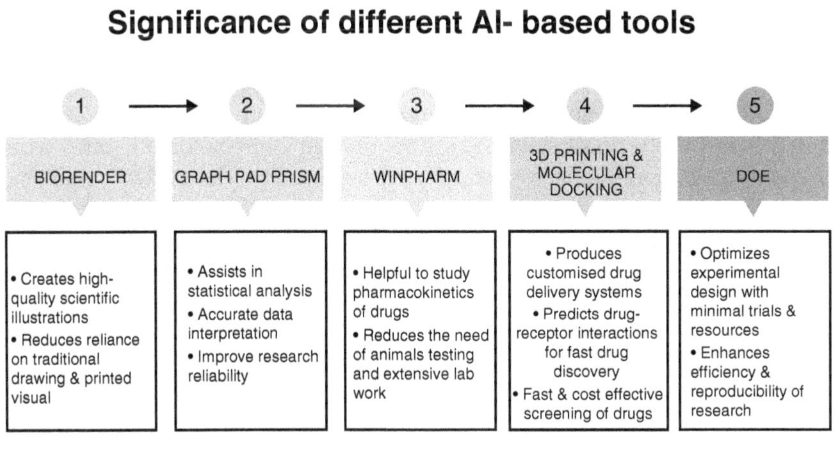

Figure 6.2 Significance and applications of different AI-based tools.

reported that it is the latest and unique tool to enhance the publication visuals and quality of research papers or reports. If we talk about its value in sustainability, then it is accurate to say that BioRender has the ability to replace the traditional handmade or pen-and-paper-based figures with editable and paper-free diagrams. It is able to enhance the clarity and beauty of images as well as be helpful to make complex cycles, reactions, and processes easier and clearer. It also decreases the cost of printing; therefore, BioRender is an eco-friendly tool in pharmaceutical research.

Apart from BioRender, different other AI-based tools are utilized frequently in the pharma field to achieve precision in drug delivery systems. These tools are helpful to achieve an accurate dose at the desired receptor site to achieve an essential therapeutic effect. Moreover, these tools are helpful to prevent drug toxicity as well as facilitate drug safety. In the educational sector, students learn about dose calculation and personalized treatment and dose calculation with the help of this tool. It is also a sustainable approach toward patient care.

Furthermore, the most significant advanced technology that is enabling pharma research to meet the current demand of the healthcare sector is nanotechnology. Nanotechnology is the most important field nowadays, and it is a powerful tool, especially in combination with AI. On the basis of AI-generated data, results analysis, or evaluations, different nanoformulations can be prepared with better efficacy and safety. These nanoformulations have excellent bioavailability. AI is helpful to maintain uniformity and sustainability in nanoformulations too. WinPharm is an important advanced instrument used to study pharmacokinetic parameters of drugs, i.e., drug absorption, distribution, and excretion without using animals. It is an AI-based study of drug absorption that replaces the human trials as well as in vivo studies. It is a cost-effective, fast, and cruelty-free method to study the efficacy of drugs. DOE (Design of Experiments) is a statistical technique, in combination with AI, employed to analyze experimental data and to design scientific studies in pharmaceutical research. This is a planned and systemic technique used by scientists to prevent or minimize footprints in laboratories. Molecular docking and 3D printing are also an integral tool used to enhance the quality of research. 3D printing is helpful to create realistic models of different organs and to minimize animal requirements for different drug-oriented studies. It facilitates resource sustainability. Molecular docking is a virtual and digital platform used to create new or novel drug compounds without wastage of chemicals. Therefore, it is also an environmentally friendly AI-based smart tool used to create relationships of receptors and binders. These techniques are paper-free, clutter-free, eco-friendly, and sustainable methods. Similarly, GraphPad Prism is another AI-based software useful for statistical analysis of obtained results to ensure research sustainability and quality. It is a digital platform to obtain fast, accurate interpretations of results that ultimately boost pharmaceutical research and development. Regenerative medicines and robotic surgeries are also AI-based unique sectors of the health sector that enhance the quality and sustainability of human beings.

3.1 Biologics and Biosimilars in Sustainable Healthcare

A biosimilar is essentially a biological medication that has been shown to be very similar to an original medication, with no meaningful differences in quality, safety, or effectiveness. When biologics are made from living things, they undergo a number of biological and natural changes. The first European biosimilar approval came in 2006, and the very first regulatory pathway for biosimilars to be launched was established in Europe in 2005. The European Medicines Agency approved 94 biosimilars as of June 2023. As biologics in novel therapeutic areas get closer to patent expiration, the biosimilar pipeline in various nations will keep changing. Understanding how policies might enhance the sustainability of biosimilar marketplaces is crucial for a number of reasons. First, different nations have different rates of biosimilar adoption. By 2021, biosimilars will account for 10% of Europe's biologic pool, with 7% of that share coming in the previous five years (Alnaqbi et al., 2023). Biological medicines are larger and more complex in structure than small-molecule drugs. Currently, biological medicines can be grouped into three main categories:

a Products that are closely related to natural body factors and are often used as substitution therapies.
b Monoclonal antibodies (mAbs) that target specific soluble or cell surface proteins, disrupting cell signaling pathways and their responses.
c Engineered proteins that act like soluble receptors, receptor antagonists, or fusion proteins.

To be more specific, biological medicines come in various forms, including hormones like insulin and growth hormones for hormone deficiencies, mAbs for treating autoimmune diseases and cancer, blood products for individuals with hemophilia, immunomodulators like interferon beta for managing multiple sclerosis, enzymes for dissolving blood clots, and vaccines for preventing certain diseases. The characteristics of biological medicines, which include biosimilars, have been branded complex and highly heterogeneous. It is thus realized that these products may contain certain differences between reference products (RPs) and biosimilars. However, any small differences between the reference product and the biosimilar are unlikely to have significant impacts on the quality and safety of the biosimilar, thanks to the rigorous processes they undergo before receiving approval. Biosimilars actually undergo massive comparability exercises to show high similitude to the reference product in relation to efficacy, safety, and quality. This will include the chemical, biological, and physical compositions of the product and their clinical trials for safety and effectiveness in human beings. The increasing divergence and complexity of the biosimilar market create new strategic opportunities for innovation and growth in the pharmaceutical industry. At the same time, biosimilars have a more direct and greater impact on healthcare system sustainability while also promoting population health (Mascarenhas-Melo et al., 2024). Utilization of biosimilars, ratified by the US Food and Drug Administration as highly similar to their predecessor biologics, can transform the healthcare environment in the biologic sector by saving a significant amount of dollars for both payors and patients. With the biosimilar launch, there is an emergence of the question of how organizations are going to transition patients off originator biologics and switch to biosimilars. Although it is possible to find in the publications the results of patients when switching biologic originators to biosimilars, there is a lack of publications regarding the mechanism by which healthcare systems have made this transition and switched patients on biosimilars (Bhardwaj et al., 2022).

3.2 Innovations in Vaccine Development

Immunization is one of the traditional pillars of community healthcare, offering a lot to both the prevention and management of infections. The conventional means of developing a vaccine like an inactivated or weakened pathogen have been instrumental in defining the impending immunization pattern. But the changing adversity of emerging infectious diseases, the necessity of quick reactions to pandemics, and developments of biotechnology have embraced the requirements of next-generation platforms. It then examines the paradigm shift into innovative methods such as the mRNA vaccines, viral vector vaccines, and nanoparticle technologies. Nanoparticles serve as yet another branch of vaccine development, which has with it several distinct delivery and targeting benefits. Looking forward to the future of vaccine production, imagine how to foresee and fully utilize the trends of the increasing scientific and technological capabilities as applied to prepare and respond to the threat of the emerging infectious diseases at a worldwide level. In the field of vaccine development, the revolution is imminent because researchers and scientists are taking a stride toward the emergent infectious diseases. Over the past few years, the world has been faced with several emerging novel pathogens causing a real challenge to the global healthcare fraternity. This has seen renewed efforts in the production of state-of-the-art vaccines not only to counter the present menace but also to predict and contain future pandemics. To develop effective drugs and vaccines with new designs, it is necessary to understand the target biology as well as have the relevant tools and technologies needed to achieve the intended outcome (Prigodich et al., 2021). Vaccines have given a big contribution to the prevention of infectious diseases since the 18th century, the first known example being the preventive method of Edward Jenner, who used to process the cowpox vaccine against smallpox in 1796. Vaccines have efficacy in that they trigger certain immune responses to effectively eliminate the spread of various communicable diseases, and they conserve the well-being of both an individual and a population group. Nevertheless, traditional vaccine technologies are associated with some challenges, including reverting to virulence and long production processes. New vaccine technologies, such as mRNA, DNA, nanoparticle, and mosaic, have emerged within the past years through rapid development of biotechnology. Such experimental technologies should increase the safety and effectiveness of vaccines and reduce the development times. Such cutting-edge technologies do not only demonstrate significant potential to both increase the safety and efficiency of vaccines but also speed up both the development and production processes as well as offer new ways of dealing with emerging infectious diseases in the future. Designing and formulating novel vaccines is critical in addressing the drawback of previous vaccines and improving our capacity to deal with the infectious diseases that emerge in the future. Although traditional vaccines are effective to a certain degree, they normally face problems of unwarranted immune response, reversion into the virulent state, and time-consuming development. These issues motivate scientists to discover and come up with new vaccine technologies. There have been new vaccine technologies that are unique in their advantages; these technologies emerged in recent years. As an example, mRNA vaccines proved their quick creation and response ability in connection to the COVID-19 pandemic. Stable vaccines: stable and durable immune responses are present with DNA vaccines, making them more prominent. Mosaic vaccines are designed to give general and multi-strain protection against different strains of a pathogen, whereas personalized vaccines adapt immune response by taking into consideration individual genetic factors, giving more effective protection. It is in the process of possible prevention and control of the infectious diseases that these new vaccine technologies promise a large step forward (Dou, 2024; Hoodbhoy, 2024).

3.3 Continuous Manufacturing Technologies

The pharmaceutical market has changed by a tremendous extent over the last ten years due to a number of rather diverse reasons and ever-growing pressure. Among these changes is a continuous process being applied in the production of new therapies that are still under development. Continuous manufacturing in the pharmaceutical industry is not something new in the industry, but what is different about its application currently is compared to the past times. The high-volume products were the motivation to use continuous processing in earlier times, and it is quite the same factor as continuous processing use in the commodity chemicals industry (Burcham et al., 2018). A longstanding limit on innovation in the pharmaceutical industry has restricted such efforts to the research and development of new active compounds; to this day no change has occurred to the structure of the production, which to a large degree relied upon the use of batchwise technologies. As it has already been shown in a number of other industrial sectors, continuous manufacturing (CM) is far more beneficial than batches. The production thus can be made at higher speed, lesser cost, and with adaptability much easier and with so much flexibility of quality management. During the past years, the core regulatory agencies realized the necessity to implement a change in the production of drugs and began to support and advertise continuous technologies and make pharmaceutical companies implement and transfer this kind of production. Therefore, nowadays extensive research has been done in the diverse areas of pharmaceutical technologies, such as drug substance to drug product production (Domokos et al., 2021). Active pharmaceutical ingredients are also being designed using CM followed by the manufacturing of solid oral dosage forms (Adamo et al., 2016). Ceaseless production of pharmaceuticals is one of the advanced manufacturing initiatives that, as indicated by the Subcommittee for Advanced Manufacturing of the National Science and Technology Council, can achieve sustained prosperity and growth (Subcommittee for Advanced Manufacturing of the National Science and Technology Council, 2016). Patients and the investment community will also get an advantage since the CM will reduce the time required in product development (Vargas et al., 2018). CM is likely to offer economically priced, high-quality drug products with yield and cost-effectiveness over time to the pharmaceutical industry. Besides, cheap scale-up, compact manufacturing facilities, and online/inline process monitoring and control are other advantages of CM. Proper guidelines that pass through the regulating authorities are leading to the implementation of CM by the pharmaceutical manufacturers. Nevertheless, a series of difficulties of this technology application in the pharmaceutical industry are manifested in process design and control, as well as quality control. As it is evident, there has been some reluctance in taking the CM approach, as much investment has been put in the batch process, which remains high, and the staff is well trained using this process. Competent firms will not mind undergoing a transition from batch to continuous schemes of operations provided the perks gained are readily attainable, and these are in the form of huge profits, fast rates of development, and process safety to attain the desired product quality. Major companies in the pharmaceutical industry want to make the shift in solid oral dosage products to CM, and they include Novartis, GSK, Pfizer, Lilly, and Abbott. It is primarily explained by the necessity of the high capital and expertise investment. However, the generics industry can make headway in this transition only when it is viewed as a small-scale change but with amazing advantages (Helal et al., 2019).

3.4 Biodegradable and Recyclable Packaging

Packaging of pharmaceutical preparations, usually known as drug packaging, includes both the packaging and the packaging process (Kumar et al., 2023). Packaging is a science, art, and technology applied to protect the product, facilitate distribution and storage of the product, convey nutritional information, and present the product to the consumer. The Indian Brand Equity Foundation indicates that consumption of packaging is larger in the food packaging field than in non-food and tobacco products. Glass, paper, synthetic plastic, cardboard, co-extruded films, and laminates are presently the key materials used in packaging. Flexible packaging and various synthetic plastic laminates form a major part of packaging in India and nearly all the world. The environmental effect of such intractable synthetic plastic as waste is increasing the overall international interest. Since the available method of disposal has some limitations and acceptable landfills, they end up in incineration, which leads to the production of hazardous air pollution, and costly techniques of recycling are increasing the urge to create packing material that is biodegradable and can serve all functions needed by food without posing any risk to the environment. The other major reasons that have led to the development of biodegradable packaging are the rise in crude oil prices, the rise in demand by consumers, the expansion of consumer packaging, the creation of new applications of bioplastics, and higher economic feasibility (Meena et al., 2017). In the world, plastic packaging enjoys the biggest market, followed by packaging representing nearly half of all plastic wastes. According to Defruyt, only 2% of the plastic package materials are recovered to be used as packages in the world, with the rest being burned or landfilled or washed off to water bodies and the environment. Besides, sustainability is a more complicated issue than merely enhancing material collection and recycling but trying to look more closely at what types of materials are present in the market. The author points out that three out of ten packaging products made of plastic are either so complex or small to be recycled; these products include multi-layered plastic material and small sachets/wrappers, respectively. It does not mean that packaging materials will never be in our lives because this is the case in spite of the challenges. Packaging materials form an important aspect of our lives, owing to the fact that we use them on a daily basis at grocery shops and supermarkets, restaurants, reputable pharmaceuticals, etc. Packaging has been found to be critical in the preservation of byproducts or contents, whether during transportation, storage, or handling. It also contributes toward the shelf life of the products (Ibrahim et al., 2022).

3.5 Energy and Water Efficiency in Production Plants

The pharmaceutical sector uses a lot of water and has different water purity levels. The current trend of SDGs takes into account water reuse, which is deemed to be among the primary ways to reduce water use in manufacturing plants. Nonetheless, the recycling of the water in the manufacture of pharmaceuticals raises concerns for the regulatory authorities dealing with product quality and drug safety, and therefore the new strategies may adequately balance the opposing interests of quality water reuse in the production of pharmaceuticals and the fact that used water cannot contaminate pharmaceutical production by reusing water. The zero liquid discharge technologies allow virtually the entire avoidance of wastewater releases, with a maximum possible reuse of water in the manufacturing industry. Severe requirements on the quality of water and the dangers to human health from contaminated products can be regarded as the key obstacles to recycling water in the pharmaceutical industry (Strade et al., 2020). The issue of sustainability in the pharmaceutical industry has received increased consideration in the last few years, with a simultaneous consideration of the wonderful progress that the industry still has the capacity of realizing. The pharmaceutical sector is fierce in energy, which explains the trend of expanding curiosity in environmental sustainability and the awareness of the potential for improving energy performance. Nevertheless, diversity of the processes and inadequacy of data concerning production and the use of energy render the computation of Energy Performance Indicators (EnPIs) as well as enumeration of Energy Performance Improvement Actions (EPIAs) almost equivalent to each other. Although the amount of data provided was not very high, the authors came to the conclusion that a number of sustainability practices might result in a less environmental outcome in the sphere. Among those exercises, the application of sub-metering, metering, and energy performance symbols can save 10% of energy use and 18% of waste. In accordance with the increased level of interest in energy transition, more literature studies are dedicated to energy efficiency in various industries, among which there is the pharmaceutical industry. Although the pharmaceutical industry has certain estimations regarding the CO_2 energy intensity, this sector in general does not have information concerning final energy consumption or resource consumption; consequently, it is not possible to analyze the pharmaceutical industry's sustainability performances. This entails also that the sector does not have an energy performance index as well as the knowledge of how energy use occurs within the plants, thereby compromising the identification of what can be considered the line of action in energy saving. A recent study on the energy performance of the Swiss chemical and pharmaceutical industry serves as a suitable illustration. The authors highlight the absence of Specific Energy Consumption (SEC) indexes, which are conventionally defined as the ratio of energy utilized to a factor of production, such as the production of goods, because production-related statistics are confidential. They also mention that the absence of public industrial databases is a hindrance to the development of energy efficiency analysis, the purpose of which is to point at energy efficiency schemes. In this respect, they say that a bottom-up one, founded on actual case studies, may be more confident concerning other approaches analyzing the entire sector on the statistical level: the information was based on energy audits given to individual firms. Because a section of the pharmaceutical market deals with bulk manufacturing, the entire sector is typically included in the larger chemical industry, which presents another challenge when evaluating the energy outputs of the pharmaceutical sector. The chemical industry falls under the NACE code 20, with the pharmaceutical having the code NACE 21, with the production of bulk identified as 21.10 and drug production as 21.20 based on the Statistical Nomenclature of Economic Activities inside the European Community (Bruni et al., 2023).

3.6 Pharmaceutical Waste Reduction Strategies

According to the World Health Organization (WHO), pharmaceutical waste is defined as unwanted pharmaceuticals, and they are mainly medications, vaccines, sera, and pharmaceutical products that are expired, unused, spilled, and infected and not essential, and their disposal should be done with care and regard. An increase in the amount of pharmaceutical waste has been mostly caused by the rise in the patient/prescription base and the prescription, use, and overmanufacture of drugs. A rise in the number of unused, expired, and misplaced medicines has served to aggravate the scarcity of medicine, increase the percentage of pharmaceutical waste levels, and reduce the cost of medicine disposal, and it is an emerging challenge in the beyond-saver world that needs a comprehensive approach in terms of solving the problem. The final stage in the life cycle of pharmaceutical waste is the disposal stage; either conventional burning or a non-burning method is used. Here it is important to mention that the pharmaceutical waste majorly contains only 15% potentially harmful waste and 85% general waste. The quantities of the prescribed pharmaceutical waste in the water courses, streams, and underground water have also been known to be very high, and it has also been proved that a percentage of the waste has been found to pose some effects on water and the climate. A system of resource management and preservation, or what we would call being useful for as long as feasible through recovery and reuse, is the foundation of the circular economy (CE), a comprehensive ideology. The lifetime of the natural ecosystem, where people rely on physical and business existence, is bridged by the CE approach. It serves as a guide on how to dispose of waste, distinguish between biodegradable and non-biodegradable waste, and promote recycling and reuse. One can distinguish between multiple circularity possibilities in CE, such as the 3R, 4R, or even 9R models. The 9R model is the best application of CE and takes into consideration the following: Rethink, Refuse, Reduce, Repair, Recover, Reuse, Refurbish, Repurpose, Remanufacture, and Recycle. CE is rapidly growing as an alternative strategy for company improvement and in an effort to meet the SDGs of the United Nations. The CE goods and services are designed to work in harmony with the environment and have closed loops, meaning they are created and then released for reuse. One of the primary objectives of the CE is to encourage and facilitate increased sustainability. A supply chain that manages assets, operations, finances, and data to boost supply chain output while lowering environmental impacts and enhancing social welfare is said to be sustainable. According to the European Union (EU) parliament, EU organizations could potentially save around €600 billion by implementing sustainable waste management methods in general. These activities include minimizing waste, eco-friendly product development, and reuse. Furthermore, it could help cut greenhouse gas emissions by 4% annually. Among the advantages of the CE are enhanced economic growth, enhanced environmental quality, increased raw material safety, and accelerated innovation. Pharmaceutical waste management is officially a highly specialized subject that requires knowledgeable, experienced, and trained personnel at both the administrative and ground levels. A large amount of waste is generated at healthcare institutions as a result of inadequate training, a lack of proper protocols, and disparity between demand and supply in the hospital inventory management system. This can make financial and environmental issues worse. To enhance the waste reduction and supply chain, appropriate steps should be made, particularly with regard to the management, assessment, quantification, purchase, and use of medical stocks.

There are many excellent examples of practices that try to reduce, reuse, and recycle medications, as this study highlights. However, more work is needed to maximize these efforts and offer precise guidelines on standardized techniques that can be used and incorporated into pharmacy practice. As mentioned previously in the paper, incorrect prescribing, repeated medicine requests, noncompliance with medication regimens, and stockpiling are some of the ways that patients and healthcare providers can both worsen and improve pharmaceutical waste management.

Actions can be taken to determine and tackle the sources of waste formation in addition to optimizing product utilization while it is in the system as completed items. By employing proper disposal techniques, this will reduce the amount of danger posed to patients, their family in their homes, and the environment. It is important not to undervalue the patient's contribution to efficient pharmaceutical waste management. From a comprehensive standpoint, implementing the CE and associated principles can aid in waste reduction across the pharmaceutical supply chain. Although recycling and reusing medications reduces pharmaceutical waste from an economic and environmental standpoint, their use requires additional development, government and economic authorities' approval, and support from all supply chain participants. Thus, by employing CE as a binding mechanism for ongoing and future waste reduction initiatives, pharmaceutical waste disposal can be improved (Alshemari et al., 2020). Active pharmaceutical ingredients (APIs) are chemical-based compounds that are mostly produced in China, India, Europe, and the United States. Because of their pharmacological activity, APIs are mostly used in combination with other ingredients to diagnose, treat, cure, and mitigate illnesses. However, several pharmaceutical companies have started importing these medications from countries that manufacture active ingredients back to their own countries in recent years. Modern drugs have been used by people to identify, treat, prevent, and cure diseases. The primary ingredient, the API, is biologically and chemically active and must function in your body. Other ingredients, known as excipients, like lactose or mineral oil, are chemically unusable and give the pill properties like volume, sweet flavor, or color. These excipients facilitate the absorption of APIs by the bodily systems. An API is made by a multi-step synthesis using a range of chemical compounds and raw materials (Kumar et al., 2022).

3.7 Reverse Logistics and Drug Take-Back Programs

Moving products back to their starting place or to a location for recycling, repair, or disposal is known as reverse logistics. Reverse logistics in the pharmaceutical sector is mainly concerned with gathering, moving, and securely getting rid of unwanted, expired, or recalled drugs. It includes a variety of actions intended to guarantee the safe, effective, and legal return of pharmaceutical products following use or when they are no longer required. Traditional logistics, however, is concerned with getting commodities from producers to customers. Reverse logistics' capacity to lessen the negative environmental effects of pharmaceutical waste is one of its main advantages. When pharmaceuticals are disposed of inappropriately, particularly when flushed down toilets or dumped in landfills, they can contaminate drinking water, rivers, and lakes. Antibiotics, hormones, and chemotherapy treatments are among the medications that might upset aquatic ecosystems and cause bacteria to become resistant. Reverse logistics also makes it possible to dispose of prohibited substances safely, which lowers the possibility of abuse or diversion for illegal purposes. Reverse logistics keeps unwanted drugs from being mishandled and lowers the risk of public health issues by making sure they are sent back to the right facilities for secure disposal. Furthermore, by giving hospitals, pharmacies, and customers the means to properly return unneeded prescription drugs, reverse logistics makes it easier to comply with national and local laws. For instance, customers can return unneeded prescriptions to pharmacies, hospitals, or specified drop-off locations through take-back programs, which are frequently made possible by reverse logistics systems. Because it helps reduce the threats to the environment and public health that come with inappropriate drug disposal, pharmaceutical reverse logistics is an essential component of waste management. Prescription drugs can contaminate water systems, lead to antibiotic resistance, and expose people and wildlife to dangerous compounds when they are disposed of inappropriately, such as flushing them down the toilet or putting them in the garbage. In order to ensure that pharmaceuticals are not abused, misdirected, or disposed of inappropriately, reverse logistics offers a methodical way to collect and dispose of them in an environmentally friendly way (Adeyemo et al., 2024).

4 Digital Transformation and Smart Technologies

The OECD predicts that the need for raw resources will increase from 90 gigatons in the present to 167 gigatons in 2060. The United Nations created 17 plans of action and SDGs, focusing on attaining global sustainable growth and sustainable development. Every nation's primary objective is creating corporate systems and procedures that will lead to sustained growth. The importance of creating contemporary, forward-thinking business systems with the goal of achieving sustainable manufacturing is emphasized by the 12th Sustainable Development Goal, "Responsible Production and Consumption." Additionally, stakeholders are more interested in sustainable practices that preserve ecological balance and shield the environment from contamination. A nation's economy, political stability, cultural and legal aspects, and general social environment all play a role in the successful transition to sustainable growth. Institutional, technological, and business strategy changes are necessary to give organizations the ability to meet the new challenges and contribute to sustainable growth. Therefore, the inclusive engagement with digitally enhanced stakeholders is essential to achieving sustainable supply chain growth and related SGDs. Communication methods have changed as a result of digitalization. Every sector and daily life have been completely transformed by modern technologies, such as smartphones, smart automobiles, and other devices. The use of digital goods and services rises as a result of industry digitalization. Digital transformation (DT) is essential for improving customer interactions because it promotes flexibility, agility, and real-time transparency. As a result, sustainable development depends on cost reduction, improved efficiency, resource optimization, and on-time delivery. Through the adoption and development of digital competences including big data analytics (BDA), machine learning, B2B learning networks, the Internet of Things, robots, DT, and AI refers to a transformation of the business development paradigm and significant changes in its ecosystem. It was emphasized that although DT is dangerous because of its high initial operational costs and costs, it still has long-term advantages for the business and is essential in controlling organizational performance. DT has an impact on the supply chain. DT helps firms reengineer their business development models, prepares them to tackle future difficulties, and changes the relationship between supply chain stakeholders. DT gives businesses the tools they need to integrate gadgets and activate intelligence into their systems in order to enhance supply chain efficiency. The smart gadgets that were made available as a result of DT implementation are intelligent, communicative, programmable, and perform better (Rehman Khan et al., 2022).

4.1 Internet of Things in Pharma Supply Chains

The phrase "Internet of Things" (IoT) is a catchphrase in the information technology industry. The Internet of Things is a network of networked computers with unique identifiers (UIDs) that may transmit data. Throughout the pharmaceutical product's manufacturing process, IoT may be useful in tracking and optimizing different unit operations for real-time surveillance and control to increase production efficiency. In order to boost operational effectiveness, IoT can be utilized to monitor the real-time storage conditions of pharmaceutical products and enhance transparency in pharmaceutical supply chain management and warehousing. The Internet of Things is an innovative mover in the realm of information technology. In order to create the acronym "Internet of Things," or IoT, the words "Internet" and "Things" are joined. Millions of people around the world are connected by the Internet, a global network of interconnected computer systems that employ the standard Internet protocol suite (Internet Protocol/Transmission Control Protocol). Numerous enterprises worldwide have been significantly impacted by the IoT. IoT hasn't yet had a significant effect on the medical device and pharmaceutical industries, though, because the pharmaceutical business has become quite pragmatic in its embrace of technological advancements. IoT, however, has a lot of promise to help pharmaceutical businesses increase the efficiency of their manufacturing, reduce costs, and alter the way they distribute drugs to consumers. IoT connects the patient, the pharmaceutical company, and the physician by tracking patient adherence to prescribed medication in the cloud. The pharmaceutical business may leverage IoT to discover treatments and deliver better care while saving more lives by utilizing sensors and smart devices. IoT offers the pharmaceutical business increased profitability, resilience, and efficiency, but it also has tremendous breakthrough potential that might lead to a new age of transformation. Even though the Internet of Things is still in its infancy, smart devices and machine-to-machine technologies for communication have gained popularity as instruments for digitizing data and processes in the pharmaceutical industry. By upending the long-standing, traditional structures in the highly regulated pharmaceutical sector, from medicine production to distribution, IoT is fostering innovation. Pharmaceutical companies are now far more willing to experiment with IoT technology to enhance quality, boost productivity, reduce production errors, and elevate stakeholder expectations about medicine efficacy. The use of IoT in clinical development, pharmaceutical production, patient contacts, and supply chain management, not only reduces the time to market for pharmaceuticals but also enhances regulatory compliance by using real-time data flow to identify flaws along the value chain. Numerous industries regularly make investments in the use of IoT in manufacturing and supply chain management. Common Internet of Things applications that are particularly well-suited for many pharmaceutical organizations include connected materials, cold chain monitoring, sample lifecycle management, equipment, people, and smart packaging. The IoT is a new paradigm that is gaining traction in the pharmaceutical sciences, namely in supply chain management, manufacturing, and warehousing. Because IoT enables smart technologies for anywhere, anytime, anything, and any media communication, it has the ability to contribute new elements to pharmaceutical operations. IoT is developing into a crucial field that is seeing a notable increase in the creative application of technology in pharmaceutical operations to raise consumer satisfaction levels (Sharma et al., 2020). Digitalization has altered how people interact with their surroundings and communicate. New devices and technology, like computers, cell phones, autonomous cars, and smart wearables, have fundamentally altered how we access and share information. These developments and digital shifts affect all industries, and supply chains are no exception. In companies undergoing these rapid changes, supply chain digitalization increasingly encompasses digital products and services as well as the management of supply chain operations (Nasiri et al., 2020).

4.2 Blockchain for Transparent and Ethical Sourcing

With its decentralized and unchangeable ledger, blockchain technology offers an optimistic way to tackle the problems of guaranteeing efficiency as well as transparency in sustainable supply chains. The decentralized feature of blockchain technology is also essential for improving supply chain effectiveness. Conventional supply chains frequently depend on centralized systems, which are susceptible to bottlenecks, data breaches, and single points of failure. By distributing the ledger among several nodes, blockchain's decentralized architecture, however, makes sure that no one party controls the entire system. By lowering the chance of interruptions and guaranteeing uninterrupted operation even in the face of technological problems or cyberattacks, this decentralization improves the resilience and security of supply chains. Furthermore, data silos—a prevalent problem in conventional supply chains—can be eliminated with the aid of blockchain's capacity to offer a cohesive and transparent record of transactions. A distributed ledger technology (DLT) called blockchain keeps track of transactions across several computers and makes sure that once they are registered, they cannot be changed later. Each block of a blockchain has a timestamp, transaction information, and a cryptographic hash of the previous block, forming a secure and visible chain of events. Because blockchain technology offers significant improvements in efficiency, transparency, and traceability, so it has the potential to completely transform supply chain management. Blockchain guarantees that every movement and transaction in the supply chain is precisely documented and verifiable by offering an immutable and decentralized ledger, which increases stakeholder trust. However, there are many obstacles in the way of widespread adoption, such as the difficult and expensive integration with current legacy systems, scalability problems that can raise costs and slow processing times, and the requirement to manage multiple regulatory environments to guarantee adherence to trade, environmental, and data privacy standards. (Nwariaku et al., 2024). The successful implementation of the data structure in the Bitcoin application is the main foundation for the new application development paradigm brought about by blockchain technology. Similar to a linked list, the basic idea behind the blockchain data structure is that all nodes in the network share it, and each node maintains a local copy of every block (connected with the longest chain) beginning with its genesis block (Musamih et al., 2021).

4.3 Digital Twins for Process Optimization

The creation of virtual copies of items or procedures that mimic the behavior of their real counterparts is known as digital twin technology. In order to increase its efficacy, the goal is to examine its behavior or efficacy in specific situations. When applied to machines, goods, or even entire company ecosystems, the digital twin concept may optimize the present, uncover information from the past, and even forecast how well the various sectors under analysis will perform in the future. Digital twins are revolutionizing supply chains by offering a variety of solutions to support data-driven decision-making, collaborative settings, and more reliable business operations (Marmolejo-Saucedo, 2020). For the past few decades, digital twins, or DTs, have become a standard in the engineering sector. In recent years, it has gained attention in the health sectors. This chapter extends a comprehensive analysis of DT and its pivotal function in revolutionizing several aspects of healthcare (Ritu et al., 2024).

5 Challenges and Barriers to Sustainable Innovation

Globally, industrial activity has affected the environment and taken human lives. The increasing negative environmental difficulties around the world have forced many stakeholder groups, including environmental activists and policy professionals, to support additional government regulations. Governments have responded to these demands by enacting stricter laws and regulations that mandate that industries and enterprises adhere to specific sustainability standards. Sustainability is a significant global concern. The industrial sector is one that makes a substantial contribution to the growing global sustainability issue. Manufacturing companies need to find innovative solutions to this complex and growing worldwide environmental problem. However, when trying to innovate for sustainability, manufacturing companies—particularly those in emerging economies like India—face numerous obstacles, some of which are organizational in nature and others of a technological kind. In order to address this problem, the barriers that prevent the manufacturing sector from adopting and implementing sustainable innovation should be accurately recognized, assessed, and prioritized in order to give some guidance on how to approach and plan for these obstacles according to their severity. Some techniques that are in line with the barriers are necessary to overcome them. No one tactic can assist in getting beyond every obstacle. Technological, cultural, social, and economic hurdles are the most noticeable in the contemporary growing economy and require immediate action from organizations and policymakers. Investing in the newest technologies and offering incentives to staff members who think creatively and embrace sustainable practices within the company are two effective ways to get past these obstacles. Additionally, governmental support—such as favorable rules and low tax slabs—is crucial for businesses implementing sustainable and green practices. Support can also take the form of training organizations to instill a sustainable culture in them and granting access to facilities and technologies that are available in other wealthy nations (Gupta et al., 2020).

6 Personalized Medicine and Precision Pharma

Personalized medicine refers to the tailored, individualized management strategy that ensures the correct patient receives the right medication at the right dosage. Numerous concerns, such as the unjustified bad effects of drugs in many patients and the lack of consistency in treatment efficacy—which can range from 25% to 80% depending on the drug class—were the driving forces behind the strategy. Personalized medicine includes environmental factors, specific patient health challenges, epigenetic, proteomic, and genomic research. The utilization of a precise, customized diagnosis of an individual's genetic profile and targeted treatment of that ailment is a new field of research in personalized/precision medicine. It takes into account a patient's or a group of related patients' genetic, phenotypic, and environmental factors that may affect the safety and effectiveness of a specific medication (Alghamdi et al., 2022). Personalized medicines enable the creation of flexible treatment formulations that consider a medical history, genetic composition, individual's physiology. Precision drugs, which use state-of-the-art 3D printing technology, have become popular in the pharmaceutical sector (BG et al., 2023).

6.1 Sustainable Nanotechnology in Drug Delivery

Nanotechnology is a rapidly developing field of science and technology that will revolutionize every field with its groundbreaking discoveries and scientific breakthroughs. It's the study of minuscule particles. Nanotechnology is used in every aspect of our daily lives, including food safety, agro science, water purification, pharmaceuticals, disease treatment, drug delivery systems, catalysis, energy conservation, and cosmetics. Because nanotechnology is interconnected with every branch of science, including engineering, chemistry, physics, and biology, its benefits in our daily lives are surprisingly high. This technology's advancements are groundbreaking. For example, the use of nanotechnology has significantly improved the old traditional methods of food packaging, diagnosis, water purification, and electrical appliances. All branches of research and technology are connected to the vast field of nanotechnology. Many scientists, engineers, and researchers are currently developing novel applications of this technology for the benefit of humanity. Chemical engineering, biochemistry, and electronics are among the many fields in which this technique finds use. Nanotechnology offers creative ways to filter water and make it drinkable as our natural resources, including drinkable water, deteriorate. In addition to being utilized in water treatment techniques, it also produces high-quality food, improves the quality of food packaging, extends food shelf life, detects viruses in food, and makes several other contributions to the field of food science. Doctors may now diagnose ailments earlier and detect diseases at an early stage thanks to technology, and many severe diseases can be cured with simple and quick treatments. Since many aspects of nanotechnology are still in need of development, this technology will require more concentrated research. Researchers and scientists have concentrated on nanotechnology in all branches of science and technology, allowing for a plethora of new chances for scientific investigation into NPs (Raghav et al., 2020).

6.2 Collaborative Models and Open Innovation

While open innovation (OI) signifies a shift toward more open and dispersed methods of invention, opportunities refer to the increasing importance of digital platforms as a site for value creation and distribution. The OI paradigm states that in order to accelerate internal innovation; companies are increasingly sourcing information and technologies from beyond their boundaries (in-flows) and searching for external markets to commercialize or monetize their internal knowledge assets and techniques (outflows). OI contradicts earlier paradigms of innovation that emphasized internalizing knowledge and maintaining total control over the creation process. A wide range of organizations, including universities, federal labs, and other innovation intermediaries, as well as new and established businesses, have benefited from the development of creative approaches to collaboration and partnerships in the fields of innovation and commercialization thanks to this emphasis on transparency. Most of the research that has been done on platforms and OI has focused on how they help businesses expand or how they encourage entrepreneurship. In a broad sense, OI refers to the collaboration of companies, individuals, and other types of organizations in the creation of novel goods and services, as well as the exchange of the advantages and disadvantages of R&D and commercialization. The OI framework is based on the notion that companies can benefit greatly from sharing knowledge and creating new concepts with partners and cannot rely solely on their own investigations in a world filled with dispersed knowledge. As the world becomes more interconnected, OI offers a means of lowering risks, saving money on research, and swiftly bringing discoveries to market (Nambisan et al., 2018).

7 Conclusion

Sustainable development is currently a basic need of pharmaceutical sector to deal with different global challenges. Pharmaceutical research and education field is focusing on greener manufacturing practices, waste minimization, water purification and saving, and eco-friendly procedure to save environmental owing our social and economic responsibility. Different innovative tools, i.e., graph pad prism, BioRender, molecular docking etc. are used to enhance the efficiency of pharmaceutical sector as well as to maintain sustainability in the field. Traditional methods of research and innovation are replaced with modern one to get prompt and superior results. Different collaborations are essential to achieve sustainability in education and research field of pharmaceutical sciences. By involving AI-based tools and smart tools, ecological footprints can be decreased and an eco-friendly environment can be created.

References

Adamo, A., Beingessner, R.L., Behnam, M., Chen, J., Jamison, T.F., Jensen, K.F., Monbaliu, J.C.M., Myerson, A.S., Revalor, E.M., Snead, D.R. and Stelzer, T., 2016. On-demand continuous-flow production of pharmaceuticals in a compact, reconfigurable system. *Science*, 352(6281), pp.61–67.

Adeyemo, K.S., Mbata, A.O. and Balogun, O.D., 2024. Pharmaceutical waste management and reverse logistics in the US enhancing sustainability and reducing public health risks. *Significance*, 4(6):1720–1729.

Agrawal, M., Bansal, A., Khandelwal, V.K. and Bansal, N., 2024. Sustainable pharma: The need, current status and mission for the future. *Scripta Medica*, 55(4), pp.489–499.

Alghamdi, M.A., Fallica, A.N., Virzì, N., Kesharwani, P., Pittalà, V. and Greish, K., 2022. The promise of nanotechnology in personalized medicine. *Journal of Personalized Medicine*, 12(5), p.673.

Alim, M. and Sulley, S., 2024. Beyond healing: Embracing the triple bottom line approach in post-pandemic healthcare. *Cureus*, 16(2), e54019 [online]

Alnaqbi, K.A., Bellanger, A., Brill, A., Castañeda-Hernández, G., Clopés Estela, A., Delgado Sánchez, O., García-Alfonso, P., Gyger, P., Heinrich, D., Hezard, G. and Kakehasi, A., 2023. An international comparative analysis and roadmap to sustainable biosimilar markets. *Frontiers in Pharmacology*, 14, p.1188368.

Alshemari, A., Breen, L., Quinn, G. and Sivarajah, U., 2020. Can we create a circular pharmaceutical supply chain (CPSC) to reduce medicines waste? *Pharmacy*, 8(4), p.221.

Banik, B.K., Sahoo, B.M., Kumar, B.V.V.R., Panda, K.C., Jena, J., Mahapatra, M.K. and Borah, P., 2021. Green synthetic approach: An efficient eco-friendly tool for synthesis of biologically active oxadiazole derivatives. *Molecules*, 26(4), p.1163.

BG, P.K., Mehrotra, S., Marques, S.M., Kumar, L. and Verma, R., 2023. 3D printing in personalized medicines: A focus on applications of the technology. *Materials Today Communications*, 35, p.105875.

Bhar, S., 2023. Role of drug repurposing in sustainable drug discovery. In *Drug Repurposing-Advances, Scopes and Opportunities in Drug Discovery*. IntechOpen, 163–175.

Bhardwaja, B., Klocke, S., Ekinci, E., Jackson, A., Kono, S. and Olson, K.L., 2022. Switching from biologic to biosimilar products: Insight from an integrated health care system. *BioDrugs*, 36(1), pp.1–11.

Bruni, G., Martini, C., Martini, F. and Salvio, M., 2023. On the energy performance and energy saving potential of the pharmaceutical industry: A study based on the Italian energy audits. *Processes*, 11(4), p.1114.

Burcham, C.L., Florence, A.J. and Johnson, M.D., 2018. Continuous manufacturing in pharmaceutical process development and manufacturing. *Annual Review of Chemical and Biomolecular Engineering*, 9(1), pp.253–281.

Domokos, A., Nagy, B., Szilágyi, B., Marosi, G. and Nagy, Z.K., 2021. Integrated continuous pharmaceutical technologies—A review. *Organic Process Research & Development*, 25(4), pp.721–739.

Dou, X., 2024. Modern innovations in vaccine development: Exploring new trends and technologies. *Theoretical and Natural Science*, 61, pp.1–9.

Gupta, H., Kusi-Sarpong, S. and Rezaei, J., 2020. Barriers and overcoming strategies to supply chain sustainability innovation. *Resources, Conservation and Recycling*, 161, p.104819.

Gupta, R., Srivastava, D., Sahu, M., Tiwari, S., Ambasta, R.K. and Kumar, P., 2021. Artificial intelligence to deep learning: Machine intelligence approach for drug discovery. *Molecular Diversity*, 25, pp.1315–1360.

Helal, N.A., Elnoweam, O., Eassa, H.A., Amer, A.M., Eltokhy, M.A., Helal, M.A., Fayyaz, H.A. and Nounou, M.I., 2019. Integrated continuous manufacturing in pharmaceutical industry: Current evolutionary steps toward revolutionary future. *Pharmaceutical Patent Analyst*, 8(4), pp.139–161.

Hoodbhoy, P., 2024. Innovations in vaccine development: From traditional approaches. *Multidisciplinary Surgical Research Annals*, 2(1), pp.11–25.

Ibrahim, I.D., Hamam, Y., Sadiku, E.R., Ndambuki, J.M., Kupolati, W.K., Jamiru, T., Eze, A.A. and Snyman, J., 2022. Need for sustainable packaging: An overview. *Polymers*, 14(20), p.4430.

Kim, S., Ga, S., Bae, H., Sluyter, R., Konstantinov, K., Shrestha, L.K., Kim, Y.H., Kim, J.H. and Ariga, K., 2024. Multidisciplinary approaches for enzyme biocatalysis in pharmaceuticals: Protein engineering, computational biology, and nanoarchitectonics. *EES Catalysis*, 2(1), pp.14–48.

Kumar, R., Sadeghi, K., Jang, J. and Seo, J., 2023. Mechanical, chemical, and bio-recycling of biodegradable plastics: A review. *Science of the Total Environment*, 882, p.163446.

Kumar, V., Bansal, V., Madhavan, A., Kumar, M., Sindhu, R., Awasthi, M.K., Binod, P. and Saran, S., 2022. Active pharmaceutical ingredient (API) chemicals: A critical review of current biotechnological approaches. *Bioengineered*, 13(2), pp.4309–4327.

Marmolejo-Saucedo, J.A., 2020. Design and development of digital twins: A case study in supply chains. *Mobile Networks and Applications*, 25(6), pp.2141–2160.

Martinengo, B., Diamanti, E., Uliassi, E. and Bolognesi, M.L., 2025. Medicinal chemistry: A key driver in achieving the global sustainable development goals. *Journal of Medicinal Chemistry*, 68(7), pp.6916–6931.

Mascarenhas-Melo, F., Diaz, M., Gonçalves, M.B.S., Vieira, P., Bell, V., Viana, S., Nunes, S., Paiva-Santos, A.C. and Veiga, F., 2024. An overview of biosimilars—Development, quality, regulatory issues, and management in healthcare. *Pharmaceuticals*, 17(2), p.235.

Meena, P.L., Goel, A., Rai, V., Rao, E., Singh Barwa, M., Manjeet, C., Barwa, S., Vinay, A., Goel, V., Rai, E. and Rao, S., 2017. Packaging material and need of biodegradable polymers: A review. *International Journal of Applied Research*, 3(7), pp.886–896.

Milanesi, M., Runfola, A. and Guercini, S., 2020. Pharmaceutical industry riding the wave of sustainability: Review and opportunities for future research. *Journal of Cleaner Production*, 261, p.121204.

Mittal, N. and Mittal, R., 2021. Repurposing old molecules for new indications: Defining pillars of success from lessons in the past. *European Journal of Pharmacology*, 912, p.174569.

Musamih, A., Salah, K., Jayaraman, R., Arshad, J., Debe, M., Al-Hammadi, Y. and Ellahham, S., 2021. A blockchain-based approach for drug traceability in healthcare supply chain. *IEEE Access*, 9, pp.9728–9743.

Nambisan, S., Siegel, D. and Kenney, M., 2018. On open innovation, platforms, and entrepreneurship. *Strategic Entrepreneurship Journal*, 12(3), pp.354–368.

Nasiri, M., Ukko, J., Saunila, M. and Rantala, T., 2020. Managing the digital supply chain: The role of smart technologies. *Technovation*, 96, p.102121.

Nwariaku, H., Fadojutimi, B., Lawson, L.G.L., Agbelusi, J., Adigun, O.A., Udom, J.A. and Olajide, T.D., 2024. Blockchain technology as an enabler of transparency and efficiency in sustainable supply chains. *International Journal of Science and Research Archive*, 12(2), pp.1779–1789.

Pal, P., 2018. Treatment and disposal of pharmaceutical wastewater: Toward the sustainable strategy. *Separation & Purification Reviews*, 47(3), pp.179–198.

Prigodich, A.E., Wang, S., Verhoest, P., Warne, N., Allerton, C., Burkhardt, J., Fernando, K. and Dolsten, M., 2021. Innovation in breakthrough drugs and vaccines: Development risk, patient impact, and value. *Drug Discovery Today*, 26(10), pp.2232–2237.

Raghav, S., Yadav, P.K. and Kumar, D., 2020. Nanotechnology for a sustainable future. In C.M. Hussain (Ed.), *Handbook of Nanomaterials for Manufacturing Applications* (pp.465–492). Elsevier.

Rehman Khan, S.A., Ahmad, Z., Sheikh, A.A. and Yu, Z., 2022. Digital transformation, smart technologies, and eco-innovation are paving the way toward sustainable supply chain performance. *Science Progress*, 105(4), p.00368504221145648.

Ritu, T.H., Nag, A., Bairagi, A.K. and Rahman, A., 2024. Digital twins for healthcare in industry 5.0: Fundamentals, pharmaceutical manufacturing applications, diagnostic precision, digital patient innovations, and drug discovery impact. In C.K.K. Reddy, T. Sithole, M. Ouaissa, Ö. Özer and M.M. Hanafiah (Eds.), *Soft Computing in Industry 5.0 for Sustainability* (pp.357–376). Springer Nature Switzerland.

Sharma, A., Kaur, J. and Singh, I., 2020. Internet of things (IoT) in pharmaceutical manufacturing, warehousing, and supply chain management. *SN Computer Science*, 1(4), p.232.

Sharma, R., Bhardwaj, I., Grima, S., Sachdeva, T., Sood, K. and Özen, E. eds., 2024. *Sustainable Development Goals: The Impact of Sustainability Measures on Wellbeing*. Emerald Publishing Limited.

Shin, J., Kim, C. and Yang, H., 2018. The effect of sustainability as innovation objectives on innovation efficiency. *Sustainability*, 10(6), p.1966.

Soltys, L., Olkhovyy, O., Tatarchuk, T. and Naushad, M., 2021. Green synthesis of metal and metal oxide nanoparticles: Principles of green chemistry and raw materials. *Magnetochemistry*, 7(11), p.145.

Srivastav, A.L., Grewal, A.S., Tiwari, M. and Pham, T.D. eds., 2023. *Role of Green Chemistry in Ecosystem Restoration to Achieve Environmental Sustainability*. Elsevier.

Strade, E., Kalnina, D. and Kulczycka, J., 2020. Water efficiency and safe re-use of different grades of water-Topical issues for the pharmaceutical industry. *Water Resources and Industry*, 24, p.100132.

Tessema, F.B., Asfaw, T.B., Tadesse, M.G., Gonfa, Y.H. and Bachheti, R.K., 2025. In silico studies as support for natural products research. *Medinformatics*, 2(1), pp.11–21.

Tseng, M.L., Chang, C.H., Lin, C.W.R., Wu, K.J., Chen, Q., Xia, L. and Xue, B., 2020. Future trends and guidance for the triple bottom line and sustainability: A data driven bibliometric analysis. *Environmental Science and Pollution Research*, 27, pp.33543–33567.

Vargas, J.M., Nielsen, S., Cárdenas, V., Gonzalez, A., Aymat, E.Y., Almodovar, E., Classe, G., Colón, Y., Sanchez, E. and Romañach, R.J., 2018. Process analytical technology in continuous manufacturing of a commercial pharmaceutical product. *International Journal of Pharmaceutics*, 538(1–2), pp.167–178.

Winterton, N., 2021. The green solvent: A critical perspective. *Clean Technologies and Environmental Policy*, 23(9), pp.2499–2522.

7 Metrics for Implementing and Assessing the Environmental Impact of Healthcare and Other Products

Shivam Sharma, Diksha Gulati, Bhawna Chopra, and Gagandeep Kaur

1 Introduction

The primary focus of healthcare evaluation is directly on health outcomes and financial analysis; however, the environmental aspects are yet to be ignored. These include various pollutants and environmental harms that have an unintended but negative impact on the healthcare system (Pichler et al., 2019). Medical devices (MDs) are some important health instruments, encompassing an enormous and diversified product range, ranging from simple ligatures to pacemakers, grafts, or auxiliary support machines. Metrics are some powerful tools utilised for tracking the determinants of community health and outcomes (L & CM, 2004). These indicators are measurable, sophisticated, robust, unambiguous, accountable and reflective of community values (*Environmental Health Indicators: Framework and Methodologies*, n.d.; Hancock et al., 1999).

The metrics identify community problems and prioritize policy development, while allowing leaders to monitor progress and compare results over time. An important component of the community health information base is environmental measurements. Environmental variables have a significant impact on human health, both "upstream" (such as the energy sources used by a society) and directly (such as the quality of the air individuals breathe). Both harmful exposures, such as pollution, and "salutogenic" exposures, like parks and green areas, may be measured using environmental measures (Jakubowski & Frumkin, 2010).

Three initiatives provide guidance when considering environmental measurements for community health. First, starting in the 1980s, several towns began to identify liveability indicators, commonly called quality of life indicators (Dluhy & Swartz, 2006). These often represent health-related environmental issues. Second, sustainability metrics have been popular in recent years. Numerous sustainability metrics focus on ecological aspects that are related to human health. Third, environmental public health indicators have been discussed by the Council of State and Territorial Epidemiologists in partnership with the Centres for Disease Control and Prevention (CDC), with a focus on drinking water, air quality, asthma, and climate change. In this chapter, we will discuss various matrices for the assessment of the environmental impact of various healthcare products, such as life cycle assessment (LCA) of healthcare products, which will impart some major insights regarding the

DOI: 10.4324/9781003640486-7

environmental hazards caused by a particular healthcare product throughout its life cycle; other matrices, such as eco-design, carbon footprint, energy consumption, waste generation, toxicology, and ecological impact, are also useful in the assessment of environmental effects of various healthcare products. Medical waste is considered to be harmful and injurious due to its high level of toxicity and ability to harm the environment (Eckelman & Sherman, 2016).

2 Matrices for Assessing Environmental Impact

2.1 Life Cycle Assessment

LCA aids in measuring the environmental effect of a product at every stage of its life cycle, from raw material extraction to disposal at the end of its useful life. In addition to identifying important environmental hotspots, it offers information to help decision-making. This is an elaborate approach for the assessment of the effect of various MDs throughout their life cycle (Gavilán-García et al., 2015; Moultrie et al., 2016).

The possibilities of MDs causing global warming, acid rain, human health risks, toxicity in marine ecosystems, depletion of the ozone layer, and production of smog, along with fossil fuel depletion, are some key indicators that are assessed by LCA. It also includes some tools like TRACI and SimaPro, which use databases such as Ecoinvent that can be used to analyse inventory data of the life cycle of medical products. These tools can also help in the quantification of these parameters. According to data generated after the research work carried out on LCA, single-use MDs have a major negative impact on the environment because of their disposable nature and their requirement of more number of resources, as well as the production of a large quantity of waste (S. Unger & Landis, 2016). However, if we talk about reusable MDs, they have less negative impact on our environment if we adopt a recycling and reprocessing approach as a final alternative. Material switching, for example, from petroleum-based plastics to biopolymers, is also known to have fewer negative consequences, especially respiratory toxicity and carcinogenesis. Considering all the above-mentioned factors, LCA is overall an effective metric and instrumental approach that helps in the assessment and reduction of MDs' induced environmental impact, which can further help us to shift towards a more sustainable healthcare industry (Sharma et al., 2024).

MDs' LCA studies are essential for understanding the impact of MDs on the environment and people at every stage of their life cycle, from the origin of raw materials to disposal. These investigations usually utilise databases like Ecoinvent and technologies like SimaPro and TRACI to analyse the stages, including manufacturing, use, transportation, and end-of-life management. According to LCA study results, reusable devices often have lower environmental impacts, albeit sterilisation procedures may increase emissions, whereas disposable MDS typically have higher environmental impacts because of their short life cycles and substantial waste creation. The choice of material is crucial; research shows that using biopolymers instead of traditional materials like PVC and thermoplastic polyurethane might lessen environmental damage (Jones & Halamka, 2013). Although CO_2 emissions may differ depending on energy sources, recycling mercury thermometers has been demonstrated to minimise environmental impacts when compared to landfill disposal, and switching to reusable anaesthetic equipment can cut expenses. LCA studies give manufacturers and healthcare organisations important information that helps them evaluate disposable and reusable equipment, find environmental hotspots, choose the best materials, and create sustainable procedures (C. L. Thiel et al., 2015). There aren't many LCA studies for MDs, though, and further investigation is required to examine a larger variety of tools and materials, such as metals and ceramics. LCA studies may significantly contribute to the advancement of sustainability in the healthcare industry by filling these gaps (McGain et al., 2017).

2.2 Eco-Design Studies

Beyond LCA, eco-design principles and sustainability-focused approaches serve as the foundation for additional metrics used to evaluate the environmental effects of MDs. To reconcile ecological and financial needs, eco-design places a strong focus on incorporating environmental factors into the product creation process (PDF; Life Cycle Management: A Bridge to More Sustainable Products, n.d.). Selection of material and use of products that are based on the principle of recycling, reuse, or remanufacturing, reducing the use of materials like PVC and mercury, are some examples of the ecological design matrix. Reducing the product's bulk and volume, extending the product life, and optimising the packing material are some of the important measures to lower the production of waste and balance resource usage. Production efficiency by reducing the release of pollutants and consumption of energy during the process of manufacture is also a crucial approach. The evaluation of these indicators is done with tools like "maturity grids and systemic design frameworks." These will help the designer to spot any scope for environmental enhancements throughout the life cycle of a medical device. Survey and engagement of stakeholders are also important to enhance the ecological design further by incorporating insights from various professionals involved in design, manufacturing and usage of MDs (Bocken et al., 2016). Together, all these criteria will help in the overall sustainable use of MDs by tracking issues such as expertise required for transdisciplinary requirements, regulatory obstacles, and single-use business models. By focusing on these matrices, the shift of the healthcare sector towards more ecological production and design methods will overall reduce the total negative impact of medical products and devices (Moultrie et al., 2015).

To reduce the negative environmental effects of medical devices throughout the life cycle, eco-design metrics focus on the incorporation of environmental factors to be included in the design and development process (Sutcliffe et al., 2009). These indicators highlight the importance of considering sustainability in the product design process for the optimisation of financial and environmental advantages before using a device practically. In contrast with LCA, eco-design studies involve the creation of frameworks, tools, and various approaches that can direct manufacturers, along with designers, to develop more environmentally friendly products and medical equipment. For example, to find important sustainability concerns while enhancing the accessibility and usage. A systematic method for dialysis equipment was developed. These studies show how important it is for people from different fields to work together and communicate better with each other to find important environmental stages, look into eco-design ideas that might work, and successfully put solutions into action Even though eco-design is still in its early stages in the medical device business, these efforts show (*PDF; Life Cycle Management: A Bridge to More Sustainable Products*, n.d.) that it has the potential to make healthcare more innovative and environmentally friendly. These studies show how important it is for people from different fields to work together and communicate better with each other to find important environmental stages, look into eco-design ideas that might work, and successfully put solutions into action. Even though eco-design is still in its early stages in the medical device business, these efforts show that it has the potential to make healthcare more innovative and environmentally friendly (S. Unger & Landis, 2016).

2.3 Combination Studies

Researchers who combine eco-design and LCA methods are trying to make medical devices (MDs) that are better for the environment by using the best parts of both. Usually, LCA is used to find the most environmentally harmful parts of present devices. Then, eco-design ideas are used to make the devices more sustainable or better. Unger et al. (2017) looked at single-use MDS made of petroleum-based plastics and those made of biopolymers. They found that biopolymers had less of an impact on respiratory and cancer-causing effects, but they also caused problems like smog from transportation and farming (S. R. Unger et al., 2017). Likewise, researchers assessed the long-term environmental impacts of a regular plastic emesis bowl and compared it to a version that had improvements made to the way it was made. They showed that pollution control methods usually had less of an effect on the environment, except for emissions from transportation (Gabriel et al., 2009). Campion et al. (2015) used LCA and eco-design to rethink disposable custom packs that are used during delivery. They found that cotton and polypropylene were the biggest environmental problems and made a greener pack with the best materials (Campion et al., 2015). Hanson and Hitchcock (2009) used LCA and functional analysis to improve the design of single-use dialysers, which made them more durable without losing their ability to do their job. These studies show that combining LCA and eco-design helps people make smart choices, which lets makers reduce the damage they do to the environment over the whole life cycle, make production processes better, and get rid of harmful materials. But issues like pollution from transportation and the need for farming inputs for biopolymers show how important it is to do thorough assessments before putting eco-design ideas into action. All in all, these combined ways give us useful information for making medical equipment that is better for the environment (Hanson & Hitchcock, 2009).

2.4 Other Metrics for Environmental Impact Assessment

2.4.1 Carbon Footprint

The emission of greenhouse gases, which is produced throughout the lifespan of a healthcare product from its extraction, production, transportation, use, and disposal. Various manufacturing units and organisations may determine how these healthcare goods contribute to climate change by measuring emissions and adopting initiatives to reduce the level of carbon footprint by switching to clean techniques of production and streamlining the transportation logistics (Rodríguez-Jiménez et al., 2023).

2.4.2 Energy Consumption

It measures the amount of energy that is required during the production, distribution, and usage of healthcare products. It highlights the importance of the integration of renewable sources of energy in the manufacturing process, which will ultimately improve the efficiency of energy and reduce its consumption, lowering the cost and reducing the impact of fossil fuels on the environment (Bawaneh et al., 2019).

2.4.3 Water Usage

This matrix is used to measure the amount of water used by various manufacturing companies to produce or discard medical products. This matrix carries an importance, especially in those places where water scarcity exists, because the overuse of water can impart stress on the environment, and by measuring the water use, we can also adopt water-saving methods and various technologies to ensure justified use of water sources in a sustainable manner (Dixit & Pradeep Kumar, 2023).

2.4.4 Waste Generation

It indicates the amount of waste and garbage produced throughout the life of a medical device, which includes packaging and end-of-life disposal after a product's useful life. It can be measured by measuring the amount of trash produced. This matrix tells the importance of recycling, reuse, and proper disposal of products with proper waste management to reduce environmental pollution, along with a reduced landfill contribution. We can use environmentally friendly product packaging and biodegradable materials, which are very good alternatives to reduce the garbage output (Eker & Bilgili, 2011).

2.4.5 Toxicity

This matrix is used to analyse the amount of release of various hazardous materials and pollutants during various phases, such as production, use, and disposal of medical goods and services. These contaminants have the potential to impact the ecosystem and human health. By ensuring this matrix, manufacturers or producers can prioritise a safe material and process, ensuring that medical and healthcare products and supplies do not pollute our environment (Brausch & Rand, 2011).

2.4.6 *Resource Depletion*

The usage of non-renewable sources such as raw materials, which are utilised in manufacturing healthcare goods, is measured by resource depletion. To lower the dependence on resources, which are already limited in quantity, this matrix will promote the usage of renewable sources of energy along with sustainable options. Moreover, it will encourage sustainable and circular economic activities such as the reuse, reduction, and recycling of materials and products. (Geissdoerfer et al., 2017).

2.4.7 *Ecological Impact*

The impact on ecology helps in the evaluation of healthcare goods and services, along with their impact on the ecosystem, including biodiversity and habitat loss. This indicator matrix promotes some actions to preserve and build an ecosystem that will guarantee that goods and services do not impact the natural areas. The negative ecological effects of healthcare products can be lowered by decreasing the quantity of pollutants and utilising eco-friendly products and materials, as depicted in Figure 7.1 (Vatovec et al., 2013).

If we take all these matrices together, they all offer a strong foundation for the evaluation of healthcare goods and services affecting the ecosystem. Healthcare

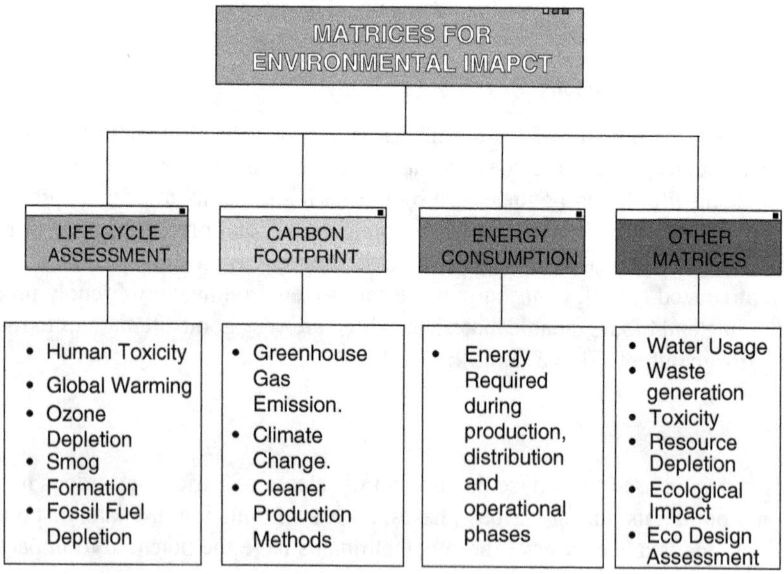

Figure 7.1 Matrices for environmental impact.

companies and factories can reduce their environmental impact, and they can also support worldwide sustainability initiatives by analysing these factors when making any choice (McGinnis et al., 2021).

3 Environmental Performance Benchmarks

Benchmarks and indicators are useful in the measurement of environmental performance at the hospital level. They are commonly known as measurable standards or reference points, which are useful in the evaluation and comparison of environmental impact along with sustainable efforts in healthcare operations. They help various healthcare settings to assess their ongoing performance, set goals and targets and track progress towards an improved environmental impact and practices (Hensher & McGain, 2020).

3.1 Global Reporting Initiative Dimensions

The Global Reporting Initiative (GRI) elements give us a basic way to judge how well hospitals take care of the world (Ortiz & Marin, 2014). It includes many things, like keeping an eye on both dangerous and non-dangerous items that are used in hospitals. Looking at how much energy is being used and putting plans in place to lower that use. Evaluate how water is used and make sure it is managed in a way that is viable. Protecting and restoring ecosystems that have been damaged by hospital operations. Putting limits on solid trash, liquid discharges, and air emissions can help protect the environment. Looking at how the products and services that healthcare organisations offer affect the environment. Making sure that environmental laws and rules are followed (McGlynn, 1997). Getting transportation processes to leave less of an environmental impact. Judging sellers based on how environmentally friendly they are. Putting in place ways for people to report environmental problems (Bradley et al., 2009).

3.2 Legal Compliance

It is important for Indian hospitals to follow the Biological Waste Management Rules, 2016, so that biological waste is handled, treated, and thrown away safely. The State Pollution Control Board (SPCB) or the Pollution Control Committee (PCC) must give permission to all healthcare facilities (HCFS), such as hospitals, clinics, blood banks, labs, and animal hospitals. When it comes to bedded hazardous chemical facilities (HCFS), approvals are good for as long as the Water Act of 1974 and the Air Act of 1981 allow them to be. However, non-bedded HCFS only needs a one-time authorisation. The SPCB or PCC must permit healthcare centres in rural or remote areas that want to use deep burial pits. Regulations say that pharmaceutical waste has to be put into colour-coded groups at the source (yellow, red, white, and blue), and businesses that are within 75 km of a Common Biomedical Waste Treatment Facility (CBWTF) have to take their trash to the CBWTF. With the SPCB/PCC's permission, facilities outside of this area may set up captive treatment facilities. Waste must be kept in certain places so that it does not get stolen, spread out, or contaminated by animals. All trash bags or bins must have barcoded labels on them so that they can be tracked.

Hospitals must send an annual report to SPCB/PCC by June 30 each year, including waste creation, treatment, disposal, training, accidents, and compliance. Spills, fires, and other major incidents must be reported to the SPCB or PCC within 24 hours. However, smaller incidents, like needle stick injuries, should be recorded privately. Anything that goes wrong with garbage pickup or storage for more than 48 hours needs to be recorded. To make sure workers are safe on the job, hospitals must do yearly health checks on people who handle biological waste, vaccinate them against Hepatitis B and Tetanus, and make sure they have enough personal protective equipment (PPE). All employees must go through training in how to handle biological waste when they first start working there and every year after that. Records of this training are kept and included with the yearly report (Singh et al., 2017).

Hospitals with 30 beds or more must set up a biomedical waste management committee to make sure they follow the rules. Smaller hospitals must hire a supervisor. The state of permissions, the amount of waste made per bed, incidents, and training completed are all things that are monitored. Under the Environment Protection Act, 1986, not following the rules could lead to legal consequences such as stopping activities, fines of up to ₹1 lakh, or jail time. Hospitals must follow these rules to stay out of trouble with the law, protect public health, and protect the earth (Pandey et al., 2016).

3.3 Indicators

These are metrics that can be used to measure how well the world is doing. Indicators help organisations keep track of their progress towards their goals by giving them data-driven insights for strategic planning and operational improvements, making more people aware of environmental problems, and comparing their performance to industry standards (*Prepare for EU Sustainability | Reporting CSRD Readiness*, n.d.). Examples include the following:

3.3.1 Quantitative Metrics

These matrices are used globally to benchmark a healthcare facility's efficiency in management and reduction of waste generation. A large proportion of waste comes from the single-use MDs, disposable kits and packaging. Monitoring this statistic metric can closely connect operational procedures to resource conservation by giving initiatives like waste segregation training and surgical product reprocessing a measurable goal. It also includes a matrix for tracing low-value and high-volume single-use plastic consumables. Examples include kilograms of solid waste generated per patient bed/day and monthly usage of plastic cups and office supplies (Cheng et al., 2009).

3.3.2 Strategic Indicators

It includes two matrices. The reduction in energy consumption (10% reduction goal) and the reduction in material usage (20% reduction goal). The first metric monitors a facility's progress in lowering its energy consumption, which is a major contributor to Scope 1 and Scope 2 GHG emissions in the healthcare industry. It is strategic since it calls for long-term planning and financial commitment (e.g. transitioning to renewable energy sources, improving heating, ventilation and air conditioning (HVAC) systems, and designing green buildings). Although it doesn't specifically address specific medical items, cutting back on consumption frees up funds that may be wisely allocated towards purchasing more costly but ecologically friendly green medical products (such as locally grown vegetables or solar-powered diagnostic equipment). The second metric tackles the significant environmental effect ingrained in the supply chain by concentrating on reducing the overall amount of items consumed (Scope 3). This is accomplished for medical items by focusing on "dematerialisation" and moving away from a linear consumption model towards a circular one. This involves requiring suppliers to decrease packaging (source reduction) and putting in place reprocessing procedures for single-use gadgets. The organisation is forced to thoroughly examine its whole procurement and usage lifecycle when it sets a percentage reduction objective for materials (Li et al., 2024).

3.3.3 Monitoring Indicators

Measurability, validity, and controllability of actions taken to achieve goals (Tawfik-Shukor et al., 2007). In the context of this chapter, measurability refers to the requirements that the metrics selected be measurable, readily obtainable, and reliably reported over an extended period of time. This entails putting in place a dependable mechanism (such as IT-based logging or scheduled manual weighing) to record information on medical goods and waste, such as the number of MDIs prescribed, the kilogrammes of trash produced, or the kW/h (kilowatt per hour) of energy used. Measurability guarantees that advancement may be impartially monitored in relation to a reference point. The degree to which the measure faithfully captures the desired result or strategic objective is known as validity. Since it targets the specific environmental stressor, measuring the volume of high global warming potential (GWP) anaesthetic gases used is a more valid measure of climate impact than simply counting the number of surgeries performed. This is an example of how a valid metric for healthcare sustainability should capture the intended environmental impact. Controllability indicates that the organisation has the direct power, means, and sway to change the indicator's result. When it comes to medicinal items, the health system has direct control over the packaging (PCR content) and building energy efficiency (a strategic indicator). However, they solely affect emissions from patient transport. Controllability is essential for establishing attainable, responsible goals (Saviano et al., 2018).

3.3.4 Operational Indicators

These indicators include existence of revised standard operating procedures (SOPs) and number of training sessions conducted for staff. The official control system that incorporates sustainability into routine clinical and logistical tasks is

SOPs. Regarding medical items, updated SOPs guarantee proper, required procedures such as using reusable or reprocessed medical equipment, properly disposing of sharps to avoid needlestick accidents, and separating regulated medical waste (RMW) from municipal garbage. Their presence offers an auditable compliance standard and communicates institutional commitment (Garg, 2023). Number of training sessions conducted for staff: Since the majority of healthcare waste is generated at the moment of patient care, this statistic is crucial for staff capacity and cultural change. Training guarantees that employees understand how to use the new sustainable SOPs, such as recognising recyclable product packaging or prescribing a lower-carbon alternative. The best sustainability policies fall short at the bedside without training (Barakat et al., 2023).

3.4 Best Practices

Best practices identified in the study include the following:

- **Environmental Training Plans**: Training staff on sustainable practices and waste management.
- **Internal Communication Systems**: Establishing systems to share environmental goals and progress.
- **Hospital Sanitisation Procedures**: Standardising cleaning and disinfection processes to improve environmental performance.
- **Sustainable Food Purchasing**: Procuring healthy and sustainably grown food as part of the "Green Hospitals Agenda."
- **Waste Management Initiatives**: Implementing plans to handle, sort, and dispose of healthcare waste effectively. (Pasqualini Blass et al., 2017).

4 Innovations and Stakeholder Dynamics in Sustainable Product Development

4.1 Precycling Strategies

For the healthcare industry, where a lot of throwaway items are used every day, lowering trash production before it happens is especially important. For instance, switching from things to single-use items. For instance, hospitals can switch from single-use items like plastic needles and some gloves to others that can be used more than once and to environmentally friendly products. Prior to recycling, things with minimal packaging are designed, and recycled or biodegradable materials are used in medicines and health products. This method not only has less of an impact on the environment, but it also pays less for managing waste (Kaewunruen et al., 2020).

4.2 Dematerialisation

It includes cutting down on the amount of real materials used in the health business while still keeping them useful and functional. Patients can check on their health online thanks to improvements in smart tech and telemedicine. This means they will not have to go to a healthcare centre as often. (Merchant et al., 2015). In the same way, using digital healthcare data will get rid of the need for paper-based systems, which saves time and money. Dematerialisation also applies to medical tools, where small and light designs use less material and cost less to ship.

4.2.1 Circular Economy

In a circular economy plan, waste is turned into resources by creating a closed-loop system that has less of an effect on the environment. In the healthcare business, this means using used and recycled products and turning old things into new ones (Steward, 2012). Some surgery tools, for instance, can be cleaned and fixed up so they can be used again, and pharmaceutical waste can be processed to get rid of the useful chemicals. This way cuts down on waste, costs less, and encourages the smart use of resources.

4.2.2 Climate-Smart Healthcare

It uses a mix of methods to lessen the effects of climate change on the healthcare industry. To do this, we need to use technologies that use less energy, energy that comes from green sources, and make MDs that use fewer resources and cause less damage to the world. For example, installing solar cells to cut down on fossil fuel use, using lightning systems, and developing technologies that save water. Making healthcare products and services with low carbon input is also part of it.

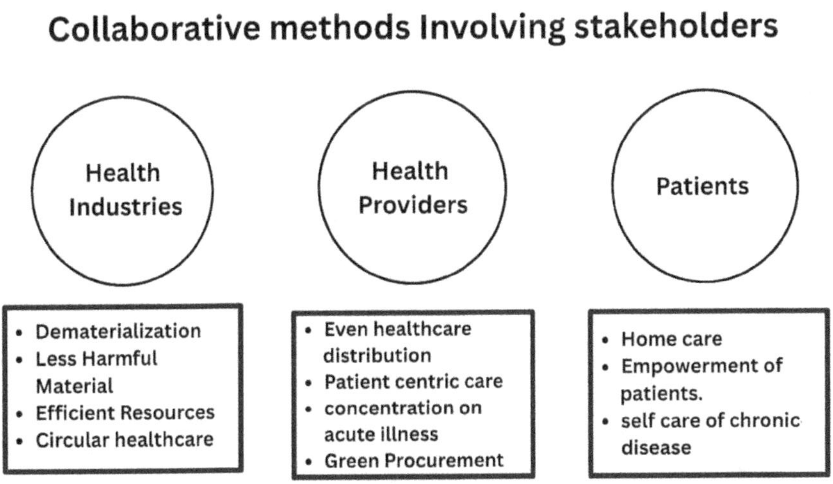

Figure 7.2 Collaborative methods involving stakeholders for the identification of best practices.

4.2.3 Stakeholder Dynamics

An open method is built into sustainable healthcare when new ideas and community interactions come together. Distributed healthcare systems are one example. Telehealth and smart devices are two new technologies that have made it possible for healthcare to move from hospital-based models to distributed systems, where care is given in people's own homes or nearby. This makes people stronger and lessens the damage that fixed services do to the world. Dynamic Supply Chains: Groups working together make better use of resources and less waste, and the principles of the circular economy make sure that things are reused or returned. Collaboration across sectors: Forums and shared areas allow partners to work together to come up with solutions, making sure that ideas fit the needs of the healthcare system and its users (Pereno & Eriksson, 2020). Different collaborative methods have been displayed in Figure 7.2.

5 Recent Trends and Strategic Outcomes

Recent trends and strategic outcomes after implementing sustainable practices in the healthcare industry and other products show a strong move towards reducing environmental impact, primarily focusing on decarbonisation, the circular economy, and green innovation. The strategic implementation programme of sustainable practices is rapidly evolving, driven by consumer demand, regulatory pressure, and the recognition of long-term cost benefits. This is resulting in tangible reductions in the environmental impact across various sectors, particularly healthcare and consumer products.

5.1 Recent Trends in Sustainable Implementation

Recent trends emphasise holistic, data-driven, and circular approaches to sustainability:

- Circular Economy Integration: A big change from the "take-make-dispose" approach to one that puts more emphasis on making goods and materials last longer, be reused, be fixed up, and be recycled. This is becoming an important part of cutting down on trash and raw material use (Ghisellini et al., 2016).
- Decarbonisation of Supply Chains (Scope 3 Focus): Companies are paying more attention to Scope 3 emissions, which are secondary emissions from the value chain, such as producers and the use and disposal of products. These emissions often make up the biggest part of a company's carbon footprint. This is making sellers work together on projects like renewable energy, improving transportation, and environmentally friendly buying.
- Green Procurement and Standards: Buying teams are taking environmental factors into account when making decisions, especially in healthcare. Regulatory bodies and medical groups are changing treatment standards to support options that are better for the environment (Perry, 2023).
- Digital Traceability and Transparency: Technologies like AI, IoT, and blockchain are being used to make it possible to see the environmental and social

effects of goods from where the raw materials come from to who uses them, which helps stop "greenwashing" (Rejeb & Rejeb, 2020).

5.2 Current Outcomes and Examples

5.2.1 Healthcare Sector

The healthcare sector, a significant contributor to global carbon emissions, is seeing targeted interventions yield measurable environmental and operational benefits (Table 7.1).

5.2.2 Other Products (Consumer Goods and Manufacturing)

Sustainable practices in manufacturing and consumer goods are shifting from simple compliance to a source of **competitive advantage**, with positive impacts on resource use and customer loyalty (Table 7.2).

6 Current Global Perspective on Environmental Impact Assessment

The recent global perspective on the requirement of implementation and assessment of the environmental impact of healthcare and other products is considered one of the urgent steps. It requires regulatory integration, which is driven by recognition of some severe consequences of healthcare products on planetary and human health.

6.1 Global Perspectives on Environmental Impact Assessment

The necessity for rigorous environmental impact assessment (EIA), particularly for products, stems from several critical global realities:

- **Significant Sectoral Footprint:** Important Sectoral Footprint: The healthcare business is known all over the world for polluting the environment; its actions are to blame for 5.2% of all greenhouse gas (GHG) pollution. This number can go up to 10% in countries with lots of money. This effect includes more than just carbon. It also includes air pollution like sulphur dioxide and nitrogen fumes, water use, and the production of a lot of medical waste. Making and throwing away things is a big part of the healthcare supply chain, which has a world effect of 60–70% (Karliner et al., 2020; Lenzen et al., 2020).
- **Mitigation of Health Risks:** It's a vicious cycle: Pollution and climate change make people's health worse, which means more people need medical care, which causes even more emissions. This is why it is socially and strategically important to test and lessen the effects of goods to cut down on direct health risks like breathing problems, heart diseases, and the spread of infectious diseases (Romanello et al., 2024).

Table 7.1 Impactful sustainable practices with their outcomes and examples in healthcare settings

S. No.	*Sustainable Practice*	*Current Outcomes and Environmental Impact Reduction*	*Examples*	*Source*
1	Anaesthetic gas reduction	A big drop in greenhouse gas (GHG) pollution; desflurane, which is a strong GHG, is being taken out	The English National Health Service (NHS) promised to shut down desflurane and replace it with options that are lower in global warming potential. This will greatly reduce the NHS's total carbon footprint	Moonesinghe (2024)
2	Waste management and circularity	A smaller amount of trash going to dumps; resource saving. Getting rid of trash lowers operating costs	Through strong recycling and composting programmes, Kaiser Permanente (USA) was able to keep a lot of trash out of landfills. Single-use medical devices (SUDs) are being reprocessed, which means that fewer new devices are being made	C. Thiel et al. (2025)
3	Energy efficiency and renewables	Less reliance on fossil fuels and less energy use, which lowers carbon pollution and running costs	As a result of adding solar panels, HVAC systems that use less energy, and LED lights, hospitals are saving a lot of energy. Some hospitals have set goals to get all of their energy from clean sources	C. Thiel et al. (2025)
4	Sustainable prescribing	Lowering the carbon impact of pharmaceuticals and improving patient health through better control of medications	When it makes practical sense, dry powder inhalers (DPIs) or soft mist inhalers (SMIs) should be preferred over metered dose inhalers (MDIs) that use high global warming potential propellants (HFCs)	Maughan et al. (2016)

Table 7.2 Impactful sustainable practices with their outcomes and examples in other technical sectors

S. No.	*Sustainable Practice*	*Current Outcomes and Environmental Impact Reduction*	*Examples*	*Sources*
1	Eco-design and manufacturing	Less loss of materials and energy during production; it's easier to fix things and recover them. Not as much use of new materials	Companies that make clothes are using recovered plastic bottles or materials like organic cotton to make their clothes. The "Made to be Remade" idea tells designers how to make products that last and can be used again and again	Geissdoerfer et al. (2017)
2	Sustainable packaging	Less plastic trash, especially single-use plastics, and lower emissions from shipping because the materials are lighter	Companies are switching their packing materials to ones that are simple, biodegradable, or made from 100% post-consumer recycled (PCR) materials. This cuts down on pollutants and trash going to landfills	Yuen et al. (2025)
3	Green logistics and supply chain	Transportation and storage pollution will go down, and the supply chain will be more resilient	Brands are investing in electric or low-emission car fleets for "last-mile" transport, optimising delivery routes and combining shipments to cut down on greenhouse gas emissions	McKinnon et al. (2015)
4	Product-as-a-service (PaaS) models	Products last longer, don't need to be made as often, and there is less trash	To keep gadgets in use longer and make sure they are properly disposed of at the end of their useful lives, tech and electronics companies are giving repair programmes, take-back plans, and subscription services (leasing instead of buying)	Hidalgo-Crespo et al. (2024)

- **Regulatory Integration and Standards**: Environmental duty is being asked for more and more by global regulators all the way through the life of a product. The Circular Economy Action Plan and REACH rules for chemicals in the European Union (EU) push companies to make products that last longer, can be recovered, and have fewer dangerous materials in them (eco-design). Extended Producer Responsibility (EPR) programmes also make businesses answerable for how their products are thrown away and remade. Companies can report on their environmental impact in a way that is dependable and easy to compare thanks to international standards such as ISO 14040/44 for LCA and the GRI Standards (Losa, 2025) (*ISO 14040:2006 – Environmental Management – Life Cycle Assessment – Principles and Framework*, n.d.).
- **Shift to Proactive Assessment:** LCA methods that look ahead are being used more and more to find "hot spots" and help with design before a product even comes out on the market. More and more, Health Technology Assessment (HTA) is being used to check new technologies for harms to the environment, such as gases with a high GWP or parts that are harmful to the environment, such as diclofenac. This makes sure that the safety of the patient, the cost, and the value to the world are all thought about (McGinnis et al., 2021).
- **Health and Environmental Feedback Loop:** People who work in workplaces or use a lot of energy pollute the air, and natural stresses like not having enough water can also make people sick. These stresses can cause heart disease, stroke, and breathing problems. As more people get sick, health services are put under more stress. This makes the surroundings worse and people's health worse (Watts et al., 2018).
- **Integration with Decision-Making:** It's getting more and more important for big businesses to take steps to protect the environment. Its main goal is to look at things that are harmful on their own, such as drugs like diclofenac that are ecotoxic or numbing gases with a high GWP. This protects both the safety of the patients and the value of the surroundings. Also, more than 80 countries have said they will build health systems that can react to climate change and don't use a lot of carbon (Pinho-Gomes et al., 2022).

6.2 Case Studies

The key environmental outcome/metric is discussed in Table 7.3.

7 Challenges and Opportunities

While these innovations and dynamics offer significant benefits, they also face some challenges.

7.1 Challenges

Fragmentation: The healthcare field is characterised by numerous "silos" that hinder communication and collaboration among individuals. To break down these silos, we need new ways of organising things and tools that everyone can use together.

Regulatory Barriers: Laws need to be changed for environmentally friendly practices to be put into place, which can take time and be hard to understand. Policymakers need to find a mix between short-term economic worries and long-term goals that will be sustainable (Geels, 2005).

Resource Constraints: Creating and expanding sustainable solutions often needs a lot of money, which can be hard to get. Stakeholders need to work together to find ways to fund and promote projects that are good for the environment.

Knowledge Gaps: A lot of people do not know about or have the skills to use sustainable healthcare methods. To build skills and bring about change, education

Table 7.3 Case study with initiatives taken in the healthcare sector along with assessment area and key focus

S. No.	*Initiative*	*Organisation/ Industry*	*Assessment Focus*	*Key Environmental Outcome/Metric*	*Source*
1	BD ecoFinity® life cycle solution	Becton Dickinson (Acute Care/ medical)	Single-use medical sharps disposal	Provides an environmentally preferable disposal solution for single-use medical sharps, reducing the environmental impact of medication delivery	Clark et al. (2022)
2	Green chemistry packaging (nPulp)	YFY Group (China/ packaging)	Paper packaging production	Utilises a bio-based pulp product (nPulp) from straw waste, which addresses air pollution by finding an alternative to burning crop residue	Bajpai (2015)
3	Suction waste management	Serres (Healthcare products)	Suction bag disposal	Their Nemo system allows hospitals to save up to 97% CO_2 from waste transportation to incineration for suction bags	Webb (2024)

and training programmes are important. Even with these problems, the move to sustainable healthcare opens up a lot of doors (Chiarini & Vagnoni, 2016).

Cost Savings: Sustainable habits like using less energy and throwing away less trash can help healthcare workers lower their costs.

7.2 Opportunities

7.2.1 Improved Patient Outcomes

People can take charge of their own health with patient-centred care methods, which leads to better outcomes and fewer hospital stays (Karamat et al., 2019).

Environmental Benefits: Getting healthcare products and services to use less carbon helps protect the earth and slow down climate change.

Innovation and Growth: Sustainable healthcare leads to improvements in drugs, medical tools, and clean energy, which opens up new markets and business opportunities.

Stakeholders can work together to make a healthcare system that is physically, socially, and economically sustainable by promoting teamwork, driving innovation, and building understanding. This complete method makes sure that healthcare systems are strong, flexible, and able to meet the needs of people in the future (Charlesworth & Jamieson, 2019).

8 Conclusion

In conclusion, figuring out how healthcare products affect the environment is an important part of both sustainable healthcare methods and protecting the environment. Metrics like LCA, eco-design studies, and the combination of both LCA and eco-design methods give us a lot of information about how MDs affect the environment. This information helps us make smart decisions and create products that will last. Along with other important indicators like carbon footprint, energy consumption, water usage, waste generation, toxicity, resource depletion, and ecological impact, these metrics are a big part of figuring out how harmful healthcare products are to the environment and how to make sure that operations are done responsibly. Also, environmental performance benchmarks like the GRI dimensions, legal compliance, and indicators make it possible to measure and improve healthcare operations' environmental impact and efforts to be more sustainable. This encourages a culture of accountability and constant improvement. Also, new ideas in environmentally friendly product development like precycling, dematerialisation, the circular economy, and climate-smart healthcare offer big chances to lower the healthcare industry's environmental impact and encourage eco-friendly practices. To fully integrate sustainable healthcare practices and make sure they are widely used, it is important to deal with problems like fragmentation, regulatory barriers, limited resources, and information gaps. Stakeholders can overcome these problems by working together and coming up with new ideas for sustainable healthcare. This will save money, help patients, be better for the environment, and lead to general growth, which will ensure a strong and long-lasting healthcare system in the future.

References

Bajpai, P. (2015, June 23). Green chemistry and sustainability in pulp and paper industry. *Green Chemistry and Sustainability in Pulp and Paper Industry*, (pp-65–84). Cham: Springer International Publishing; 2015 Jun 23. https://doi.org/10.1007/978-3-319-18744-0

Barakat, B., Milhem, M., Naji, G. M. A., Alzoraiki, M., Muda, H. B., Ateeq, A., & Abro, Z. (2023). Assessing the impact of green training on sustainable business advantage: Exploring the mediating role of green supply chain practices. *Sustainability 2023, 15*(19), 14144. https://doi.org/10.3390/SU151914144

Bawaneh, K., Nezami, F. G., Rasheduzzaman, M., & Deken, B. (2019). Energy consumption analysis and characterization of healthcare facilities in the United States. *Energies 2019, 12*(19), 3775. https://doi.org/10.3390/EN12193775

Bocken, N. M. P., de Pauw, I., Bakker, C., & van der Grinten, B. (2016). Product design and business model strategies for a circular economy. *Journal of Industrial and Production Engineering, 33*(5), 308–320. https://doi.org/10.1080/21681015.2016.1172124

Bradley, E. H., Curry, L. A., Ramanadhan, S., Rowe, L., Nembhard, I. M., & Krumholz, H. M. (2009). Research in action: Using positive deviance to improve quality of health care. *Implementation Science : IS, 4*(1). https://doi.org/10.1186/1748-5908-4-25

Brausch, J. M., & Rand, G. M. (2011). A review of personal care products in the aquatic environment: Environmental concentrations and toxicity. *Chemosphere, 82*(11), 1518–1532. https://doi.org/10.1016/J.CHEMOSPHERE.2010.11.018

Campion, N., Thiel, C. L., Woods, N. C., Swanzy, L., Landis, A. E., & Bilec, M. M. (2015). Sustainable healthcare and environmental life-cycle impacts of disposable supplies: A focus on disposable custom packs. *Journal of Cleaner Production, 94*, 46–55. https://doi.org/10.1016/J.JCLEPRO.2015.01.076

Charlesworth, K. E., & Jamieson, M. (2019). Healthcare in a carbon-constrained world. *Australian Health Review : A Publication of the Australian Hospital Association, 43*(3), 241–245. https://doi.org/10.1071/AH17184

Cheng, Y. W., Sung, F. C., Yang, Y., Lo, Y. H., Chung, Y. T., & Li, K. C. (2009). Medical waste production at hospitals and associated factors. *Waste Management (New York, N.Y.), 29*(1), 440–444. https://doi.org/10.1016/J.WASMAN.2008.01.014

Chiarini, A., & Vagnoni, E. (2016). Environmental sustainability in European public healthcare. *Leadership in Health Services (Bradford, England), 29*(1), 2–8. https://doi.org/10.1108/LHS-10-2015-0035

Clark, J., Fera, T., Fortier, C., Gullickson, K., Hays, A., Murdaugh, L., Ogden, R., O'Neal, B., Rush, J., & Vest, T. (2022). ASHP guidelines on preventing diversion of controlled substances. *American Journal of Health-System Pharmacy : AJHP : Official Journal of the American Society of Health-System Pharmacists, 79*(24), 2279–2306. https://doi.org/10.1093/AJHP/ZXAC246

Dixit, M. K., & Pradeep Kumar, P. (2023). Analyzing water use embodied in the initial construction and life cycle management of healthcare facilities. *IOP Conference Series: Earth and Environmental Science, 1176*(1). https://doi.org/10.1088/1755-1315/1176/1/012011

Dluhy, M., & Swartz, N. (2006). Connecting knowledge and policy: The promise of community indicators in the United States. *Social Indicators Research, 79*(1), 1–23. https://doi.org/10.1007/s11205-005-3486-2

Eckelman, M. J., & Sherman, J. (2016). Environmental impacts of the U.S. Health care system and effects on public health. *PLOS ONE, 11*(6), e0157014. https://doi.org/10.1371/journal.pone.0157014

Eker, H. H., & Bilgili, M. S. (2011). Statistical analysis of waste generation in healthcare services: A case study. *Waste Management & Research : The Journal of the International*

Solid Wastes and Public Cleansing Association, ISWA, *29*(8), 791–796. https://doi.org/10.1177/0734242X10396755

Environmental health indicators: Framework and methodologies. (n.d.). Retrieved October 8, 2025, from https://www.who.int/publications/i/item/WHO-SDE-OEH-99.10

Gabriel, C. A., Bortsie-Aryee, N. A., Apparicio-Farrell, N., & Farrell, E. (2009). How supply chain choices affect the life cycle impacts of medical products. *Journal of Cleaner Production, 182*, 1095–1106. https://doi.org/10.1016/J.JCLEPRO.2018.02.107

Garg, A. (2023). *Monitoring Tools for Setting up the Hospital Project: Initial Planning, Building and Equipment*, 1–622. Springer Nature 2023. https://doi.org/10.1007/978-981-99-6663-9

Gavilán-García, I. C., Fernández-Villagomez, G., Gavilán-García, A., & Alcántara-Concepcion, V. (2015). Alternatives of management and disposal for mercury thermometers at the end of their life from Mexican health care institutions. *Journal of Cleaner Production, 86*, 118–124. https://doi.org/10.1016/j.jclepro.2014.08.013

Geels, F. (2005). Co-evolution of technology and society: The transition in water supply and personal hygiene in the Netherlands (1850–1930) - A case study in multi-level perspective. *Technology in Society*, *27*(3), 363–397. https://doi.org/10.1016/J.TECHSOC.2005.04.008

Geissdoerfer, M., Savaget, P., Bocken, N. M. P., & Hultink, E. J. (2017). The circular economy – A new sustainability paradigm? *Journal of Cleaner Production, 143*, 757–768. https://doi.org/10.1016/J.JCLEPRO.2016.12.048

Ghisellini, P., Cialani, C., & Ulgiati, S. (2016). A review on circular economy: The expected transition to a balanced interplay of environmental and economic systems. *Journal of Cleaner Production, 114*, 11–32. https://doi.org/10.1016/J.JCLEPRO.2015.09.007

Hancock, T., Labonte, R., & Edwards, R. (1999). Indicators that count! Measuring population health at the community level. *Canadian Journal of Public Health = Revue Canadienne de Santé Publique*, *90*(Suppl 1), S22. https://doi.org/10.1007/BF03403574

Hanson, J. J., & Hitchcock, R. W. (2009). Towards sustainable design for single-use medical devices. *Annual International Conference of the IEEE Engineering in Medicine and Biology Society. IEEE Engineering in Medicine and Biology Society. Annual International Conference, 2009*, 5602–5605. https://doi.org/10.1109/IEMBS.2009.5333495

Hensher, M., & McGain, F. (2020). Health care sustainability metrics: Building a safer, low-carbon health system. *Health Affairs (Project Hope)*, *39*(12), 2080–2087. https://doi.org/10.1377/HLTHAFF.2020.01103

Hidalgo-Crespo, J., Riel, A., Golinska-Dawson, P., Peeters, J. R., Werner-Lewandowska, K., & Duflou, J. R. (2024). Facilitating circularity: Challenges and design guidelines of Product-as-a-Service (PaaS) business model offers for electrical and electronic equipment. *Procedia CIRP*, *128*, 567–572. https://doi.org/10.1016/J.PROCIR.2024.03.037

ISO 14040:2006 - Environmental management — Life cycle assessment — Principles and framework. (n.d.). Retrieved October 8, 2025, from https://www.iso.org/standard/37456.html

Jakubowski, B., & Frumkin, H. (2010). Environmental metrics for community health improvement. *Preventing Chronic Disease*, *7*(4), A76.

Jones, P. H., & Halamka, J. D. (2013). *Design for Care : Innovating Health Care Experience*. Rosenfeld Media.

Kaewunruen, S., Sresakoolchai, J., & Zhou, Z. (2020). Sustainability-based lifecycle management for bridge infrastructure using 6D BIM. *Sustainability 2020, 12*(6), 2436. https://doi.org/10.3390/SU12062436

Karamat, J., Shurong, T., Ahmad, N., Afridi, S., Khan, S., & Khan, N. (2019). Developing sustainable healthcare systems in developing countries: Examining the role of barriers, enablers and drivers on knowledge management adoption. *Sustainability 2019, 11*(4), 954. https://doi.org/10.3390/SU11040954

Karliner, J., Slotterback, S., Boyd, R., Ashby, B., Steele, K., & Wang, J. (2020). Health care's climate footprint: The health sector contribution and opportunities for action. *European Journal of Public Health, 30*(Supplement_5). https://doi.org/10.1093/EURPUB/CKAA165.843

L, G., & CM, C. (2004). Environmental health indicators: Bridging the Chasm of public health and the environment. *Environmental Health Indicators*. https://doi.org/10.17226/11136

Lenzen, M., Malik, A., Li, M., Fry, J., Weisz, H., Pichler, P. P., Chaves, L. S. M., Capon, A., & Pencheon, D. (2020). The environmental footprint of health care: A global assessment. *The Lancet. Planetary Health, 4*(7), e271–e279. https://doi.org/10.1016/S2542-5196(20)30121-2

Li, N., Dong, Y., & Zhang, G. (2024). County-level integrated healthcare practice in China: A Kaiser permanente-inspired approach. *International Journal of Integrated Care, 24*(4). https://doi.org/10.5334/IJIC.8610

Losa, R. (2025). Public policies on circular economy: A systematic review. *Ecological Economics, 228*, 108452. https://doi.org/10.1016/J.ECOLECON.2024.108452

Maughan, D. L., Patel, A., Parveen, T., Braithwaite, I., Cook, J., Lillywhite, R., & Cooke, M. (2016). Primary-care-based social prescribing for mental health: An analysis of financial and environmental sustainability. *Primary Health Care Research and Development, 17*(2), 114–121. https://doi.org/10.1017/S1463423615000328

McGain, F., Story, D., Lim, T., & McAlister, S. (2017). Financial and environmental costs of reusable and single-use anaesthetic equipment. *British Journal of Anaesthesia, 118*(6), 862–869. https://doi.org/10.1093/BJA/AEX098

McGinnis, S., Johnson-Privitera, C., Nunziato, J. D., & Wohlford, S. (2021). Environmental life cycle assessment in medical practice: A user's guide. *Obstetrical & Gynecological Survey, 76*(7), 417–428. https://doi.org/10.1097/OGX.0000000000000906

McGlynn, E. A. (1997). Six challenges in measuring the quality of health care. *Health Affairs (Project Hope), 16*(3), 7–21. https://doi.org/10.1377/HLTHAFF.16.3.7

McKinnon, A. C., Browne, M., Whiteing, A. E., & Piecyk, M. (2015, Feb 3). *Green Logistics : Improving the Environmental Sustainability of Logistics*. Kogan Page Publishers.

Merchant, K. A. S., Ward, M. M., Mueller, K. J., Rural Health Research & Policy Centers, & Rural Policy Research Institute, R. C. for R. H. P. A. U. of I. C. of P. H. D. of H. M. and P. (2015). Hospital views of factors affecting telemedicine use. *Rural Policy Brief, 2015 5*, 1–4.

Moonesinghe, S. R. (2024). Desflurane decommissioning: More than meets the eye. *Anaesthesia, 79*(3), 237–241. https://doi.org/10.1111/ANAE.16219

Moultrie, J., Sutcliffe, L., & Maier, A. (2015). Exploratory study of the state of environmentally conscious design in the medical device industry. *Journal of Cleaner Production, 108*, 363–376. https://doi.org/10.1016/J.JCLEPRO.2015.06.014

Moultrie, J., Sutcliffe, L., & Maier, A. (2016). A maturity grid assessment tool for environmentally conscious design in the medical device industry. *Journal of Cleaner Production, 122*, 252–265. https://doi.org/10.1016/J.JCLEPRO.2015.10.108

Ortiz, E., & Marin, S. (2014). Global Reporting Initiative (GRI) as recognized guidelines for sustainability reporting by Spanish companies on the IBEX 35: Homogeneity in their framework and added value in the relationship with financial entities. *Intangible Capital, 10*(5). https://doi.org/10.3926/ic.492

Pandey, A., Ahuja, S., Madan, M., & Asthana, A. K. (2016). Bio-medical waste managment in a tertiary care hospital: An overview. *Journal of Clinical and Diagnostic Research : JCDR, 10*(11), DC01–DC03. https://doi.org/10.7860/JCDR/2016/22595.8822

Pasqualini Blass, A., da Costa, S. E. G., de Lima, E. P., & Borges, L. A. (2017). Measuring environmental performance in hospitals: A practical approach. *Journal of Cleaner Production, 142*, 279–289. https://doi.org/10.1016/J.JCLEPRO.2016.07.213

(PDF) Life Cycle Management: A Bridge to More Sustainable Products. (n.d.). Retrieved October 8, 2025, from https://www.researchgate.net/publication/237254414_Life_Cycle_Management_A_Bridge_to_More_Sustainable_Products

Pereno, A., & Eriksson, D. (2020). A multi-stakeholder perspective on sustainable healthcare: From 2030 onwards. *Futures, 122*. https://doi.org/10.1016/J.FUTURES.2020.102605

Perry, T. (2023). Reducing the adverse environmental impacts of prescribing. *Therapeutics Letter*. https://www.ncbi.nlm.nih.gov/books/NBK608179/

Pichler, P.-P., Jaccard, I. S., Weisz, U., & Weisz, H. (2019). International comparison of health care carbon footprints. *Environmental Research Letters, 14*(6), 064004. https://doi.org/10.1088/1748-9326/ab19e1

Pinho-Gomes, A. C., Yoo, S. H., Allen, A., Maiden, H., Shah, K., & Toolan, M. (2022). Incorporating environmental and sustainability considerations into health technology assessment and clinical and public health guidelines: A scoping review. *International Journal of Technology Assessment in Health Care, 38*(1). https://doi.org/10.1017/S0266462322003282

Prepare for EU Sustainability | Reporting CSRD Readiness. (n.d.). Retrieved October 7, 2025, from https://www.csrdreadiness.com/?utm_term=sustainability%20reporting%20directive&utm_campaign=Website+traffic-Search-csrdreadiness-1&utm_source=adwords&utm_medium=ppc&hsa_acc=8049917490&hsa_cam=21799253197&hsa_grp=174334210531&hsa_ad=716504436475&hsa_src=g&hsa_tgt=kwd-1418806075643&hsa_kw=sustainability%20reporting%20directive&hsa_mt=p&hsa_net=adwords&hsa_ver=3&gad_source=1&gad_campaignid=21799253197&gbraid=0AAAAAovX5IG4MPatkVotbSzN4jpTEGjXk&gclid=Cj0KCQjw9JLHBhC-ARIsAK4PhcpeLcD304ZCCFqDuYUqJXBD-yzlhMV-6dPNQyLoAUDJ9E3gEskiXK0aAtGrEALw_wcB

Rejeb, A., & Rejeb, K. (2020). Blockchain and supply chain sustainability. *Logforum, 16*(3), 363–372. https://doi.org/10.17270/J.LOG.2020.467

Rodríguez-Jiménez, L., Romero-Martín, M., Spruell, T., Steley, Z., & Gómez-Salgado, J. (2023). The carbon footprint of healthcare settings: A systematic review. *Journal of Advanced Nursing, 79*(8), 2830–2844. https://doi.org/10.1111/JAN.15671

Romanello, M., Walawender, M., Hsu, S. C., Moskeland, A., Palmeiro-Silva, Y., Scamman, D., Ali, Z., Ameli, N., Angelova, D., Ayeb-Karlsson, S., Basart, S., Beagley, J., Beggs, P. J., Blanco-Villafuerte, L., Cai, W., Callaghan, M., Campbell-Lendrum, D., Chambers, J. D., Chicmana-Zapata, V., … Costello, A. (2024). The 2024 report of the Lancet Countdown on health and climate change: Facing record-breaking threats from delayed action. *Lancet (London, England), 404*(10465), 1847. https://doi.org/10.1016/S0140-6736(24)01822-1

Saviano, M., Bassano, C., Piciocchi, P., Di Nauta, P., & Lettieri, M. (2018). Monitoring viability and sustainability in healthcare organizations. *Sustainability 2018, 10*(10), 3548. https://doi.org/10.3390/SU10103548

Sharma, B., Swanton, B., Kuo, J., Sysawang, K., Yagyu, S., Motala, A., Tolentino, D., Meshkati, N., & Hempel, S. (2024). Use of life cycle assessment in the healthcare industry: Environmental impacts and emissions associated with products, processes, and waste. *Use of Life Cycle Assessment in the Healthcare Industry: Environmental Impacts and Emissions Associated with Products, Processes, and Waste*. https://www.ncbi.nlm.nih.gov/sites/books/NBK610172/

Singh, A., Joshi, H. S., Katyal, R., Singh, R., & Singh, H. (2017). Biomedical waste management rules, 2016: A brief review. *International Journal of Advanced and Integrated Medical Sciences*, *2*(4), 201–204. https://doi.org/10.5005/JP-JOURNALS-10050-10107

Steward, F. (2012). Transformative innovation policy to meet the challenge of climate change: Sociotechnical networks aligned with consumption and end-use as new transition arenas for a low-carbon society or green economy. *Technology Analysis and Strategic Management*, *24*(4), 331–343. https://doi.org/10.1080/09537325.2012.663959

Sutcliffe, L. F. R., Maier, A. M., Moultrie, J., & Clarkson, P. J. (2009). Development of a framework for assessing sustainability in new product development. In *DS 58–7: Proceedings of ICED 09, the 17th International Conference on Engineering Design*, Vol. 7, Design for X/Design to X, Palo Alto, CA, USA, 24.-27.08. 2009 (pp. 289–300).

Tawfik-Shukor, A. R., Klazinga, N. S., & Arah, O. A. (2007). Comparing health system performance assessment and management approaches in the Netherlands and Ontario, Canada. *BMC Health Services Research*, *7*. https://doi.org/10.1186/1472-6963-7-25

Thiel, C., Collins, A., & Vukelich, D. (2025). The case for hospitals to boost single-use device reprocessing programs. *NAM Perspectives*, *2025*, 10.31478/202506c. https://doi.org/10.31478/202506C

Thiel, C. L., Eckelman, M., Guido, R., Huddleston, M., Landis, A. E., Sherman, J., Shrake, S. O., Copley-Woods, N., & Bilec, M. M. (2015). Environmental impacts of surgical procedures: Life cycle assessment of hysterectomy in the United States. *Environmental Science & Technology*, *49*(3), 1779–1786. https://doi.org/10.1021/ES504719G

Unger, S., & Landis, A. (2016). Assessing the environmental, human health, and economic impacts of reprocessed medical devices in a Phoenix hospital's supply chain. *Journal of Cleaner Production*, *112*, 1995–2003. https://doi.org/10.1016/J.JCLEPRO.2015.07.144

Unger, S. R., Hottle, T. A., Hobbs, S. R., Thiel, C. L., Campion, N., Bilec, M. M., & Landis, A. E. (2017). Do single-use medical devices containing biopolymers reduce the environmental impacts of surgical procedures compared with their plastic equivalents? *Journal of Health Services Research & Policy*, *22*(4), 218–225. https://doi.org/10.1177/1355819617705683

Vatovec, C., Senier, L., & Bell, M. (2013). An ecological perspective on medical care: Environmental, occupational, and public health impacts of medical supply and pharmaceutical chains. *EcoHealth*, *10*(3), 257–267. https://doi.org/10.1007/S10393-013-0855-1

Watts, N., Amann, M., Arnell, N., Ayeb-Karlsson, S., Belesova, K., Berry, H., Bouley, T., Boykoff, M., Byass, P., Cai, W., Campbell-Lendrum, D., Chambers, J., Daly, M., Dasandi, N., Davies, M., Depoux, A., Dominguez-Salas, P., Drummond, P., Ebi, K. L., … Costello, A. (2018). The 2018 report of the Lancet Countdown on health and climate change: Shaping the health of nations for centuries to come. *The Lancet*, *392*(10163), 2479–2514. https://doi.org/10.1016/S0140-6736(18)32594-7

Webb, C. M. J. (2024). *Sustainable solutions for respiratory and airway biomedical devices*. https://bura.brunel.ac.uk/handle/2438/29285

Yuen, C. B., Chong, H. L., Kwok, M. H., & Ngai, T. (2025). Natural polymer-based food packaging: Paving the way to a greener future – a review. *Sustainable Food Technology*, *3*(4), 908–929. https://doi.org/10.1039/D5FB00021A

8 Policy Guidelines for Sustainable Practices Regarding Biomedical Waste Management and Emissions

Vikas Sharma, Shikha Aggarwal, Anil Kumar, Parul Sood, and Gagandeep Kaur

1 Background

Medical waste, also known as healthcare waste, is defined by the World Health Organization (WHO) as any form of waste generated by healthcare facilities (HCFs) and used in diagnosis, treatment, or vaccination. This includes items such as used syringes, needles, metal sharps, dressings, blood samples, body parts, pharmaceutical, chemical, radioactive, and device materials (Ananth et al., 2010). Medical waste poses a significant risk to both human and environmental health if not properly treated. Poor waste management leads to a variety of problems, such as injuries from sharp equipment, infectious agent-related illnesses in humans, and chemical contamination of the environment (Ghanimeh et al., 2019). The United States generates more than 3.5 million metric tonnes of medical waste annually, with a disposal cost of $790 per metric tonne, making it the leading nation in the world in this regard (Lee et al., 2004). In the late 1970s, syringes, bandages, and other medical garbage began to wash up on the eastern coast of the United States, marking the beginning of a distinct category of medical waste within the municipal waste stream. After much public pressure, the United States Medical Waste Tracking Act (MWTA) was drafted and came into effect on November 1, 1988. HCFs initially installed 6,500 small, unregulated medical waste incinerators on-site as a response to this problem. It wasn't long before it became clear that these little burners were a bigger pollution problem than medical waste alone and that they also gave people carte blanche to produce ever-increasing amounts of trash, much of which was single-use plastic (Das et al., 2025). According to WHO (1999), healthcare waste might be solid, liquid, or gaseous and may be contaminated by organic and inorganic substances, including pathogenic microorganisms and radionuclides produced from in vitro studies. The tissues and fluids found in hospital trash are quite dangerous. About 85% of hospital waste, public and airborne, is not harmful to health workers; 10% is infectious; and 5% is posed by non-infectious but toxic flora in the environment (WHO, 1999).

2 Introduction

Medical waste in hospitals refers to products generated during patient diagnosis, treatment, immunization, and biological research (Rutala & Weber, 2014).

DOI:10.4324/9781003640486-8

Hospitals, research centres, healthcare education programmes, clinics, labs, blood banks, animal homes and veterinary colleges create biomedical waste (BMW). Since the publication of the BMW (Management and Handling) Rules 1998, the problem of hospital waste management in India has become more prominent. HCFs are required by the rule to practise environmentally conscious waste management by properly sorting, disinfecting, and disposing of waste. The proper handling and disposal of biological waste, particularly in HCFs like hospitals, is essential for protecting both public health and the environment from the potential toxicity and contamination that this material can cause. Biomedical waste includes a wide range of products resulting from medical procedures, research activities, and patient care, and its improper handling poses major risks. Common disposal techniques including incineration have been linked to environmental pollution and the generation of dangerous gases (Omo & Hassan, 2024). The way hospital waste is disposed of can be rather dangerous; this increases environmental pollution as well as major public health threats, including AIDS, hepatitis, plague, cholera, and other such illnesses. The harmful elements in BMW could damage the land, bodies of water, and atmosphere, thereby affecting the neighbouring population's health. Poor treatment of medical waste causes contamination, a bad smell, and the proliferation of bugs, rats, and worms, as well as the spread of diseases like typhoid, cholera, and hepatitis through injuries resulting from contaminated sharp objects (Soliman & Ahmed, 2017; Rayan et al., 2021). In recent times, one of the fastest expanding worldwide sectors is healthcare. Healthcare is a rapidly growing industry due to the increasing availability of medical treatments, a growing number of chronic diseases, and the high demand for innovative treatments. This expanding sector is also producing more garbage than ever before; hence, the treatment and disposal of this waste is becoming essential. Among the several ways used in healthcare waste (HCW) disposal includes chemical treatments, landfilling, and incineration. These basic techniques and their increasing application create their own issues that harm the environment, thereby affecting public health and causing the worldwide healthcare crisis. An increasing amount of HCW involves an increase in use of HCW disposal strategies, including landfilling, composting, and the most recommended method: incineration, as well as other paths, including source reduction and reprocessing and recycling (Kenny & Priyadarshini, 2021). Although these issues might be quite harmful for the environment, their influence on individuals is broad. The release of pollutants such as sulphur, acid gases, metals, particulate matter, and oxides of nitrogen can occur when incineration is properly used as a disposal method. In addition to increasing the chance of cancer and chronic diseases, these pollutants have obviously damaged human health by interfering with the endocrine and respiratory systems (Khobragade, 2019; Sharma et al., 2013).

2.1 Current Situation of Biomedical Waste Management

Looking at the data on biomedical waste management (BMWM) in various Indian states reveals a diverse array of scenarios. Use of the Common Biomedical Waste Treatment Facility (CBWTF) capacity varies greatly, with percentages falling anywhere from 17% to 86%. The disparity between the two points highlights how ineffective the facilities' waste management procedures are compared to BMW's management systems. Arunachal Pradesh, Goa, Mizoram, and Nagaland are among the states that require improvements to their infrastructure because to a lack of CBWTFs or insufficient capacity. States such as Chhattisgarh, Haryana, Maharashtra, and Punjab are struggling to utilize their CBWTF capacity at a rate below 60%, which suggests that there may be problems in completely utilizing approved capacity. In contrast, other regions can learn from the examples set by states like Assam, Jammu and Kashmir, Kerala, and Tamil Nadu when it comes to efficient exploitation of CBWTF capacity. While the approved CBWTF capacity is greater than the actual BMW generation, several states would still need more capacity or new infrastructure. In order to create a more unified and efficient national waste management system, it is essential to tackle these difficulties and encourage states to work together, sharing knowledge and resources (Costa et al., 2023; Banerjee et al., 2023).

There is an estimated 7–8% yearly increase in the amount of BMW produced by the nation, which reaches over 600 tonnes per day in 2022. Approximately 20% of HCFs do not follow the correct protocols for disposing of BMW, according to alarming data (Saxena et al., 2022). Problems with public and environmental health are worsened since only a small portion of BMW is being processed using eco-friendly technologies. The healthcare industry can significantly lessen its impact on the environment by adding recycling and reusing initiatives (Jacob et al., 2021). The purpose of a circular economy is to make resources last longer by minimizing the number of products and materials used, reusing them, recycling them, and recovering them. The traditional linear economy follows a "take, make, dispose" model, while a circular economy tries to reduce waste and keep goods, materials, and resources in use for as long as feasible. Contributing to environmental protection and reducing negative impacts on ecosystems, this method encourages the continued use and regeneration of resources (Saha, 2023). In order to reduce waste and environmental damage, the concepts of a circular economy emphasize reducing, reusing, and recycling resources. In particular, SDG 12 (Responsible Consumption and Production) is supported by this strategy, which promotes sustainable activities. Adopting a circular economy model guarantees effective usage of resources and reduces adverse impacts on public health and the environment in the context of BMW (Mahjoob et al., 2023). In order to reduce, reuse, and recycle, the 3R system promotes these practices to those who produce waste. In order to create a better and cleaner environment, everyone needs to be familiar with the 3R (Jibril et al., 2012).

Biomedical waste is any waste that comes from diagnosing, treating, or vaccinating people or animals or from research. To keep healthcare workers and the community safe from infection, contamination, and other threats, biological waste must be properly separated and disposed of. Biomedical waste is sorted into groups, and each group of waste is put in special colour-coded bags or containers to keep it safe. Table 8.1 shows that BMW is sorted using a colour-coded approach (Kanyal et al., 2021).

Table 8.1 Biomedical waste classifications

Types of Waste	*Colour-Coded Container*	*Type of Bag to Be Used*
• Human anatomical waste • Animal anatomical waste • Soiled waste • Discarded or expired medicine Laboratory waste • Chemical waste • Chemical liquid waste	Yellow	Plastic bags that are yellow and not chlorinated and are thicker than 50 microns or containers
Contaminated waste	Red	Red plastic bags that don't contain chlorine and are thicker than 50 microns or containers
Waste sharps including metals	White	Containers that are white, transparent, puncture-proof, leak-proof, and tamper-proof
Glassware metallic body implants	Blue	Blue-marked cardboard boxes or blue-coloured containers that are puncture-proof and temper-proof

During a June 2007 meeting in Geneva, key guidelines for the safe and sustainable management of healthcare waste were established by the WHO. The harmful consequences of healthcare waste on both people and the environment can be minimized with the right selection of resources and unwavering commitment. The cost of effectively managing BMW should be shared by every individual involved because they are all legally obligated to ensure the safety of others. Furthermore, manufacturers have a duty to manufacture medical equipment that are safe for the environment in order to assure their proper disposal. WHO emphasized the importance of investing funds to set up, fund, and maintain an effective system for managing healthcare waste. Some examples of these include innovative and creative methods that decrease the amount of harmful medical waste and its damaging effects (Salkin & Kennedy, 2004).

The separation, packing, transportation, and archiving of BMW is another point of distinction. The number of categories has been minimized to four in order to provide better identification. It is essential to segregate BMW at the point of generation, which is one of the primary principles of BMW disposal. All HCWs are going to find it easy to use and comprehend, as a huge number of categories has been reduced. The current system associates each waste category and treatment choice with the bag or container's colour code, such as yellow, red, white, or blue (Yadav & Mittal, 2023).

2.2 *Classification of Medical Waste*

Estimates by the WHO indicate that, given their infectivity, toxicity, and occasionally radioactivity, 15–20% of medical waste could be categorized as

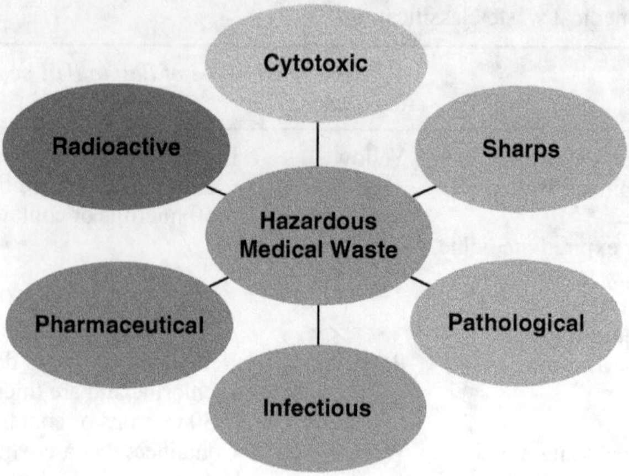

Figure 8.1 Different types of hazardous medical waste.

hazardous materials. Medical waste management techniques, however, vary among nations since this classification is not very clear or consistent (Tsai, 2021; Windfeld & Brooks, 2015; Komilis et al., 2017). Figure 8.1 shows that medical waste can be a direct or indirect reference to HMW which can be contagious, poisonous, or otherwise dangerous. Examples of this kind of waste include infectious, pathological, harmful, pharmacological, and chemical materials produced by HCFs as a result of providing treatment or doing preventative measures. In contrast, MSW and all other common, non-infectious types of waste are categorized as non-hazardous medical waste (NHMW). Most of the time pathogens are present in HMW. Consequently, it is highly contagious and can spread many diseases and infections if not properly handled and disposed of. Additionally, it has the potential to pollute land, water, plants, animals, and air, which can in turn induce disease transmission due to inadequate management (Yoon et al., 2022).

2.3 Sources of Biomedical Waste

Urban solid trash has captured the interest of many, including civic administrators, environmentalists, and town planners. However, certain unique waste sources have received comparatively less attention. An example of this type of trash is BMW, which is mostly produced by HCFs such as hospitals, clinics, veterinary hospitals, general practitioners' offices, blood banks, animal houses, and research organizations. Households, businesses, educational institutions and research centres, blood banks and clinical labs, and HCFs (for people and animals) constitute the other sources of BMW (Babu et al., 2009). Figure 8.2 shows all the various kinds of waste mentioned under the BMW.

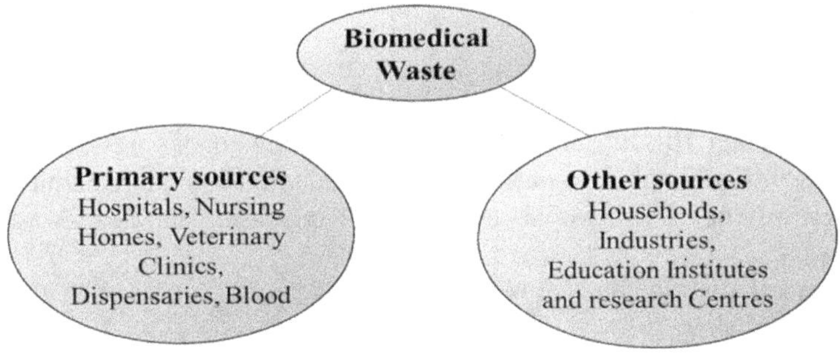

Figure 8.2 Source of biomedical wastes.

3 Medical Waste Management Process

Waste from HCFs must be collected, treated, and disposed of in accordance with the guidelines of BMWM. This BMWM, which can be infectious or otherwise dangerous if not managed correctly, is a huge risk to people and the planet. From the point of generation all the way to proper disposal, medical waste (MW) undergoes several types of treatments as part of medical waste management.

3.1 Segregation

Segregation of the waste at the site of generation comes first. This implies sorting the several kinds of garbage into several containers. This guarantees that every kind of waste is handled and disposed in the suitable manner. The sharp items should usually be separated exactly at the source. Medical staff members handle the segregation; they need training to properly dispose of garbage and prevent infections. Should a mistake arise during waste separation, it should not be fixed in order to contaminate the other garbage. Safe storage of MW helps to prevent unapproved human contact, which might lead to illnesses (Azmal et al., 2014; Thakur, 2024).

3.2 Waste Collection and Transportation

To prevent the accumulation of trash which can transmit diseases, MW collection should occur once daily at a high frequency. Furthermore, the staff members in charge of collecting should have safety equipment to avoid contaminations and diseases that ought to be properly disposed of afterwards. The waste is collected from the healthcare centre and transported to the treatment site using secondary transportation for the purposes of disposal, recycling, and treatment. Treatment facilities either exist off-site in another location or inside a different healthcare institution (Attrah et al., 2022).

3.3 Waste Treatment

Waste may require treatment before it can be discarded based on its nature. Some common approaches include:

Autoclaving: This kills microbes by means of steam under pressure.

Incineration: To destroy waste, this involves high-temperature burning of it.

Microwaving: This involves the killing of organisms and heats waste using microwaves.

Chemical disinfection: This involves destroying microbes with the use of chemicals (Thakur, 2024).

3.4 Disposal

After treatment, the waste can be disposed of at another suitable facility or a landfill. Careful choice of the disposal technique indicates that the waste is not harmful to the environment or human health. Effective infectious waste prevention measures help to protect the medical care workers from health hazards. Along with safeguarding the safety of staff, these management strategies safeguard the environment and public health from the risks produced by the hospital's waste. Effective management promises that infectious waste is handled in compliance with accepted and approved practices from the moment of production until waste is treated and finally disposed (Thakur, 2024).

4 Emission Control Strategies

Incineration is the treatment of choice for most healthcare systems due to its ability to quickly reduce waste volume by 95–96% and inactivate infectious biological elements at high temperatures. The generation of electricity, the incineration of trash, the manufacture of minerals, ferrous and non-ferrous metals, and chemicals, and the open burning of solid waste are the main sources of dioxins. The most effective method for dealing with BMW, also known as clinical or healthcare waste, and other hazardous materials is to heat them to a point where they no longer contain any infectious agents. Only then may they be disposed of in secure landfills. Nevertheless, according to several national inventories worldwide, incinerator emissions are a major source of PCDDs, PCDFs, and dl-PCBs (dioxin-like polychlorinated biphenyls). The main type of incineration facility in nations that are developing is biomedical waste incinerators (BMWIs) (Ajay & Prathish, 2024).

4.1 Non-Incineration Methods for Biomedical Waste Treatments

Within 1 hour, 5–3,000 kg of BMW may be processed using autoclave-based technology. Also, this method has rather minimal operational expenses and environmental pollutants. This method is thought fit for treating sharps, microbiological waste, and throwaway items. Like the autoclave technique, microwave-based treatment releases rather less pollution. Waste is sterilized in BMW using electromagnetic waves with a wavelength between 1 and 1,000 mm and frequency between 900 and 2,500 MHz in microwave treatment (Thind et al., 2021). The BMW is sterilized at high temperatures using pyrolysis, a thermal method similar to the one used for conventional incineration. In pyrolysis, however, treatment occurs devoid of oxygen. Waste combustion is so minimal, and emissions are thus reduced. Still, waste volume reduction suffers compromise. Likewise in plasma pyrolysis, BMW is treated at high temperature and without oxygen. MW burns broken petrol and coke using high-temperature pyrolysis technology. Compared to conventional incineration, the operational cost of pyrolysis can be reduced by using combustible petrol as fuel. In comparison with conventional incineration, pyrolysis with a lower air coefficient results in less flue gas production and less equipment required to purify that gas, leading to a less expensive total cost. Due to the high oxygen combustion rate, dioxins are easily formed during incineration. Pyrolysis reduces dioxin production compared to normal burning since it can eliminate acid gases and operate without oxygen. Fuel for the furnace can be supplied directly from high-temperature pyrolysis MW (Zhu et al., 2008; Messerle et al., 2018). It is also necessary to assess if chemical disinfection is applicable for the treatment of infectious waste. When compared to alternative treatment options, chemical therapy has a moderate operational cost. Chemical treatment has been acknowledged as a preliminary or preventative technique due to its ineffectiveness in reducing waste volume and its effectiveness in disinfection. Nevertheless, there have been recent reports of their use in reprocessing and reusing personal protective equipment (PPE), a type of COVID waste. Vaporized hydrogen peroxide's disinfection capabilities have been advanced for use in PPE kit treatment due to its compatibility with polymer-based products and decreased treatment time. Its usage in the controlled disinfection of old N95 masks has also demonstrated promising results (Barcelo, 2020; Chin et al., 2020; Xu et al., 2020).

4.2 Substitution

Healthcare equipment may have its harmful emissions from incinerators drastically cut if particular raw materials weren't used in their production. A good example would be the fact that the burning units primarily release chlorine due to medical equipment and products made of PVC. Even more concerning is the fact that medical items containing PVC release dioxins and furans when burnt. As a result, it is recommended to promote the use of bio-based plastics in place of PVC in medical items, in addition to focusing on effective separate handling of the BMW. Masks are also made of polypropylene and polyethylene, which can increase the amount of microplastics in freshwater bodies and cause various health problems. Specifically, the polypropylene and polyethylene masks can be replaced with cloth masks. The present healthcare system also makes use of a number of items that depend on the use of mercury, including sphygmomanometers and thermometers. When these products reach the end of their useful life, they are burnt, which releases mercury into the air. The use of healthcare items containing mercury is currently prohibited in several countries. It is now possible to phase out mercury thermometers from India's healthcare system due to the widespread use of contactless infrared radiation thermometers (Thind et al., 2021).

4.3 Biomedical Waste Segregation

Proper segregation is essential for identifying MW, managing BMW effectively, and minimizing hazardous waste. An important first step in managing MW effectively is segregation. For this, biological waste must be separated from general hospital waste materials. Using colour-labelled bags to efficiently separate infectious waste from non-infectious waste is a crucial step in MW segregation, which also helps reduce hazardous waste volume and allows for correct composition assessment (Kalaivani, 2009; Longe & Williams, 2006). It is recommended to segregate biological waste at its source, which includes patient care areas, diagnostic services, operating rooms, labour rooms, and treatment spaces, as part of proper BMWM. Therefore, it is the responsibility of medical professionals to properly manage these wastes from formation to disposal. Inadequate segregation procedures at the medical centre led to inadequate waste classification estimations. To avoid health risks it is important to properly handle the various waste streams that are produced, and the process of segregation serves as a helpful guide for this task. Healthcare hazardous waste should be collected in appropriate containers based on its classification and then treated and disposed of in a safe manner. The amount of BMW that needs treatment or that ends up in landfills untreated is increased by poorly segregated trash. The public health system benefits from BMW segregation since it reduces health threats to the general public following exposure to disposed waste, and the waste management budget benefits from less MW (Okechukwu et al., 2022).

4.4 Installation of Emission Control Systems

Studied the way that cutting-edge cleaning and filtering technology mitigated emissions of pollutants from an incinerator system for medical laboratory waste. In order to ensure a combustion efficiency of 99.93% and increase the average incineration temperature to over 950°C, liquid waste solvent could be added to the main combustion chamber. The results demonstrate the impurities were effectively removed by utilizing advanced scrubbing and filtering equipment. As a result, the amounts of pollutants in the chimney stack flue gas were found to be within the permitted emission requirements. As the system HCl removal rate exceeds 99.99%, it effectively shields the fabric screen from chemical degradation. This two-stage scrubbing procedure involves reducing the flue gas temperature to 70°C, which in turn reduces condensable particulate matter (CPM) to filterable particulate matter (FPM). The FPM was effectively eliminated in a sequential manner by the fabric filter. Separate from one another, particles that can be filtered and those that can be condensed make up particulate matter. Controlling FPM is possible with the use of modern approaches to managing air pollution. Containing CPM in flue gas keeps it in the vapour phase, but when discharged into the environment, it changes into particulate matter or aerosols (Liao et al., 2024). When it comes to air pollution control devices (APCDs), CPM is a major cause for alarm because it can bypass them. In their solid form, particles or aerosols can reduce visibility in the sky and add significantly to air pollution. Because of this, we must immediately begin working on a way to eradicate CPM (Li et al., 2019; Wang et al., 2020, 2022).

4.5 Policy Recommendations for Sustainable Practices

4.5.1 Using Hydrogen Peroxide Vapour

During the current coronavirus outbreak, reusing PPE is a temporary but promising solution. There is increasing evidence that various reprocessing methods, such as dry heat, hydrogen peroxide vapour, ozone, and ultraviolet light at 2,000 mJ/cm^2 (254 nm), can be effective. The majority of these methods involve the use of hydrogen peroxide vapour (VH_2O_2). Transformation of structural elements, such as an outer envelope, an RNA genome, and a protein capsid, is associated with the aforementioned ways of disinfection and viral inactivation. Maintaining the integrity of PPE, particularly its fit and filtering capacity, as well as its non-toxicity and safety, is another critical aspect of efficient PPE disinfection (Rowan & Laffey, 2021; Pinon & Vialette, 2019).

4.5.2 Pre-sorting and Disinfection

The possibility of disease transmission or an increase in plastic and MW makes waste management a major concern during a coronavirus pandemic. It is imperative that governments enhance their waste management strategies with the goal of maximizing collection, reuse, and recycling capacities. It is essential to pre-sort and clean MW in order to increase its recyclability. In addition, ultraviolet (UV), ozone and volatile organic compound (VOC) decontamination technologies can propose a long-term plan for treating wastewater and trash.

Considerations such as waste volume, budget, waste kind, and frequency of maintenance are essential when deciding on appropriate decontamination equipment because it completely destroys microorganisms at temperatures exceeding 800°C; incineration is often the best solution related to pathogenic waste in large quantities. Moreover, if the daily MW quantity is not deemed excessive, methods such as physical disinfection using microwaves or chemical decontamination, including the application of disinfectants, could be considered. In the end MW treatment facilities should be more automated so that they require less personnel (Prata et al., 2019; Silva et al., 2021).

4.5.3 Improvement in Modern Sustainable Technology

Recycling goals, waste management efficiency, and carbon footprint can all be improved with bio-based plastics. So, conventional and fuel-based plastic substrates put less strain on the economy and the environment. Decomposition by biological or enzymatic processes in open air is an additional advantage of bio-based biodegradable polymers. Biological polymers, including sugar, cotton, straw, cane, potato, starch, and cellulose, are used in bioplastics, either partially or completely. Sustainable and innovative ways to reuse mixed and complicated plastic packaging can be developed through investments in research on plastic alternatives. One example is the production of high-quality chemicals and resins from plastic waste by chemical reprocessing, a new applied science that gets funded through investments. It has already been stated that bioplastic is not an ideal or ultimate solution. The quality of bioplastics should be thoroughly tested for degradability or recyclability before they hit the market. Additionally, there needs to be an effort to simplify infrastructure for practical bioplastic waste disposal. The Centres for Disease Control and Prevention have also suggested that people make their own fabric masks to wear. A multi-layer face mask manufactured at home can effectively prevent the spread of COVID-19 by respiratory droplets in the event of a pandemic or a mask shortage. Washable and reusable face masks made of materials like cotton can help lessen the environmental impact of commercially available, single-use masks that aren't biodegradable (Napper & Thompson, 2019; Teymourian et al., 2021).

4.5.4 Public Awareness Campaigns

By promoting sustainable behaviours, giving up old habits, and adapting to new ones, people need to change the way people think about plastic usage. It is equally important to encourage researchers to reach this goal for an effective communication strategy and to help decision-makers identify relevant communication channels so that society's environmental knowledge and information can be improved. The key to save humanity from successive disasters lies in government policy, individual accountability, and commercial enterprises. By separating recyclables at home, people may help reduce the recycling load. Additionally, authorities could launch campaigns, run ads, use social media, etc. to raise public knowledge of the problems inside the waste management sector. Additionally, it must establish a system for mutually beneficial information exchange to guarantee that all parties are adequately prepared to handle potentially dangerous biological waste (Teymourian et al., 2021).

4.5.5 Promote a Circular Economy within HCFs

Circular economy (CE) directly affects the created and obtained items. If items are produced in a CE, waste reprocessing rises and resource extraction from the environment declines. Since GHGs are released both in their manufacture and transit, acquired commodities also significantly contribute to the carbon footprint of healthcare. By selecting minimal hazardous trace medical supplies and gadgets and substituting reusable ones for single-use ones, one can help to reduce healthcare waste. Hospitals have been employing somewhat large quantities of throwaway things during the past few years; many reusable products have been replaced by disposable ones. For instance, buying reusable sharp containers rather than throwaway ones helps to significantly lower the carbon footprint of the sharps waste stream. Consequently, healthcare institutions can reduce their greenhouse gas (GHG) emissions through sustainable procurement and purchasing. This can be achieved by hospitals influencing their suppliers to supply goods and services in a sustainable manner. Procurement should incorporate criteria that promote eco-friendly products, buy from local suppliers to reduce and reuse packaging whenever possible and invest in long-lasting equipment or devices to prolong the life of products.

The life cycle assessment approach might help hospitals to better comprehend the financial and environmental expenses of bought goods or procedures. Reducing the carbon footprint and GHG emissions is another crucial environmental concern. CE naturally lowers GHG emissions since it requires lowering and reusing resources, which reduces the manufacturing of commodities, thus lowering the GHG emissions by up to 70%. Though it may be seen as a separate idea from CE. Furthermore, if we consider the fuels generating the GHG emissions as "Resources", then restricting the use of these resources (R-Reduce) will help us to see that the CE idea incorporates the decrease in GHG emissions (Soares et al., 2023).

4.5.6 *Incentives for Hospitals and Laboratories*

The BMWM process is unique in several respects, including sorting, packing, transportation, and storage. The segregation of BMW must occur at the point of generation, which is one of the fundamental principles of BMW disposal. This has been made simpler so that all HCWs may easily navigate it and avoid the confusion caused by the high number of categories. The bags or containers are now colour-coded (yellow, red, white, and blue) according to the kind of garbage and the treatment option for that waste. Only authorized recyclers will receive the BMW supplied in the red/blue recycling bags or containers. As a result, the recycler will remain within the jurisdiction of the relevant government bodies. In recent years, recycling has received more attention as a means to reduce pollution and preserve resources. The new regulations reduce the process of obtaining an HCF and establish new standards for its authorization. Based on the colour code, type of waste, and treatment methods, BMW has been divided into four groups (Datta et al., 2018).

4.5.7 *Use of Bioremediation in Biomedical Waste Management*

Bioremediation involves utilizing naturally occurring organisms, such as microorganisms and plants, to convert harmful waste into less harmful or non-toxic components. Microorganisms are more commonly used as bioremediation agents than plants because of their rapid growth and versatility. The use of diverse microbial communities, including bacteria, fungi, and algae, has proven effective in the removal of numerous environmental contaminants. Biomedical waste is a combination of solid or liquid materials that contains a high concentration of organic contaminants; as a result, it is amenable to biological treatment. Bioremediation is one of the promising biological treatments. As mentioned earlier, this method is seen as a substitute for the physical processes and hazardous chemicals that are currently employed in remediation. Compared to the present techniques of waste disposal, bioremediation is both more cost-effective and environmentally friendly (Azubuike et al., 2016; Ayilara & Babalola, 2023; Dixit et al., 2015). Microorganisms are ideally suited to remove contaminants from soil and groundwater because of their unique genetic, physiological, and biochemical characteristics. Modern bioremediation sites have their microbial populations studied using a variety of cutting-edge molecular approaches. There is hope in a promising new technique called phytoremediation, which uses plants and rhizospheric microorganisms to clean up a variety of contaminants found in MW. For the purpose of disposing of sediments and waters affected by nuclear waste, scientists have discovered promising possibilities in plants and bacteria. Thus, it is critical to develop a bioremediation process-based research strategy that provides low-cost, high-efficiency solutions for dealing with solid and liquid biological waste from hospitals (Khan, 2024).

4.6 World Health Organization Guidance

According to the policy document of WHO "Safe health-care waste management", nations should evaluate their options for healthcare waste management systems before settling on one. Government organizations are encouraged to implement the following methods by WHO:

Short-Term Strategies

- Every single component of the syringe is made from the same plastic in order to make recycling easier.
- Selecting healthcare devices that do not include polyvinyl chloride.
- Identifying and developing recycling options whenever feasible, such as for plastic and glass.
- Research into and promotion of innovative technologies or alternatives to small-scale incineration.
- Incineration, when performed effectively, can be an acceptable option for health-care waste management in developing nations until more environmentally and health-friendly alternatives become available. Incinerators must be operated in a certain way to ensure proper waste reduction and segregation, proper placement away from populated areas, a well-engineered design, construction according to appropriate dimensional plans, management and staff training, and proper operation.

Medium-Term Strategies

- Additional measures that reduce the frequency of unnecessary injections to minimize the quantity of potentially dangerous MW that must be handled.
- Investigations address the potential health consequences of long-term exposure to trace amounts of dioxin and furan.
- Risk evaluation that compares the health hazards linked to combustion and coming into contact with MW.

Long-Term Strategies

- To reduce the health risks associated with (a) improper disposal of MW and (b) exposure to carcinogens like dioxins and furans, it is necessary to promote non-incineration solutions for final disposal on a large scale.
- Support countries to establish a national standard for how to safely handle healthcare waste.

- Help nations design and execute comprehensive policies and laws to combat healthcare waste.
- Promote environmentally sound handling of healthcare waste in accordance with the Basel Convention (Chartier, 2014).

4.7 Identification of Key Biomedical Waste Management Factors

BMWM needs to be systematic, as a single error could harm the people in control. There are six steps for operating BMW: observing the waste that was made; segregating, collecting, and categorizing the waste; storing, transporting, and treating the waste (Endris et al., 2022). In order to lessen the potential consequences of improper BMWM, segregation, the process of separating various forms of waste, is utilized. It is more likely that sharps and other types of waste will be mixed up with typical waste when waste simply gets dumped out. Any person who handles waste could contract an infectious disease from these sharps. Another concern is the high likelihood of reusing discarded syringes and needles in hospitals due to improper segregation. Sorting materials by kind helps keep this from happening and moves us closer to our aim of recycling all of the metal and plastic waste we produce (Singhal et al., 2017). As part of the BMW collection, various coloured wastebaskets are utilized. Colour plays a crucial role in identifying and separating various types of waste into their respective bins. Hospital wards, rooms, and operating rooms are just a few examples of where they need to be appropriately labelled. In hospitals with around 250 beds, the waste must be retained for no more than 8–10 hours, whereas in nursing homes, it must be stored for 24 hours. Place an indication on the storage bag or designate the area for storage (Endris et al., 2022). Substances that pose a threat to all forms of life on Earth are known as biohazards. It was noted that the biohazard symbol is a significant public sign since it warns people about the dangers of entering the area that has been designated (Li et al., 2021).

4.8 Methods for the Treatment of BMW

The treatment of BMW can be accomplished in various ways. Incineration is a cost-effective method of waste treatment that involves using extremely high temperatures (1,800–2,000°F) to burn waste. This process reduces the overall mass of decontaminated waste by turning it into ash and gases, which are subsequently disposed of in landfills (Li et al., 2021). The common treatments are incineration, autoclave disinfection, microwave disinfection, chemical disinfection and land filling (Akter, 2000).

4.8.1 Incineration

The burning process is the most common way to treat waste because it works for any type of waste material. Furnaces that run at temperatures between 800 and 1,200°C do the incineration. The high temperatures kill the germs, get rid of 90% of the organics and change the shape and volume of waste. When any substance is burnt, it makes fly ash and gases like dioxins, furans, and mercury. These persistent environmental contaminants, which contain dioxins and furans, are thought to be cancer-causing agents. Achieving total burning of waste can reduce dioxin emissions (Giakoumakis et al., 2021). The solid byproduct of burning that is particularly heavy metal-rich is called fly ash. Chemical pre-treatment with EDTA or sodium sulphide eliminates the heavy metals from fly ash, making it suitable for recycling (Ababneh et al., 2019).

4.8.2 *Autoclave Disinfection*

One of the most efficient ways to sterilize products using heat is autoclaving (Viveksarathi & Kannan, 2015). Autoclaves are commonly used in HCFs and research facilities to sanitize reusable biomedical equipment (Panta et al., 2019). They are especially important for handling highly contagious materials, like microbial cultures or sharps, and even hospitals that are constrained in resources should have them. Multiple factors, such as the amount of moisture in the waste and the steam's penetration rate, establish the minimum contact times and temperatures. According to multiple autoclaving studies, a 60-minute cycle at 121°C is necessary to fully penetrate the waste material with steam and destroy most bacterial spores and all vegetative microorganisms with a tiny amount of waste. The installation expenses of autoclaves can range from modest to expensive, and they require energy. Additionally, there are instances where a boiler with emission control is required (Singh et al., 2024).

4.8.3 *Microwave Disinfection*

Microwave disinfection is a process that uses high-powered microwaves at low temperatures to break down organic compounds and microbes. Because the waves cause vibrations in the chemical bonds, they reduce energy consumption and emissions, making this process greener. Using electromagnetic waves with frequencies between 300 and 3,000 MHz and wavelengths between 1 mm and 1 m, the disinfection process can be carried out at temperatures ranging from 177 to 540°C. Combined with burning and autoclaving, microwave disinfection can save expenses significantly (Giakoumakis et al., 2021).

4.8.4 *Chemical Disinfection*

A common practice in hospitals is to chemically disinfect biomedical devices in order to remove pathogens. This process results in the disposal of these devices as waste (Wang, 2021). Sewage treatment chemicals are utilized to eradicate or inhibit the growth of pathogens. Disinfectants like peracetic acid and ammonium salts pose risks to both the environment and the health of individuals engaged in their use. Please refrain from using glutaraldehyde, formaldehyde, and ethylene oxide because of their carcinogenic or sensitizing characteristics. Strong disinfectants might irritate the skin, eyes, and lungs. Be careful when you handle these agents. For example, you need to wear and care for your personal protection equipment (Capoor & Parida, 2021). Since the waste is only lightly cleaned, this approach raises many safety problems. When comparing chemical disinfection versus thermal disinfection, the former is clearly superior due to sustainability and efficacy. Simple, cheap, and readily available disinfectants make chemical disinfection the superior choice (Dhama et al., 2021).

4.8.5 Land Disposal

There are two types of land-based waste management: open dumping and sanitary landfills (Idris et al., 2004). "Open dumps" are places where waste is dumped without any control or organization. They can create major pollution, fires, higher chances of disease spreading, and easy access for animals and scavengers (Khan et al., 2019). When humans come into contact with infectious substances, there is a clear risk of disease transmission. There are a number of advantages to using sanitary landfills instead of open dumping. Some of these measures include erecting geological barriers to contain garbage, following engineering protocols before accepting waste, having qualified personnel on hand to handle operations, and organizing waste dumps and daily coverage efficiently (Kamaruddin et al., 2022). To maintain efficient waste management, sanitary landfills must adhere to specific requirements. Having qualified on-site staff who can monitor and manage day-to-day operations is a crucial need. The landfill follows a systematic technique for disposing of garbage. The waste is neatly arranged in a designated location so that it may be turned over, packed down, and covered every day. In addition to minimizing the hazards connected with open garbage accumulation, this also guarantees optimal space utilization. With the completion of each stage of the landfill, a final cover is built to reduce the amount of rainwater that can seep in. An extra layer of protection from pollution is provided by this last cover (Mohamed et al., 2005).

5 Future Prospective

Due to the extreme toxicity of dioxins, there have been substantial attempts to understand their creation in response to the need for worldwide studies issued by convention rules. Processes, toxicological pathways, and the control of dioxins from known sources, leading to a significant decrease in industrial sectors up till now. Intelligent, sensor-equipped autonomous robots need further development. To guarantee correct disposal, tracking, and verifiable compliance data, the future-proof blockchain technology may set up an open ledger of trash management. The potential for BMW to be transformed into biogas or power could be investigated through the use of advanced waste-to-energy technology. In addition to helping with sustainable energy generation, this takes care of trash disposal issues. Allocating resources, intervening, and overseeing compliance may all be done in real-time using data generated by monitoring generation, collection, transport, and disposal. Factors such as population density, diseases, and healthcare activities are used by AI predictive models to forecast biological waste. This helps waste management systems to better allocate resources, optimize routes, and anticipate demands. Improved sorting through machine learning enhances recycling and waste management.

6 Conclusion

Safeguarding human and environmental health requires effective management of biological waste and control of emissions, which are both regulated and ethically important. MW must be systematically classified, segregated, and treated in order to implement sustainable practices as highlighted in this chapter. Healthcare waste management systems can be substantially improved in terms of sustainability with the implementation of policy guidelines that place an emphasis on material replacement, modern treatment techniques, and waste minimization. Policy recommendations targeted at encouraging sustainable BMWM. In order to bring hospital waste practices in line with public health and environmental objectives, these factors must be considered. These factors include technological, operational, educational, and economic aspects. Technologies that waste energy should be chosen according to the amount of MW; areas with significant volumes of waste should use mature technologies like incineration, while locations with low quantities of waste should encourage the use of environmentally friendly technologies like pyrolysis and gasification.

References

Ababneh, A., Al-Rousan, R., Gharaibeh, W., & Abu-Dalo, M. (2019). Recycling of pre-treated medical waste fly ash in mortar mixtures. *Journal of Material Cycles and Waste Management*, 22, 1–14.

Ajay, S. V., & Prathish, K. P. (2024). Dioxins emissions from bio-medical waste incineration: a systematic review on emission factors, inventories, trends and health risk studies. *Journal of Hazardous Materials*, *465*, 133384.

Akter, N. (2000). Medical waste management: a review. Research Reports in Health Studies, XXVIII, 370–394.

Ananth, A. P., Prashanthini, V., & Visvanathan, C. (2010). Healthcare waste management in Asia. *Waste Management*, *30*(1), 154–161.

Attrah, M., Elmanadely, A., Akter, D., & Rene, E. R. (2022). A review on medical waste management: treatment, recycling, and disposal options. *Environments*, *9*(11), 146.

Ayilara, M. S., & Babalola, O. O. (2023). Bioremediation of environmental wastes: the role of microorganisms. *Frontiers in Agronomy*, *5*, 1183691.

Azmal, M., Kalhor, R., Dehcheshmeh, N. F., Goharinezhad, S., Heidari, Z. A., & Farzianpour, F. (2014). Going toward green hospital by sustainable healthcare waste management: segregation, treatment and safe disposal. *Health*, *6*(19), 2632–2640.

Azubuike, C. C., Chikere, C. B., & Okpokwasili, G. C. (2016). Bioremediation techniques–classification based on site of application: principles, advantages, limitations and prospects. *World Journal of Microbiology and Biotechnology*, *32*(11), 180.

Babu, B. R., Parande, A. K., Rajalakshmi, R., Suriyakala, P., & Volga, M. (2009). Management of biomedical waste in India and other countries: a review. *Journal of International Environmental Application & Science*, *4*(1), 65–78.

Banerjee, S., Kumar, H., Sanyal, T., Mukherjee, P., & Mukherjee, D. (2023). Current landscape and future perspectives of biomedical waste management in India. In S. Roychoudhury, T. Sanyal, K. Sen, & S. Mukherjee Sanyal (Eds.), *A Basic Overview of Environment and Sustainable Development* (Vol. 2, pp. 79–93). North 24 Parganas, West Bengal, India: International Academic Publishing House (IAPH).

Barcelo, D. (2020). An environmental and health perspective for COVID-19 outbreak: meteorology and air quality influence, sewage epidemiology indicator, hospitals disinfection, drug therapies and recommendations. *Journal of Environmental Chemical Engineering*, *8*(4), 104006.

Capoor, M. R., & Parida, A. (2021). Current perspectives of biomedical waste management in context of COVID-19. *Indian Journal of Medical Microbiology*, *39*(2), 171–178.

Chartier, Y. (Ed.). (2014). *Safe Management of Wastes from Health-care Activities*. World Health Organization (WHO), Geneva.

Chin, A. W., Chu, J. T., Perera, M. R., Hui, K. P., Yen, H. L., Chan, M. C., & Poon, L. L. (2020). Stability of SARS-CoV-2 in different environmental conditions. *The Lancet Microbe*, *1*(1), e10.

Costa, J. D., Patel, H., Braganza, V., & Solanki, H. (2023). Impact of a crisis on waste management policy Adherence and practices-A narrative review of bio-medical waste management during the Covid-19 pandemic. *Current World Environment*, *18*(3), 956–967.

Das, S., Rahman, T., Adhikary, N., Roy, A., & Chakma, A. (2025). Medical Waste Management as a Pillar for Safe Urban Development: Case Studies from Satkhira, Khulna, And Jashore, Bangladesh Proceedings of the WasteSafe.

Datta, P., Mohi, G., & Chander, J. (2018). Biomedical waste management in India: critical appraisal. *Journal of Laboratory Physicians*, *10*(01), 006–014.

Dhama, K., Patel, S. K., Kumar, R., Masand, R., Rana, J., Yatoo, M. I., & Harapan, H. (2021). The role of disinfectants and sanitizers during COVID-19 pandemic: advantages and deleterious effects on humans and the environment. *Environmental Science and Pollution Research*, *28*(26), 34211–34228.

Dixit, R., Wasiullah, X., Malaviya, D., Pandiyan, K., Singh, U. B., Sahu, A., & Paul, D. (2015). Bioremediation of heavy metals from soil and aquatic environment: an overview of principles and criteria of fundamental processes. *Sustainability*, *7*(2), 2189–2212.

Endris, S., Tamir, Z., & Sisay, A. (2022). Medical laboratory waste generation rate, management practices and associated factors in Addis Ababa, Ethiopia. *PLoS One*, *17*(4), e0266888.

Ghanimeh, S., Gómez-Sanabria, A., Tsydenova, N., Štrbová, K., Iossifidou, M., & Kumar, A. (2019). Two-level comparison of waste management systems in low-, middle-, and high-income cities. *Environmental Engineering Science*, *36*(10), 1281–1295.

Giakoumakis, G., Politi, D., & Sidiras, D. (2021). Medical waste treatment technologies for energy, fuels, and materials production: a review. *Energies*, *14*(23), 8065.

Idris, A., Inanc, B., & Hassan, M. N. (2004). Overview of waste disposal and landfills/dumps in Asian countries. *Journal of Material Cycles and Waste Management*, *6*(2), 104–110.

Jacob, S., Nithianandam, S., Rastogi, S., Sakhuja, S., & Sri Laxma Alankar, S. N. (2021). Handling and treatment strategies of biomedical wastes and biosolids contaminated with SARS-CoV-2 in waste environment. *Environmental and Health Management of Novel Coronavirus Disease (COVID-19)*, 207–232. https://doi.org/10.1016/B978-0-323-85780-2.00012-3

Jibril, J. D., azimi, Sipan I. B., Sapri, M., Shika, S. A., Isa, M., & Abdullah, S. (2012). 3Rs critical success factor in solid waste management system for higher educational institutions. Procedia Social and Behavioral Sciences, 65, 626–631.

Kalaivani, K. (2009). A case study of biomedical waste management in hospitals. *Global Journal of Health Science*, *1*(1), 82–88.

Kamaruddin, M.A., Norashiddin, F.A., Yusoff, M.S., Hanif, M.H.M., Wang, L.K., Wang, MH.S. (2021). Sanitary landfill operation and management. In Wang, L. K., Wang, M. H. S., &

Hung, Y. T. (eds.), *Solid Waste Engineering and Management. Handbook of Environmental Engineering* (vol. 23). Springer, Cham. https://doi.org/10.1007/978-3-030-84180-5_8

Kanyal, D., Butola, L. K., & Ambad, R. (2021). Biomedical waste management in India-a review. *Indian Journal of Forensic Medicine & Toxicology, 15*(2), 108–113.

Kenny, C., & Priyadarshini, A. (2021). Review of current healthcare waste management methods and their effect on global health. *Healthcare (Basel, Switzerland), 9*(3), 284. https://doi.org/10.3390/healthcare9030284

Khan, B. A., Cheng, L., Khan, A. A., & Ahmed, H. (2019). Healthcare waste management in Asian developing countries: a mini review. *Waste Management & Research, 37*(9), 863–875.

Khan, M. S. A. (2024). Applications of bioremediation in biomedical waste management: current and future prospects. *Brazilian Archives of Biology and Technology, 67*, e24230161.

Khobragade, D. S. (2019). Health care waste: avoiding hazards to living and non living environment by efficient management. *Fortune Journal of Health Sciences, 2*(2), 14–29.

Komilis, D., Makroleivaditis, N., & Nikolakopoulou, E. (2017). Generation and composition of medical wastes from private medical microbiology laboratories. *Waste Management, 61*, 539–546.

Lee, B. K., Ellenbecker, M. J., & Moure-Ersaso, R. (2004). Alternatives for treatment and disposal cost reduction of regulated medical wastes. *Waste Management, 24*(2), 143–151.

Li, H., Hu, Y., Lyu, J., Quan, H., Xu, X., & Li, C. (2021). Transportation risk control of waste disposal in the healthcare system with two-Echelon waste collection network. *Mathematical Problems in Engineering, 2021*(1), 5580083.

Li, X., Zhou, C., Li, J., Lu, S., & Yan, J. (2019). Distribution and emission characteristics of filterable and condensable particulate matter before and after a low-low temperature electrostatic precipitator. *Environmental Science and Pollution Research, 26*(13), 12798–12806.

Liao, C. C., Wu, J. L., Wang, Y. F., Huang, K. L., Huang, S. W., & Kuo, Y. M. (2024). Advanced scrubbing/filtration devices for pollution control in medical laboratory waste incineration system. *Aerosol and Air Quality Research, 24*(4), 230192.

Longe, E. O., & Williams, A. (2006). A preliminary study of medical waste management in Lagos metropolis, Nigeria. *Journal of Environmental Health Science & Engineering, 3*(2), 133–139.

Mahjoob, A., Alfadhli, Y., & Omachonu, V. (2023). Healthcare waste and sustainability: implications for a circular economy. Sustainability, 15(10), 7788.

Messerle, V. E., Mosse, A. L., & Ustimenko, A. B. (2018). Processing of biomedical waste in plasma gasifier. *Waste Management, 79*, 791–799.

Mohamed, A. M. O., Maraqa, M., & Al Handhaly, J. (2005). Impact of land disposal of reject brine from desalination plants on soil and groundwater. *Desalination, 182*(1–3), 411–433.

Napper, I. E., & Thompson, R. C. (2019). Environmental deterioration of biodegradable, oxo-biodegradable, compostable, and conventional plastic carrier bags in the sea, soil, and open-air over a 3-year period. *Environmental Science & Technology, 53*(9), 4775–4783.

Okechukwu, E. C., Oparah, A. C., Aguora, S. O., & Soni, J. S. (2022). Segregation practices by health workers in urban hospitals-a step necessary to achieve minimization and effective biomedical waste management. *Texila International Journal of Public Health, 10*(2), 290–297.

Omo, Q. G., & Hassan, N. E. (2024). Biomedical waste management and their effects on the Environment: a review. *World Journal of Advanced Engineering Technology and Sciences, 11*(1), 086–095.

Panta, G., Richardson, A. K., & Shaw, I. C. (2019). Effectiveness of autoclaving in sterilizing reusable medical devices in healthcare facilities. *The Journal of Infection in Developing Countries*, *13*(10), 858–864.

Pinon, A., & Vialette, M. (2019). Survival of viruses in water. *Intervirology*, *61*(5), 214–222.

Prata, J. C., Silva, A. L. P., Da Costa, J. P., Mouneyrac, C., Walker, T. R., Duarte, A. C., & Rocha-Santos, T. (2019). Solutions and integrated strategies for the control and mitigation of plastic and microplastic pollution. *International Journal of Environmental Research and Public Health*, *16*(13), 2411.

Rayan, R. A., Choudhury, M., Kamal, M., Chakravorty, A., Devi, R. M., & Mehta, J. (2021). Biomedical waste management in healthcare. In Dutta, J., Goswami, S., & Mitra, A. (eds.), *Multidimensional Approaches to Impacts of Changing Environment on Human Health* (pp. 293–304). CRC Press.

Rowan, N. J., & Laffey, J. G. (2021). Unlocking the surge in demand for personal and protective equipment (PPE) and improvised face coverings arising from coronavirus disease (COVID-19) pandemic–implications for efficacy, re-use and sustainable waste management. *Science of the Total Environment*, *752*, 142259.

Rutala, W. A., & Weber, D. J. (2015). Disinfection, sterilization, and control of hospital waste. *Mandell, Douglas, and Bennett's Principles and Practice of Infectious Diseases*, 3294–3309.e4. https://doi.org/10.1016/B978-1-4557-4801-3.00301-5

Saha, A. (2023). Circular economy strategies for sustainable waste management in the food industry. Journal of Recycling Economy & Sustainability Policy, 2(2), 1–16.

Salkin, I. F., & Kennedy, M. E. (2004). Review of *H*ealth *I*mpacts from *M*icrobiological *H*azards in *H*ealth-care *W*astes. *Geneva: WHO.*

Saxena, P., Pradhan, I. P., & Kumar, D. (2022). Redefining biomedical waste management during COVID-19 in India: a way forward. Materials Today: Proceedings, 60, 849–858.

Sharma, R., Sharma, M., Sharma, R., & Sharma, V. (2013). The impact of incinerators on human health and environment. *Reviews on Environmental Health*, *28*(1), 67–72.

Silva, A. L. P., Prata, J. C., Walker, T. R., Duarte, A. C., Ouyang, W., Barcelò, D., & Rocha-Santos, T. (2021). Increased plastic pollution due to COVID-19 pandemic: challenges and recommendations. *Chemical Engineering Journal*, *405*, 126683.

Singh, H., YT, K., Mishra, A. K., Singh, M., Mohanto, S., Ghumra, S., & Thangadurai, D. (2024). Harnessing the foundation of biomedical waste management for fostering public health: strategies and policies for a clean and safer environment. *Discover Applied Sciences*, *6*(3), 89.

Singhal, L., Tuli, A. K., & Gautam, V. (2017). Biomedical waste management guidelines 2016: what's done and what needs to be done. *Indian Journal of Medical Microbiology*, *35*(2), 194–198.

Soares, A. L., Buttigieg, S. C., Bak, B., McFadden, S., Hughes, C., McClure, P., …& Bravo, I. (2023). A review of the applicability of current green practices in healthcare facilities. *International Journal of Health Policy and Management*, *12*, 6947.

Soliman, S. M., & Ahmed, A. I. (2017). Biomedical wastes: environmental threats and management. In Bharagava, R. N. (ed.), *Environmental Pollutants and Their Bioremediation Approaches* (pp. 427–442). CRC Press, Taylor & Francis Group

Teymourian, T., Teymoorian, T., Kowsari, E., & Ramakrishna, S. (2021). Challenges, strategies, and recommendations for the huge surge in plastic and medical waste during the global COVID-19 pandemic with circular economy approach. *Materials Circular Economy*, *3*(1), 6.

Thakur, H. (2024). Biomedical waste management in India- A review. *Journal of Population Therapeutics & Clinical Pharmacology*, *31*(01), 2222–2229.

Thind, P. S., Sareen, A., Singh, D. D., Singh, S., & John, S. (2021). Compromising situation of India's bio-medical waste incineration units during pandemic outbreak of COVID-19: associated environmental-health impacts and mitigation measures. *Environmental Pollution, 276,* 116621.

Tsai, W. T. (2021). Analysis of medical waste management and impact analysis of COVID-19 on its generation in Taiwan. *Waste Management & Research, 39*(1_suppl), 27–33.

Viveksarathi, K., & Kannan, K. (2015). Effect of the moist-heat sterilization on fabricated nanoscale solid lipid particles containing rasagiline mesylate. *International Journal of Pharmaceutical Investigation, 5*(2), 87.

Wang, H. (2021). A review of the effects of collagen treatment in clinical studies. *Polymers, 13*(22), 3868.

Wang, K., Yang, L., Li, J., Sheng, Z., He, Q., & Wu, K. (2020). Characteristics of condensable particulate matter before and after wet flue gas desulfurization and wet electrostatic precipitator from ultra-low emission coal-fired power plants in China. *Fuel, 278,* 118206.

Wang, L., Li, Y., Li, J., Zhang, H., Zhang, Z., & Ran, W. (2022). The state of the art of condensable particulate matter. *Fuel, 325,* 124807.

WHO. (1999). Guidelines for safe disposal of unwanted pharmaceuticals in and after emergencies. Essential drugs and other Medicines Department. World Health Organization, Geneva, Switzerland.180.

Windfeld, E. S., & Brooks, M. S. L. (2015). Medical waste management–A review. *Journal of Environmental Management, 163,* 98–108.

Xu, L., Dong, K., Zhang, Y., & Li, H. (2020, December). Comparison and analysis of several medical waste treatment technologies. In *IOP Conference Series: Earth and Environmental Science* (Vol. 615, No. 1, p. 012031). IOP Publishing.

Yadav, M., & Mittal, K. (2023). Bio-medical waste management. *Voyager*, 14, 51–57

Yoon, C. W., Kim, M. J., Park, Y. S., Jeon, T. W., & Lee, M. Y. (2022). A review of medical waste management systems in the Republic of Korea for hospital and medical waste generated from the COVID-19 pandemic. *Sustainability, 14*(6), 3678.

Zhu, H. M., Yan, J. H., Jiang, X. G., Lai, Y. E., & Cen, K. F. (2008). Study on pyrolysis of typical medical waste materials by using TG-FTIR analysis. *Journal of Hazardous Materials, 153*(1–2), 670–676.

9 The Role of Higher Education Institutions in Promoting Sustainable Development in Pharmaceutical Research

Mandeep Kumar Gupta, Snigdha Bhardwaj, Sushil Giri, and Rajnish Srivastava

1 Introduction

In the 21st century, the global health and medical professions are evolving rapidly. New disease emergence, antimicrobial resistance escalation, climate change health impacts, and increasing demand for fair and equitable access to healthcare have created a compelling case for sustainability in pharmaceutical research and development (Mohd et al., 2024). Sustainable Development Goals (SDGs) designed by the United Nations as a response to our global challenges in 2015 established a set of 17 interrelated goals that aim to enhance inclusive economic growth, social inclusion, and environmental protection on a global scale by 2030 (Barnett-Itzhaki, Tifferet, Berkowic et al., 2025). SDG 3: Good Health and Well-Being will play an essential role in ameliorating healthcare disparities and advancing medical science, including pharmaceuticals, through innovative approaches (Prior et al., 2025).

HEIs have become important stakeholders in facilitating the SDG agenda. As knowledge-generation and innovation entities, and in the pursuit of a skilled workforce, HEIs have the power to inform public policy, educate future leaders, and foster the importance and development of sustainable technologies. Regarding pharmaceuticals in particular, HEIs also produce qualified scientists and pharmacists and undertake clinical and other programs, not to mention the contribution of human resources via discovery research, green chemistry, and policy campaigns to individual well-being. They have a unique ability to develop academic learning and practice approaches to create policy linkages to pro forma frameworks such as global sustainability (Barnett-Itzhaki, Tifferet, Berkowic et al., 2025; Mohd et al., 2024).

As incubators of science and change agents for social impact, institutions with an emphasis on SDGs can create human resources and integrated learning and social impact approaches to develop human scientific endeavor via technological development, which is also ethical and sustainable. HEIs have the ability to contribute to adequately designed and sustainable drug formulations, the reduction of environmental externalities for contamination from pharmaceutical waste, tackling conscious consumption, furthering the requirement for greater access to essential medicines, and developing and reducing the health disparities in global health (Barnett-Itzhaki, Tifferet, Etstein et al., 2025; Oliveira & Proença, 2025).

DOI: 10.4324/9781003640486-9

In addition, numerous HEIs have already commenced changing their intent to include sustainability in their mission. With interdisciplinary research centers, partnerships with industry and non-governmental organizations, and green campus initiatives, HEIs illustrate how they are working to shape a sustainable academic and research ecosystem. The global momentum toward sustainable healthcare continues to grow—thus, HEIs now have the stewardship of sustainable pharmaceutical research to consider, not only as relevant but also as essential ("Integrating Green Chemistry and Socio-Sustainability in Higher Education: Successful Experiences Contributing to Transform Our World," 2017).

This chapter examines how HEIs might align pharmaceutical research with the SDGs. This chapter will present the context, highlight relevant SDGs in the pharmaceutical sciences, acknowledge institutional roles and global efforts, and review challenges and plans to maximize impact on sustainability leadership by HEIs. After doing this, this chapter can claim HEIs have a critical role in creating a more equitable, healthy, and sustainable world.

2 Alignment of HEIs' Mission with Sustainable Development Goals

2.1 The Strategic Role of HEIs in the 2030 Agenda

The potential impact learning and research institutes have on sustainable development is recognized and pervades the 2030 Agenda. Higher education is critical to developing informed citizens, providing innovative solutions to complex challenges, and influencing the environments within which policy and practice behaviors develop (Leal Filho et al., 2019). Universities and academic institutions are expected to be incorporating sustainability within the full spectrum of education, research, operations, infrastructure, and outreach. Globally we are seeing a number of HEIs incorporating the SDGs into their strategic mission. For example, the University of Cambridge and the University of Melbourne have sustainability offices established to facilitate campus-wide alignment with SDG-like practices while being guided by the principles of sustainability; this alignment involves education and learning in sustainability, sustainability-focused degree programs, and transdisciplinary research centers (for example, planet health and green chemistry) (Moktadir et al., 2020; Salvia et al., 2019).

HEIs also have a role as social entrepreneurs, communicating values around social justice, environmental sustainability, and economic equity through academic communication and student activism. Their association with the SDGs reinforces their relevance within society as a whole, contributes to the growing global partnerships, and grows their active engagement in improving global well-being (Findler et al., 2019).

2.2 Institutional Frameworks and Policy Integration

Incorporating SDGs into university policy means totally reformulating institutional aims, performance indicators, and funding frameworks. There are now many strategic plans that refer explicitly to the SDGs and ways in which academic staff will be recruited and sustained in order to vary forms of research funding sources and in order to design a planned approach to curricula (Findler et al., 2019).

Collaborations now take place globally to create formal frameworks for institutions like the Sustainable Development Solutions Network (SDSN) or University Global Coalitions to identify benchmarks for performance and share best practices. These frameworks encourage HEIs to think globally and act locally.

A plethora of new sustainability data and auditing, ranking, and reporting frameworks, such as the Times Higher Education Impact Rankings, all provide new avenues to assess institutional commitment to SDGs and, as a result, carry some weight, as they can assess a university's performance on health outcomes (clinical and teaching), impact of research, gender equality, and responsible consumption (Ankareddy et al., 2025).

2.3 Specific SDGs Relevant to Pharmaceutical Research

Table 9.1 summarizes the SDGs of relevance to sustainable pharmaceutical research and commitment, showing how the medical school network incorporates HEIs' contributions to each.

Table 9.1 HEI contributions to key SDGs in pharmaceutical research Hicks et al. (2015); Leal Filho et al. (2019); Pradhan et al. (2025)

SDG	*Goal Description*	*Relevance to Pharmaceutical Research*	*HEI Contributions*
SDG 3	Good health and well-being	Central to drug discovery, disease prevention, and equitable access	Clinical research, vaccine development, generics, AMR strategies
SDG 4	Quality education	Builds a skilled, sustainability-conscious pharmaceutical workforce	Curricular reforms, SDG-focused pharmacy education, online learning
SDG 6	Clean water and sanitation	Drug residues affect water quality and sanitation systems	Research on pharmaceutical pollutants, biodegradable drugs, and green disposal
SDG 9	Industry, innovation, and infrastructure	Supports sustainable industrial development and innovation ecosystems	Incubators, patents, translational research partnerships
SDG 12	Responsible consumption and production	Encourages green chemistry and waste minimization	Life cycle analysis, sustainable formulations, green labs
SDG 13	Climate action	Climate change affects drug stability. vector-borne diseases	Resilient drug supply systems, carbon footprint reduction, climate-sensitive health R&D

3 HEIs' Contribution to Achieving the SDGs

3.1 Research and Innovation

HEIs operate as an effective mechanism for pharmaceutical innovation. Notably, HEIs have a very mixed cohort of researchers producing knowledge that both extends the boundary of scientific achievement as well as productively informs public policy as well as drives change within the industry (Pushpakom et al., 2019). In fact, more HEIs are articulating their research agendas around (at least) the SDGs, for instance, in the area of drug repurposing for neglected and emerging diseases, developing targeted drug delivery systems applying nanotechnology, developing high-throughput screening for drugs applying artificial intelligence, and the pharmacology of natural products to actively support more sustainable sourcing of therapeutic agents (Schrogie, 2008). These areas not only spur and feed scientific progress, but they also address some important environmental and global health challenges. While the agency for more sustainable ways of working is gaining traction, leading funders (Wellcome Trust, NIH, and European Research Council, for example) are in fact embedding sustainability criteria into their funding priorities, with increasing aims of influencing the respective HEI research agendas for a more responsible, ethically sound, and ecological pharmaceutical innovation agenda (Chen et al., 2018).

3.2 Teaching and Capacity Building

Many of the adjuncts and faculties of higher education institutions help define and develop the competencies, skills, and values of the future generation of pharmaceutical professionals. Many HEIs have therefore considered the pragmatic and innovative mapping of their institutional competencies to the SDGs as part of the process of adopting strategies for authentic programmatic reform of their curricular offerings by developing innovative forms of pharmaceutical education (Soini et al., 2019). Such initiatives can include interdisciplinary course design that pulls together elements of pharmaceutical science courses with environmental science, public health, and ethics (Heron, 2020). As HEIs look to problem-based and experiential learning models, unique learning opportunities through internships and service learning in underserved communities increase students' direct exposure to the realities of global health (Hmelo-Silver, 2004). These forms of instructional practices enable students to learn in ways that orient them toward a more integrated and holistic understanding of health, equity, and sustainability such that graduates can inspire change in their professional practice and dispositions to sustainable pharmaceutical development (Lozano et al., 2015).

3.3 Partnerships and Knowledge Exchange

HEIs often are a mediator between research and practice as well as research and policy and research and practice. HEIs may partner with:

- Government organizations (e.g., FDA, UN, WHO)
- Non-governmental organizations (e.g., non-profit organizations, NGOs)
- Local communities and indigenous groups

These partnerships ensure the applications of their research findings are situated within the context and relevance of social change. For example, the Drugs for Neglected Diseases initiative (DNDi) and its global consortium that includes several academic institutions (Middel et al., 2017; Morel et al., 2005).

3.4 Institutional Operations and Living Laboratories

HEIs can model sustainability through their own operations. Many universities have established full green campus initiatives to create sustainable campuses, which includes employing renewable energy sources, sustainable sourcing and procurement policies, and substantial waste reduction and recycling practices. However, green campus initiatives can do more than reduce the institution's own environmental impact; they are also a learning tool for students and staff. In the field of pharmaceutical faculties, colleges and schools have also increasingly aligned protocols to green chemistry, energy-efficient lab equipment, and electronic platforms to reduce paper consumption. These operations reflect an institutional commitment to environmental sustainability and an example of how academic and institution practices can reflect sustainability (Fuchs, 2017; Kümmerer et al., 2018).

4 Education and Curriculum Development

Integration is seen as a means of linking subject areas, promoting higher-order thinking, and making the learning experience unified, meaningful, and engaging (Pearson & Hubball, 2012). Research and development (R&D) in this case is a broad term that a school can use to exist as a mechanism to develop and improve its current resources, bring in new knowledge, confirm what they already know, and create new products or technologies. R&D in pharmaceutical companies refers to the first stages of searching for or altering molecules to treat a particular disease up until the final stage of putting a product on the market (Tralau-Stewart et al., 2009).

R&D department staff members carry out lab-scale experiments to create new products, such as pre-formulation and formulation studies and scale-up and technology transfer of developed products; help troubleshoot old products and launch new ones; maintain laboratory equipment and instruments; and exhibit an awareness of operational hazards. Lastly, they carry out research and literature reviews and apply good manufacturing and laboratory practices (Yu, 2008).

One of the most important parts of drug research and development is clinical research. Clinical chemists' participation in research teams offers a unique viewpoint because they can perform pharmacokinetic, pharmacodynamic, safety, and efficacy studies on both new and existing medications (Bond & Raehl, 2007; Panchagnula & Thomas, 2000; "Standards of Practice for Clinical Pharmacists,"

2023). Clinical chemists have authored numerous articles in medical journals and have been involved in drug and development research. As a result, pharmaceutical companies are realizing the potential of clinical chemists and their importance as members of research teams (Nouri et al., 2020; "The Definition of Clinical Pharmacy," 2008).

R&D is more than just lab work. One of the most important stages of the drug journey is clinical research, where the chemist can effectively apply their expertise. As a result, chemists may be qualified to work in R&D but not yet skilled or knowledgeable. They could become more skilled in the field through post-graduation self-development, participation in training programs, and training from pharmaceutical institutions, as is the case in all professions. Nevertheless, factors other than pharmacy education alone, such as profit and career advancement, can be blamed for the low proportion of pharmacists in the industry. For sustainability and fruitful research outcomes, pharmacy academic institutions must also collaborate with government agencies, the pharmaceutical industry, and drug development units (Nouri et al., 2020).

4.1 Integrating Sustainability into Pharmaceutical Education

Pharmaceutical environmental pollution occurs when people develop, manufacture, use, and dispose of drugs. It can adversely impact ecosystems, exacerbate antibiotic resistance, and also produce large greenhouse gas emissions. The adverse environmental impacts of the healthcare sector—and the pharmaceutical industry in particular—have been gaining more attention in recent years (Belkhir & Elmeligi, 2019; Karliner et al., 2019). Pharmaceutical environmental pollution occurs when people develop, manufacture, use, and dispose of drugs and can adversely impact ecosystems, alter antibiotic resistance, and generate large greenhouse gas emissions among many other effects (aus der Beek et al., 2016). In fact, the pharmaceutical industry and healthcare sector as a whole contribute significantly to global warming. They are responsible for about 4% of the global greenhouse gas emissions, with approximately 12–40% of those emissions being attributed directly to pharmaceuticals (Karliner et al., 2019; Steenmeijer et al., 2022).

Based on the three pillars of sustainability, this holistic framework for integrated sustainability assessment of pharmaceuticals considers both footprint and handprint outcomes. The study's specific sub-goals are to (1) describe the framework's methodological development, (2) present the framework's components and structure, and (3) operationalize the framework. The social, economic, and environmental sustainability aspects of pharmaceuticals should all be improved and balanced with the use of this sustainability framework (Van Wilder et al., 2024).

4.2 Life Cycle of Framework

As shown in Figure 9.1, the life cycle of sustainability in pharmaceutical drug development illustrates key stages from discovery to disposal with a focus on environmental and social effects.

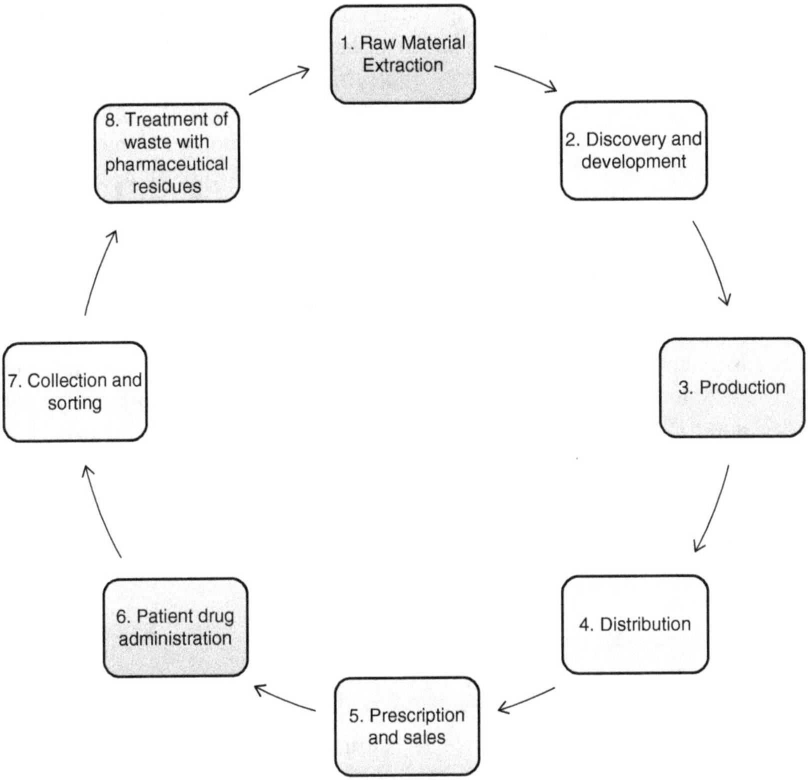

Figure 9.1 Life cycle of integrating sustainability in pharmaceutical development.

Environmental sustainability: The effects of pharmaceutical processes and products on ecosystems and biodiversity are the focus of the environmental pillar of sustainability (Morelli, 2011). Concerns about environmental sustainability in the manufacturing of pharmaceuticals are receiving more attention (Moermond et al., 2022), decreased solvent usage through microfluidics (Weaver et al., 2022), waste management for pharmaceutical products (Brechtelsbauer & Shah, 2020), and handling of pharmaceutical impurities. Finding and capturing all pertinent environmental sustainability issues is the goal of the holistic framework.

Economic sustainability: The economic pillar of sustainability describes how a pharmaceutical affects regional, national, and global economic systems (Purvis et al., 2019). Generally speaking, this pillar covers all expenses and income incurred by parties participating in the pharmaceutical life cycle, from raw material extraction to disposal. The pharmaceutical industry's primary concerns regarding economic sustainability are frequently linked to patent activity (Azad et al., 2018) and regulating spending on research and innovation, labor productivity, and human capital through systematic management, as well as new technologies (like 3D printing) (Aquino et al., 2018; Bom et al., 2019; Niño-Amézquita et al., 2017).

Social sustainability: Improving social conditions throughout the pharmaceutical life cycle is the goal of the social pillar of sustainability (SETAC, 2020). This pillar addresses a wide range of subjects, including fair competition, equality, human rights, social security, labor rights, and workplace health and safety (Moldan et al., 2012) and interested parties. The social impact along the pharmaceutical supply chain is difficult to quantify and comprehend, though. Indeed, the local context in which pharmaceuticals are produced has a significant impact on social impacts, and certain regions do not adhere to human rights and the conventions of the International Labour Organization (Van Wilder et al., 2024).

The creation of the comprehensive sustainability framework for pharmaceuticals is a significant step in the transformation of the healthcare industry into a more sustainable one. This framework might be a first step toward a more standardized way to evaluate the effects of medications. The framework can be useful in decision-making because it will enable the user to be transparent and identify data gaps, obstacles, and opportunities to achieve pharmaceutical sustainability. The framework will be operationalized in future work while taking user and stakeholder preferences into account (Van Wilder et al., 2024).

4.3 Innovative Teaching Methods and Practices and Successful Curriculum Models

Teaching teams are used in pharmacy education so that students can receive instruction from subject matter experts. Additional procedural considerations that might not arise in courses with a single instructor are provided by the implementation of team-based learning (TBL) in a team-teaching setting. Team formation, readiness assurance, prompt feedback, the order of in-class problem solving, the four "S" structure for creating team application exercises, incentive structure, and peer evaluation are the seven essential components (Haidet et al., 2012).

To build support for the team formation process, course directors should talk to all of the instructors about their plans for student teamwork. To encourage team building, productivity, and peer learning, the course director and instructors can collaborate to create the teams, which should then be utilized for the duration of the course, semester, or year (Farland et al., 2013).

In addition to offering chances for higher-order thinking and the development of non-cognitive skills like communication and teamwork, the in-class team application exercises are designed to expand on the foundational knowledge acquired during the readiness assurance process. As a result, developing these application exercises becomes essential to the TBL procedure (Farland et al., 2013).

Peer evaluation is a crucial part of TBL because it helps students cultivate the attitudes and teamwork they will need as future chemists working in collaborative healthcare settings (Persky, 2012).

Variations of team-based learning have been documented anecdotally and in the literature, and it is becoming more and more popular among colleges and pharmacy schools. Although there are chances to customize the TBL process, some essential elements ought to stay the same: immediate feedback for content, process, and student development; the readiness assurance process; and in-class team application exercises that enable simultaneous reporting that highlights key learning objectives (Farland et al., 2013).

Careful curriculum planning is necessary to promote integrative learning because it does not "just happen" for the majority of students. The sequential scheduling of related courses (e.g., a pathophysiology class, followed by a pharmacology class, followed by a therapeutics class) and the inclusion of sporadic learning activities in one discipline that draw on knowledge from other disciplines (e.g., a pharmacy practice laboratory exercise that draws on biochemistry concepts, or the inclusion of physical assessment activities in a pathophysiology course) are structural strategies for improving integration in pharmacy programs (Epstein et al., 2001; Epstein & Brosvic, 2002).

Disciplines may develop distinctive pedagogical approaches, or "signature pedagogies," as a result of this "logical connection" between teaching and learning (Shulman, 2005). To give a pharmacy-specific example, clinicians use disease states as the organizing framework for their unique knowledge, while pharmacologists use drug classes.

Crossing disciplinary boundaries in integrated curricula is made more difficult by variations in pedagogical approaches, expectations for thinking, and conceptualizations of knowledge. Nonetheless, disciplinary components are still required in integrated curricula since integrative learning requires a solid understanding of disciplinary knowledge and skills, which takes time to develop (Spelt et al., 2009). However, integrative learning also requires a significant amount of time. Time and resources are also needed to deliver and maintain integrated curricula. Even basic horizontal integration initiatives, like coordinating course topics, frequently rely on instructors being available at particular times, which may necessitate constant preparation and negotiating.

The goal of curriculum integration is to promote integrative learning, which is demonstrated in pharmacy programs by the requirement that graduates apply their knowledge and abilities from various fields to the management of patients' medication therapy in complex medical conditions.

Most students do not naturally engage in integrative learning, so integrated curricula are necessary to intentionally promote it. The process of developing an integrated curriculum is challenging, though, because it necessitates overcoming obstacles like discipline-based institutional structures, knowledge concepts, and teaching and learning traditions; it also requires developing integrative pedagogical and assessment strategies; and it has limited time and resources (Spelt et al., 2009).

5 Research and Innovation

5.1 Sustainable Research Practices in Higher Education Institutes

In the 21st century, sustainability has become a key priority for world development, especially in the fields of technology, research, and health. A key player in this change is HEIs, which serve as training grounds for aspiring scientists as well as knowledge producers and innovation incubators. Pharmaceutical sustainability—the endeavor to conduct pharmaceutical research and development that is socially, ecologically, and financially responsible—is one of the most significant areas in which HEIs contribute.

HEIs are rethinking their research ecosystems through external collaborations and internal reforms. This examines the following three aspects of this role:

1. Sustainable research practices in HEIs,
2. Collaborative research initiatives, and
3. The impact of HEI research on pharmaceutical sustainability.

5.2 Sustainable Research Practices in HEIs

The 1972 Stockholm Declaration on the Human Environment was the first to emphasize the involvement of HEIs around the world in sustainable development (SD). Since then, HEIs have participated in a number of worldwide projects and reaffirmed their dedication to SD in numerous national and international proclamations, accords, and conventions (Lozano et al., 2013).

Concerning SD in the context of higher education, the first phrase to be specified is "sustainability in higher education." The term refers to aspects of sustainability that are relevant to higher education, to put it another way. The second term to be defined is "sustainability." While these processes facilitate acknowledged or unrecognized social benefits, they advocate the warranted use of natural resources and an implicit understanding of nature in particular ways. In recent times, HEIs have seen significant growth in key areas of sustainability research. Some of the new areas include the Living Labs approach, climate change education, and the SDGs. HEIs are starting to solve social and environmental problems with the Living Labs approach as a strategy for sustainability research. Research indicates that for Living Labs projects to have transformative, sustainable outcomes, studies need to consider social and cultural processes over time in addition to technological advances (Filho et al., 2019).

HEIs will also learn about climate change through theory and practice research (Table 9.2). Climate change substantially influences science, society, the environment, and geopolitics, which has led to enormous increases in HEIs' energy, environmental, and climate change research. Colleges are using the typical approach to

Table 9.2 Sustainable research practices in HEIs

Practice Area	*Traditional Approach*	*Sustainable Approach*
Laboratory practices	High energy and chemical use	Eco-labs with low energy consumption
Drug discovery	Animal trials, high-toxicity compounds	In silico modeling, biocompatible ingredients
Research collaboration	Competitive, siloed	Open-source, interdisciplinary partnerships
Funding focus	ROI-driven	Impact- and outcome-based funding

teaching climate change, systematically including climate change studies in their courses and developing research so that these concepts can be integrated into a system (Filho et al., 2019).

In recent literature, there is rapid growth in the developing and published literature on the under-researched and rapidly growing area of study into connections, contextualized relevance, and potential actioning of the UN SDGs in higher education institutions. HEIs are looking to try and address the SDGs and incorporate the ambitious 17 goals into their plans and agendas (Leal Filho et al., 2019).

5.3 *Collaborative Research Initiatives*

LUCSUS coordinates the Lund University Center of Excellence for Integration of Social and Natural Aspects of Sustainability (LUCID) and the Lund University International Master's Programme in Environmental Studies and Sustainability Science (LUMES). To address complicated sustainability concerns, LUCID seeks to build new integrated theories and methodologies by establishing entirely new and distinctive synergies across the scientific and social sciences. It is anticipated that the study will add theoretical, methodological, and applied insights to the vast and developing field of sustainability science (Yarime et al., 2012).

5.4 *The Impact of HEI Research on Pharmaceutical Sustainability*

HEIs play a vital role in enhancing pharmaceutical sustainability through research that promotes innovation, affordability, and environmental responsibility. By applying principles of green chemistry, sustainable drug development practices, and digital transformation in pharmaceutical sciences, HEIs reduce the ecological footprint of drug production.

Case study is on holistic approach on Green Generation to implementation of green principles and practices in educational programs in pharmaceutical and medical sciences at the University of Helsinki. The primary aim of the Generation Green task force is to promote a comprehensive mindset toward overall sustainability in both current and future pharmacy professionals. Meeting this goal requires, however, systematic management of the change process. Therefore, the Generation Green task force chose to follow a previously published framework for change management by Dr. John Kotter (Kotter, 2007). The eight-step model is one of the most used ones in the area of change management.

At the Faculty of Pharmacy, the principles of green and sustainable chemistry were integrated into the pharmaceutical chemistry and pharmaceutical organic chemistry courses. On these courses, the teaching is mostly based on qualitative reasoning. Regarding the metrics of sustainable chemistry, the degree students of pharmacy become familiar with basic concepts, such as atom economy and percentage yield, whereas for green chemistry metrics (process/reaction mass intensity, reaction mass efficiency, or E-factor), the degree students of pharmacy are encouraged to deepen their knowledge in specialized chemistry courses at the Department of Chemistry, Faculty of Science (University of Helsinki).

While innovation and R&D are driving growth, they should also help society decouple growth from the exploitation of raw materials. Both resource decoupling and effect decoupling become essential components of SD when we embrace it as the development that satisfies human needs while protecting those of future generations (Sakao et al., 2024). This implies that resource-efficient use of raw materials and technological innovation are essential, as is the decoupling of resource consumption and economic growth or prosperity on the one hand and the decoupling of environmental consequences and economic growth on the other.

6 Industry Partnerships and Collaborations

The collaboration between academic institutions and industries is growing steadily. Such partnerships play a vital role in fostering a knowledge-based economy. University–Industry Collaboration (UIC) involves interactions between higher education institutions and businesses, primarily focused on promoting the exchange of knowledge and technology (Ankrah & AL-Tabbaa, 2015). Industry partnerships and collaboration have become essential rather than optional, serving as a strategic driver for progress, innovation, workforce development, and economic growth. HEIs play a crucial role in these alliances, acting as key connectors by utilizing their research expertise, skilled talent, and intellectual leadership. The Living Labs method and climate change education are two significant growing fields. These collaborations assist in bridging the gap between academic theory and practical application, ensuring that intellectual research leads to actual solutions. University–Industry Collaboration (UIC) has a long history of helping organizations improve their expertise. Recently, there has been a considerable increase in UIC across several countries, including the United States, Japan, Singapore, and states within the European Union, and in the application of SDGs (Ankrah & AL-Tabbaa, 2015).

6.1 HEIs Connecting Academia and Industry

In the rapidly changing and fiercely competitive job market of today, students who want to succeed in their professional careers must acquire skills relevant to the business. Despite providing a strong theoretical foundation, traditional academic education usually falls short in delivering the practical experience and real-world understanding that employers value. Because of these gaps between classroom instruction and the needs of business, internships and hands-on training programs have become increasingly important components of a student's educational journey.

6.1.1 Curriculum Alignment with Industry Needs

The majority of pharmacy education in India is theoretical, and out-of-date curricula don't keep up with changing industry demands. Modern processes such as IVRS/IWRS operations and pharmacovigilance reporting can be outdated in many current programs. It would be very valuable for HEIs and the industry to collaborate toward bridging this gap by:

- **Updating Course Content:** Adopting a broader range of industry-relevant modules to the course curriculum (e.g., medical writing and regulatory affairs) and the adoption of opportunities for practical learning modules (note: no practical experiences are demanded by the Pharmacy Council of India under the Pharmacy Practice Regulations (Pol et al., 2017).
- **Collaborating with Sector Skill Councils (SSCs):** Promoting and supporting skill-based initiatives, such as the Skill India Initiative, tailored to the needs of industry or to incorporate industry-specific projects.
- **Implementing International Standards**: Preparing graduates to be competitive for positions at multinational pharmaceutical companies, as articulated in the "Opportunities for Strengthening Industry Engagement" questions—BENEFIT of understanding global practices (Gawade & Sonaje, 2017).

6.1.2 Improving Training and Experiential Education Programs

Students graduating from pharmacy programs often find themselves lacking workplace skills due to outdated laboratories and minimal interaction with industry. The following suggestions could address the gap:

- **Industry-Required Internships:** Partner with pharmaceutical companies to offer stipend-based clinical training under the aegis of the National Apprenticeship Promotion Scheme (NAPS).
- **Simulation-Based Training Labs:** Set up a modern lab class to simulate processes such as clinical trials and pharmacovigilance.
- **Case-Led Teaching:** Take theoretical information and apply it to a case study drawn from real-world experience (e.g., monitoring adverse drug reactions).
- **Modular Upskilling Programs:** To enhance employability and preparedness for a workforce, provide micro-credentials in areas of pharmacy that are growing.
- **Industry–Academia Model:** Some promising developments such as Wipro's academic collaborations in engineering education and Infosys' Campus Connect might demonstrate models for similar collaborations with pharmacy education.

6.1.3 Strengthening Industry–Academia Partnerships

As HEIs and pharmaceutical companies currently are at odds, graduates often have some skills, but not all the skills they need for industry. Using the following cooperative approaches, the skills gap can be narrowed:

HEI Initiatives:

- **Curriculum Collaboration:** Development of the curriculum by working with one or more top pharmaceutical companies (e.g., Novartis and Sun Pharma) to provide tailored training courses in recent topics in regulatory compliance, as well as pharmacovigilance.
- **Faculty Enabling Programs:** Through industry-sponsored training programs, educators can upskill and align their teaching methodologies with industry practices.

- **Joint Research Projects:** Foster innovation through collaboration by creating joint research projects that address business issues and increase knowledge for academia (Palsokar & Tajne, 2018).

6.1.4 *Using Infrastructure and Policy to Improve Training*

Inadequate resources, like legacy lab equipment, restrict experiential learning in pharmacy education. Institutions should take the following strategic steps:

- **Modernize Facilities:** Involves sustainable practices such as taking advantage of Pradhan Mantri Kaushal Vikas Yojana (PMKVY) or other skill development grants to update infrastructure.
- **Regulatory Engagement:** Advocate for mandatory industry internships, akin to laws requiring medical training.
- **Global Benchmark:** The WHO's emphasis on competency-based education (2012) emphasizes how urgently academic programs need to implement organized skill-building activities (Palsokar & Tajne, 2018).

6.1.5 *Challenges Faced by Colleges in Bridging Academia and Industry*

- **Curriculum Alignment:** A key challenge involves synchronizing academic programs with the fast-changing demands of industries. Educational institutions must continuously revise their course content and instructional approaches to provide students with current, industry-relevant competencies that meet employer expectations (Bridgstock, 2009).
- **Industry Partnership Accessibility:** Many academic institutions—particularly smaller colleges or those in regions with limited industrial presence—face difficulties in developing substantive collaborations with corporate partners. The limited access to professional networks often suppresses both the variety and potential of practical training options available for the students (Engelbrecht, 2019).
- **Resource Limitations in Experiential Learning:** Numerous educational institutions face budgetary and human resource issues that limit their ability to set up extensive internship and career training programs. Enough financial resources and institutional support are still essential for creating meaningful experiential learning opportunities (Bridgstock, 2009).
- **Maintaining Program Excellence:** Ensuring practical training that is both industry-relevant and of high quality is a challenging task. Academic institutions must set up thorough evaluation procedures, provide participants with appropriate supervision during their placements, and methodically monitor outcomes to assess the effectiveness of their programs (Thakur et al., 2024).
- **Facilitating Inclusive Opportunities:** Equitable access to experiential learning is still a challenge, especially for students who are marginalized or disadvantaged groups, who often have barriers to finding valuable training placements. Creating intentional access policies for education organizations can help assure

that all students have equitable access to professional skill-building programs (Moriña, 2017).

- **Aligning Practical and Academic Objectives:** A major problem is integrating work-based learning with academic programs in an effective manner. Institutions must take care to create experiential learning opportunities that support academic objectives and give participants real, skill-building work experiences (McCafferty, 2022).
- **Keeping Pace with Innovation:** The rapid changes in working practices and technology necessitate ongoing flexibility from educational institutions. Novel methods like remote training programs and digital internships provide compelling opportunities but also present challenges for effective implementation and results outcomes (Allioui et al., 2023).

A strategy that gets the various government agencies, business partners, educational institutions, and key stakeholders working together to create an ecosystem that links the connection between professional practice and academic learning through robust internship and vocational placements.

7 Government-Led Skill Development Programs in India

The Indian government has initiated a number of programs to assist students in closing the skills gap by providing internships and vocational experience. These programs aim to improve employability and prepare the workforce.

- **National Apprenticeship Promotion Scheme (NAPS):** The Ministry of Skill Development and Entrepreneurship has implemented NAPS to financially support employers to promote apprenticeship in several sectors. The program encourages employers to take on apprentices by partially paying trainees' pay during their apprenticeship (*National Apprenticeship Promotion Scheme (NAPS) | Ministry of Skill Development and Entrepreneurship*, n.d.).
- **Pradhan Mantri Kaushal Vikas Yojana (PMKVY):** A central part to the skill development objective, PMKVY provides short-term training programs targeted at industries to equip young people with employable skills. Although internships are not the primary basis of PMKVY, it seeks to increase employability through industry-based training and competency assessment. The program also supports an apprenticeship component for a small number of sectors, which should work again to close the skills gap (*Pradhan Mantri Kaushal Vikas Yojana 4.0 (PMKVY 4.0) | Ministry of Skill Development and Entrepreneurship*, n.d.).
- **National Career Service (NCS):** NCS is a web portal that provides access to job listings, skills development programs, and apprenticeship opportunities and is an online marketplace connecting businesses, training organizations, and job seekers. NCS connects job seekers to vacancies, internships, and training paths aligned to their skills and career aspirations (*NCS|Home: National Career Service—Career Guidance and Jobs in India and Related Services*, n.d.).

- **Skill India Mission:** The government has launched a number of initiatives to foster practical learning and vocational training within this flagship program. SSCs are important components of the program that work closely with industry to provide standard training in the form of programs and vocational placements in accordance with standards defined for each sector (*Sector Skill Councils (SSC) | Ministry of Skill Development and Entrepreneurship | NSDC*, n.d.).
- **Startup India:** The government-sponsored initiative allows startups and SMEs to receive comprehensive advice, feedback, resources, and funding and builds capacity at the same time while fostering innovation and entrepreneurial development. The initiative intends to role model qualified personnel, foster practical learning, and create an entrepreneurial mindset for young professionals and students alike through a number of initiatives and benefits, including organized internship schemes (*Startup India*, n.d.).
- **Mahatma Gandhi National Rural Employment Guarantee Act (MGNREGA):** It includes skill-building elements in its framework, even though creating jobs in rural areas is its primary goal. Through a variety of development projects that need technical skills in fields including farming, building, and public works, the program gives rural kids hands-on learning opportunities. By providing focused vocational training, experiential learning opportunities, and tailored skill development programs for employers and job seekers across various industries, these government programs showcase India's all-encompassing approach to bridging the gap between academic preparation and workplace demands (*Mahatma Gandhi NREGA*, n.d.).

8 Future Prospects for the Impact of Collaboration

- **Reinforce Innovation Platform:** The recommended approach is that the shared knowledge made possible by overlapping institutional domains and interconnected ecosystems would become increasingly important for economic advancement. These cooperative relationships foster organizational agility and speed up technology advancements, creating a more dynamic and competitive company environment (Etzkowitz & Leydesdorff, 2000).
- **Encouraging Organic and Flexible Partnership Strategies**: According to research, informal professional networks usually produce greater results than strict contracts. Building deep ties between academics and corporate executives should be the top priority of academic-industry collaborations going forward. This relationship-driven approach enhances adaptability, minimizes administrative hurdles, and strengthens mutual involvement in collaborative projects (Cerych & Frost-Smith, 1985).
- **Industry–Academia Partnership Programs for Hands-on Learning:** Initiatives similar to the UK's Knowledge Transfer Partnerships (originally called the Teaching Company Scheme) provide valuable industry exposure to students. Scaling up such cooperative frameworks would better equip graduates for professional careers while simultaneously encouraging collaborative research between academia and businesses (Borah et al., 2019).

- **Continuous Learning and Workforce Development:** HEIs are anticipated to play a key role in delivering ongoing education. Partnerships may emphasize flexible training programs, digital credentials, and upskilling efforts tailored to evolving industry demands (Daher-Armache et al., 2025).
- **Policy and Institutional Backing: The** report underscores the critical role of government policies in fostering industry–academia partnerships by creating supportive frameworks and incentives. It stresses the importance of policies that:
    - Encourage collaboration between educational institutions and industries,
    - Support curriculum design that meets industry requirements, and
    - Promote research and innovation from ideation to market implementation.

    Active government engagement is vital to cultivating an environment that sustains meaningful collaborations, strengthens the research ecosystem, and ensures education remains aligned with industry needs. As an illustration, the report cites government-driven programs like the Pune Knowledge Cluster (PKC), which unites universities, businesses, and research institutions to address local challenges through science and technology initiatives (*FICCI EDUWRAP*, 2022).

9 Community Engagement and Outreach

The initiatives of higher education institutions to advance SD in pharmaceutical research rely on community participation and outreach. By bridging the gap between academia and community, programs began to not only share information for public use but also instill responsibility, inclusiveness, and beneficial action in the world. By conducting actions to leverage pharmaceutical research for people's benefit, like community programs, public awareness programs on health, health camps, and using local health professionals, the pharmaceutical science process is taken beyond the lab and article publication (Aigbe et al., 2025; Ramísio et al., 2019).

Engaging communities surrounding sustainable pharmacy practice through the involvement of activity based on public health addressing including access to affordable medicines and/or correct dose, safe and appropriate use of drugs, and consideration of antimicrobial resistance is important. Organizations can provide community training workshops, support herbal and/or green formulations, or extract local knowledge of communities, all of which attempts to promote sustainable healthcare practice overall (Jairoun et al., 2025; Mitchell et al., 2023).

Community program opportunities such as school healthy living, health promotion in villages, and mobile clinics allow students and researchers the opportunity to not only help underserved health but also gain valuable real-world experience. This encourages students to be responsible and encourages public confidence in science and education. Joint research with NGOs, government organizations, and local communities also identifies region-specific diseases and sustainable solutions, supporting a bottom-up drug development approach (Nagel et al., 2022; Shin et al., 2020).

The incorporation of community involvement in academic programs, such as service-learning modules, makes future pharmaceutical professionals sensitive to social and environmental obligations. It develops a culture in which innovation is complemented by ethical, cultural, and ecological values. Essentially, universities are catalysts in that they facilitate communities to become participatory stakeholders of pharmaceutical sustainability (Doubeni et al., 2022). By a comprehensive strategy that integrates scientific progress and human requirements, public outreach and community participation become both an ethical necessity and a utilitarian strategy in pursuing SD objectives for drug research (Rodríguez-Zurita et al., 2025).

10 Challenges and Barriers

Despite a growing recognition of the necessity for SD in drug research, higher education institutions face numerous challenges and obstacles in effectively promoting and implementing these goals (Table 9.3). A significant challenge lies in the insufficient amount of funding and funds allocated to sustainability-oriented research, especially in developing nations where institutional budgets are already strained. Students and faculty may not know or understand the principles of sustainability and how they relate to pharmaceutical sciences, which makes it harder to use sustainable practices in the classroom, in research, and in the lab. Many institutions have been slow to adopt sustainable practices because they are stuck in their ways. Traditional academic research methods focus on publication count and short-term effects over long-term environmental and social impact. A lot of the time, academics, businesses, and government officials work together at a level that doesn't exist for goals that don't work together. There are also typically legal issues, worries about intellectual property, and a lack of uniform sustainability measures to think about when deciding what sustainable practices are. Also, there is collaboration between different fields, and for sustainability to have an effect, it needs to focus on an integrative approach to learning. However, disciplines are often rigid and tied to academic disciplines, which makes sustainability practices less effective. Finally, students have very few chances to connect their academic experience to sustainability action because there aren't many platforms for it, or because the characteristics of sustainable practice are not well integrated into the learning program, or because academic experience doesn't encourage students to act for sustainability, so it doesn't have much of an impact. Higher education institutions need to be fully committed to making their schools legitimate agents of social innovation reform and sustainability action. They should promote internal capacity building and make the whole educational experience better by being inclusive in their curricular programs, forming partnerships, working with people from different sectors, and pushing for policy change. We can get rid of the hurdles so that colleges and universities may be effective agents of change in line with a unified pharmaceutical research agenda that supports global SDGs (Abo-Khalil, 2024; Al Husban, 2025; Škokić et al., 2025).

Table 9.3 Challenges and barriers in aligning pharmaceutical education and research with global sustainable development goals Abo-Khalil (2024); Al Husban (2025); Leal Filho et al. (2025); Škokić et al. (2025)

S. No.	*Challenge/Barrier*	*Description*
1	Lack of awareness and training	Many faculty and students are not adequately informed or trained on SDGs or sustainable research practices in the pharmaceutical field.
2	Limited funding and resources	Financial constraints hinder the development and implementation of sustainable research projects, green labs, and eco-friendly technologies.
3	Inadequate curriculum integration	Sustainability concepts are often not integrated into the pharmaceutical curriculum, limiting students' exposure to environmental responsibility.
4	Resistance to change	Traditional research methodologies and academic inertia often resist the adoption of new sustainable practices.
5	Lack of industry collaboration	Weak links between academic and pharmaceutical industries can limit access to real-world data, sustainable technologies, and innovation pathways.
6	Policy and regulatory barriers	Absence of supportive institutional or governmental policies for green research and sustainability can delay adoption.
7	Short-term research goals	Academic research is often focused on short-term outcomes, overlooking long-term environmental and social impacts.
8	Insufficient interdisciplinary approaches	Sustainable pharmaceutical research requires collaboration across disciplines, which is often lacking in siloed academic structures.
9	Limited infrastructure for green practices	Most institutions lack sustainable infrastructure like green labs, energy-efficient equipment, and waste disposal systems.
10	Lack of incentives and recognition	There is minimal recognition or reward for faculty and researchers who pursue sustainability-focused pharmaceutical research.

11 Future Prospectives

As worldwide demand for healthcare continues to grow and diversifies at a rapid pace, the pharmaceutical industry must adapt to the need for innovation sustainably across many segments of industry. Sustainable approaches to future pharmaceutical innovation are entering the marketplace based on advances in green chemistry, renewable feedstock, and processes for environmentally aware drug development (Colberg et al., 2025; Olawade et al., 2025; Pereira & Cotas, 2024). Emerging technologies in the drug discovery process, such as artificial intelligence (AI), machine learning, and big data analytics, are becoming tools to create a more data-driven and efficient route in exploration that will allow users to improve productivity, gaining more in return, while minimizing loss of time, money, and resources in the process of developing pharmaceuticals. The same can be said for the rise in biopharmaceutical products, personalized medicine, and 3D drug print innovations that are collectively opening up pathways for improved innovation in therapeutics toward environmental sustainability. Strategies that are becoming more common, such as life cycle assessments and environmental risk assessments, are now being used to assess quality when developing drugs and their production. Companies such as *HCL Pharma* and *Gerresheimer Device Development & Contract Manufacturing Pharmatech* are using continuous manufacturing for their tablets, while some pharmaceutical companies have designed drug products with biodegradable excipients to reduce waste. Such advancements show the move to energy-supportive and lower-waste pharmaceutical systems in the rapidly changing pharmaceutical sector (Fu & Chen, 2025; Vora et al., 2023).

In the evolving higher education landscape, HEIs serve as catalysts for sustainable transformation, characterized by their roles in engagement, policy influence, and innovation incubation. HEIs are increasingly integrating sustainability into their curricula, fostering interdisciplinary initiatives, and conducting research aimed at developing eco-sensitive pharmaceuticals and delivery systems. Institutions are establishing sustainability-focused research centers that provide students with opportunities to engage in projects aligned with the United Nations SDGs. These initiatives promote collaboration with industry and government to facilitate technology transfer and scale sustainable innovations (Basheer et al., 2025; Serrano-Bedia & Perez-Perez, 2022).

In the future, higher education institutions will be required to engage more actively and responsibly with sustainability. Institutions of higher education prepared for the future will facilitate the establishment of low-carbon laboratories, sustainable campus operations, and environmentally responsible research methodologies. Higher education institutions will contribute to the training of future scientists who will possess technical proficiency and demonstrate environmental responsibility. Digitalization, open access, and international collaborations will unlock the democratization of access to sustainable pharmaceutical education and research. It is incumbent upon higher education institutions to engage in discussions regarding policies and to advocate for regulators in the use of a more robust set of sustainability criteria during the drug development process. The future of sustainable pharmaceutical research will depend on the forthcoming roles as linked agents of change by higher education institutions at the confluence of responsibility and innovation, engaging in a shared commitment to a community of science practice for a healthier planet and society (Abdullahi et al., 2024; Lozano et al., 2013).

12 Conclusion

Higher education institutions play an important, multifaceted role in advancing sustainable pharmaceutical research. As tertiary institutions of knowledge creators, knowledge innovators, and knowledge talent developers, HEIs are ideally situated to leverage their expertise to promote the growth of the pharmaceutical sciences related to sustainability. This chapter has identified ways HEIs can further sustainability related to their research agendas, redesigning curricula, developing sustainable lab processes, and developing institute-wide policies that embrace and integrate sustainability. HEIs may reduce and replace resource use, establish effective transdisciplinary approaches, devise and execute ethical research, evaluate new technologies in a more environmentally conscious manner, and address national and global health issues while minimizing economic, environmental, and social harms.

Indeed, HEIs can support the development of technical and ethically and environmentally responsible future generations of pharmaceutical professionals. Where SDGs can be adopted as part of academic and research practices, students and researchers can be stimulated to extend and appreciate their research in relation to wider human and ecological benefits. Collaborating with industry, regulators, and international agencies can, in the best-case scenario, improve the applicability and likely real-world implications resulting from sustainable pharmaceutical studies and associated innovations from HEIs.

It is possible to address institutional leadership, faculty engagement, and funding to consider critical enablers to this change. HEIs can take sustainability seriously through governance and funding for a longer-term effect. Challenges (awareness and limited capacity and resources and resistance to change) can be addressed through policy reform, capacity building, and engagement and dialogue with stakeholders.

In conclusion, it presents a new opportunity to HEIs to embed sustainability more broadly into the fabric of pharmaceutical research and development. HEIs can make a significant contribution to the development of health sciences globally by developing a culture of responsibility, innovation, and inclusiveness. Making pharmaceutical research and development more sustainable is not simply an exercise in academia; it is a moral responsibility, and HEIs may help lead it, champion it, and sustain it—for generations to come.

Bibliography

17th FICCI Higher Education Summit 2022 (FHES 2022), themed "Global Destination for Higher Education: Advantage INDIA," was held in New Delhi from November 17–19, 2022

Abdullahi, A. M., Hussein, H. A., Ahmed, M. Y., Hussein, O. A., & Warsame, A. A. (2024). The impact of education for sustainable development on university students' sustainability behavior: A case study from undergraduate students in Somalia. *Frontiers in Education, 9*. https://doi.org/10.3389/feduc.2024.1413687

Abo-Khalil, A. G. (2024). Integrating sustainability into higher education challenges and opportunities for universities worldwide. *Heliyon, 10*(9), e29946. https://doi.org/10.1016/j.heliyon.2024.e29946

Aigbe, F., Aigbavboa, C., Ayobiojo, L., & Imoisili, P. E. (2025). Adaptive learning for inclusivity, sustainable development, and societal impact: A case study of community engagement at the University of Johannesburg. *Sustainability*, *17*(11), 4861. https://doi.org/10.3390/su17114861

Al Husban, W. (2025). The impact of integrating sustainable development goals on students' awareness and pro-environmental behavior: A case study of Jordan. *Sustainability*, *17*(6), 2588. https://doi.org/10.3390/su17062588

Allioui, H., Mourdi, Y., Allioui, H., & Mourdi, Y. (2023). Exploring the full potentials of IoT for better financial growth and stability: A comprehensive survey. *Sensors 2023, 23*(19), 8015. https://doi.org/10.3390/S23198015

American College of Clinical Pharmacy (2008). The definition of clinical pharmacy. *Pharmacotherapy*, 28(6), 816–817. https://doi.org/10.1592/phco.28.6.816

American College of Clinical Pharmacy (2014). Standards of practice for clinical pharmacists. *Pharmacotherapy*, *34*(8), 794–797. https://doi.org/10.1002/phar.1438

Ankareddy, S., Dorfleitner, G., Zhang, L., & Ok, Y. S. (2025). Embedding sustainability in higher education institutions: A review of practices and challenges. *Cleaner Environmental Systems*, *17*, 100279. https://doi.org/10.1016/J.CESYS.2025.100279

Ankrah, S., & AL- Tabbaa, O. (2015). Universities-industry collaboration: A systematic review. *Scandinavian Journal of Management*, *31*(3). https://doi.org/10.1016/j.scaman.2015.02.003

Aquino, R. P., Barile, S., Grasso, A., & Saviano, M. (2018). Envisioning smart and sustainable healthcare: 3D Printing technologies for personalized medication. *Futures*, *103*. https://doi.org/10.1016/j.futures.2018.03.002

aus der Beek, T., Weber, F. A., Bergmann, A., Hickmann, S., Ebert, I., Hein, A., & Küster, A. (2016). Pharmaceuticals in the environment-Global occurrences and perspectives. *Environmental Toxicology and Chemistry*, *35*(4). https://doi.org/10.1002/etc.3339

Azad, M. A. K., Munisamy, S., Teng, K. K., Talib, M. B. A., & Saona, P. (2018). Productivity changes of pharmaceutical industry in Bangladesh: Does process patent matter? *Global Business Review*, *19*(4). https://doi.org/10.1177/0972150918772966

Barnett-Itzhaki, Z., Tifferet, S., Berkowic, D., Arviv, T., Daya, A., Carasso Romano, G. H., & Levi, A. (2025). Strategies and challenges for green campuses. *Frontiers in Sustainable Cities*, *7*. https://doi.org/10.3389/frsc.2025.1469274

Barnett-Itzhaki, Z., Tifferet, S., Etstein, Y., Gefen, I., Ravid, O., Barokas, G., Vilnai-Yavetz, I., Carasso Romano, G. H., & Levi, A. (2025). A holistic approach to sustainability in higher education institutes: Social, economic, educational, and mobility perspectives. *Frontiers in Education*, *10*. https://doi.org/10.3389/feduc.2025.1588223

Basheer, N., Ahmed, V., Bahroun, Z., & Anane, C. (2025). Sustainability assessment in higher education institutions: Exploring indicators, stakeholder perceptions, and implementation challenges. *Discover Sustainability*, *6*(1), 252. https://doi.org/10.1007/s43621-025-01116-w

Belkhir, L., & Elmeligi, A. (2019). Carbon footprint of the global pharmaceutical industry and relative impact of its major players. *Journal of Cleaner Production*, *214*. https://doi.org/10.1016/j.jclepro.2018.11.204

Bom, S., Jorge, J., Ribeiro, H. M., & Marto, J. (2019). A step forward on sustainability in the cosmetics industry: A review. *Journal of Cleaner Production*, *225*. https://doi.org/10.1016/j.jclepro.2019.03.255

Bond, C. A., & Raehl, C. L. (2007). Clinical pharmacy services, pharmacy staffing, and hospital mortality rates. *Pharmacotherapy*, *27*(4). https://doi.org/10.1592/phco.27.4.481

Borah, D., Malik, K., & Massini, S. (2019). Are engineering graduates ready for R&D jobs in emerging countries? Teaching-focused industry-academia collaboration strategies. *Research Policy*, *48*(9), 103837. https://doi.org/10.1016/J.RESPOL.2019.103837

Brechtelsbauer, E., & Shah, S. (2020). Update on pharmaceutical waste disposal regulations: Strategies for success. *American Journal of Health-System Pharmacy*, *77*(7). https://doi.org/10.1093/ajhp/zxz360

Bridgstock, R. (2009). The graduate attributes we've overlooked: Enhancing graduate employability through career management skills. *Higher Education Research and Development*, *28*(1). https://doi.org/10.1080/07294360802444347

Cerych, L., & Frost-Smith, B. (1985). Collaboration between higher education and industry: An overview. *European Journal of Education*, *20*(1). https://doi.org/10.2307/1502999

Chen, H., Engkvist, O., Wang, Y., Olivecrona, M., & Blaschke, T. (2018). The rise of deep learning in drug discovery. *Drug Discovery Today*, *23*(6), 1241–1250. https://doi.org/10.1016/j.drudis.2018.01.039

Colberg, J., Tucker, J. L., Martínez, I., Bailey, J. D., Briddell, C., Koenig, S. G., Kopach, M. E., Michalak, S., Parsons, A., Richardson, P. F., Roschangar, F., Vestergaard, E., & Voutchkova-Kostal, A. (2025). Environmental sustainability strategy of active pharmaceutical ingredient manufacturing: A perspective from the American chemical society green chemistry institute pharmaceutical roundtable. *ACS Sustainable Chemistry & Engineering*. https://doi.org/10.1021/acssuschemeng.5c01094

Daher-Armache, G., Armache, J., & Ismail, H. N. (2025). Leadership development in U.S. Higher education: Strategies for lifelong learning and upskilling. *Journal of Innovation & Knowledge*, *10*(4), 100754. https://doi.org/10.1016/J.JIK.2025.100754

Doubeni, C. A., Nelson, D., Cohn, E. G., Paskett, E., Asfaw, S. A., Sumar, M., Ahmed, S. M., McClinton-Brown, R., Wieland, M. L., Kinney, A., Aguilar-Gaxiola, S., Rosas, L. G., & Patino, C. M. (2022). Community engagement education in academic health centers, colleges, and universities. *Journal of Clinical and Translational Science*, *6*(1), e109. https://doi.org/10.1017/cts.2022.424

Engelbrecht, M. D. (2019). Beyond the skills gap: Preparing college students for life and work. *Community College Journal of Research and Practice*, *43*(5). https://doi.org/10.1080/10668926.2018.1488552

Epstein, M. L., & Brosvic, G. M. (2002). Students prefer the immediate feedback assessment technique. *Psychological Reports*, *90*(3 PART 2). https://doi.org/10.2466/pr0.90.3.1136-1138

Epstein, M. L., Epstein, B. B., & Brosvic, G. M. (2001). Immediate feedback during academic testing. *Psychological Reports*, *88*(3 PART 1). https://doi.org/10.2466/pr0.2001.88.3.889

Etzkowitz, H., & Leydesdorff, L. (2000). The dynamics of innovation: From National Systems and "mode 2" to a Triple Helix of university-industry-government relations. *Research Policy*, *29*(2). https://doi.org/10.1016/S0048-7333(99)00055-4

Farland, M. Z., Sicat, B. L., Franks, A. S., Pater, K. S., Medina, M. S., & Persky, A. M. (2013). Best practices for implementing team-based learning in pharmacy education. *American Journal of Pharmaceutical Education*, *77*(8). https://doi.org/10.5688/ajpe778177

Filho, W. L., Mifsud, M., Molthan-Hill, P., Nagy, G. J., ávila, L. V., & Salvia, A. L. (2019). Climate change scepticism at universities: A global study. *Sustainability (Switzerland)*, *11*(10). https://doi.org/10.3390/su11102981

Findler, F., Schönherr, N., Lozano, R., & Stacherl, B. (2019). Assessing the impacts of higher education institutions on sustainable development-an analysis of tools and indicators. *Sustainability (Switzerland)*, *11*(1). https://doi.org/10.3390/su11010059

Fu, C., & Chen, Q. (2025). The future of pharmaceuticals: Artificial intelligence in drug discovery and development. *Journal of Pharmaceutical Analysis*, 101248. https://doi.org/10.1016/j.jpha.2025.101248

Fuchs, C. (2017). Critical social theory and sustainable development: The role of class, capitalism and domination in a dialectical analysis of un/sustainability. *Sustainable Development, 25*(5), 443–458. https://doi.org/10.1002/sd.1673

Gawade, S. P., & Sonaje, N. P. (2017). Designing of curriculum aspects of pharmacy undergraduate course in respect of graduate employability. *Indian Journal of Pharmaceutical Education and Research, 51*(4). https://doi.org/10.5530/ijper.51.4.78

Haidet, P., Levine, R. E., Parmelee, D. X., Crow, S., Kennedy, F., Kelly, P. A., Perkowski, L., Michaelsen, L., & Richards, B. F. (2012). Perspective: Guidelines for reporting team-based learning activities in the medical and health sciences education literature. *Academic Medicine, 87*(3). https://doi.org/10.1097/ACM.0b013e318244759e

Heron, E. (2020). Friendship as method: Reflections on a new approach to understanding student experiences in higher education. *Journal of Further and Higher Education, 44*(3), 393–407. https://doi.org/10.1080/0309877X.2018.1541977

Hicks, D., Wouters, P., Waltman, L., de Rijcke, S., & Rafols, I. (2015). Bibliometrics: The Leiden Manifesto for research metrics. *Nature, 520*(7548), 429–431. https://doi.org/10.1038/520429a

Hmelo-Silver, C. E. (2004). Problem-based learning: What and how do students learn? *Educational Psychology Review, 16*(3), 235–266. https://doi.org/10.1023/B:EDPR.0000034022.16470.f3

Idul J. J., & Walag, A. M. (2024, June, 27). Integrating green chemistry and sustainability principles to a secondary science curriculum: A mixed-methods needs assessment. *Journal of Chemical Education, 101*(7), 2765–2778. https://doi.org/10.1021/acs.jchemed.4c00341

Jairoun, A. A., Al-Hemyari, S. S., Shahwan, M., Alkhoujah, S., El-Dahiyat, F., Jaber, A. A. S., & Zyoud, S. H. (2025). Towards eco-friendly pharmaceuticals: Regulatory and policy approaches for sustainable medicines use. *Exploratory Research in Clinical and Social Pharmacy, 17*, 100576. https://doi.org/10.1016/j.rcsop.2025.100576

Karliner, J., Slotterback, S., Boyd, R., Ashby, B., & Steele, K. (2019). Health Care's Climate Footprint. *Health Care Without Harm, September.*

Kotter, J. P. (2007). Leading change: Why transformation efforts fail. In *Museum Management and Marketing*, Soldiers Field Boston, MA 02163 https://doi.org/10.4324/9780203964194-10

Kümmerer, K., Dionysiou, D. D., Olsson, O., & Fatta-Kassinos, D. (2018). A path to clean water. *Science, 361*(6399), 222–224. https://doi.org/10.1126/science.aau2405

Leal Filho, W., Shiel, C., Paço, A., Mifsud, M., Ávila, L. V., Brandli, L. L., Molthan-Hill, P., Pace, P., Azeiteiro, U. M., Vargas, V. R., & Caeiro, S. (2019). Sustainable development goals and sustainability teaching at universities: Falling behind or getting ahead of the pack? *Journal of Cleaner Production, 232*. https://doi.org/10.1016/j.jclepro.2019.05.309

Leal Filho, W., Sigahi, T. F. A. C., Anholon, R., Rebelatto, B. G., Schmidt-Ross, I., Hensel-Börner, S., Franco, D., Treacy, T., & Brandli, L. L. (2025). Promoting sustainable development via stakeholder engagement in higher education. *Environmental Sciences Europe, 37*(1), 64. https://doi.org/10.1186/s12302-025-01101-0

Lozano, R., Ceulemans, K., & Scarff Seatter, C. (2015). Teaching organisational change management for sustainability: Designing and delivering a course at the University of Leeds to better prepare future sustainability change agents. *Journal of Cleaner Production, 106*, 205–215. https://doi.org/10.1016/j.jclepro.2014.03.031

Lozano, R., Lukman, R., Lozano, F. J., Huisingh, D., & Lambrechts, W. (2013). Declarations for sustainability in higher education: Becoming better leaders, through addressing the university system. *Journal of Cleaner Production, 48*, 10–19. https://doi.org/10.1016/j.jclepro.2011.10.006

Mahatma Gandhi NREGA. (n.d.). Retrieved August 12, 2025, from https://nrega.dord.gov.in/MGNREGA_new/Nrega_home.aspx

McCafferty, H. (2022). An unjust balance: A systematic review of the employability perceptions of UK undergraduates from disadvantaged socio-economic backgrounds. *Research in Post-Compulsory Education, 27*(4). https://doi.org/10.1080/13596748.2022.2110774

Middel, K., Fehlner-Gardiner, C., Pulham, N., & Buchanan, T. (2017). Incorporating direct rapid immunohistochemical testing into large-scale wildlife rabies surveillance. *Tropical Medicine and Infectious Disease, 2*(3), 21. https://doi.org/10.3390/tropicalmed2030021

Mitchell, J., Hawkings, H., Latham, S., Fieroze, F., Arjyal, A., Barrington, D. J., Baral, S., Saify, M. B., Cooke, P., Hamade, P., Huque, R., Parajuli, A., Siddiki, A. Z., & King, R. (2023). Addressing antimicrobial resistance through community engagement: A framework for developing contextually relevant and impactful behaviour change interventions. *JAC-Antimicrobial Resistance, 5*(6). https://doi.org/10.1093/jacamr/dlad124

Moermond, C. T. A., Puhlmann, N., Brown, A. R., Owen, S. F., Ryan, J., Snape, J., Venhuis, B. J., & Kümmerer, K. (2022). GREENER pharmaceuticals for more sustainable healthcare. *Environmental Science and Technology Letters 9*(9). https://doi.org/10.1021/acs.estlett.2c00446

Mohd, S., Abdul Latiff, A. R., & Syed Azhar, S. N. F. (2024). Research impact assessment on sustainable development goals in higher education institutions: A qualitative study. *Sage Open, 14*(3). https://doi.org/10.1177/21582440241281095

Moktadir, Md. A., Ahmadi, H. B., Sultana, R., Zohra, F.-T.-, Liou, J. J. H., & Rezaei, J. (2020). Circular economy practices in the leather industry: A practical step towards sustainable development. *Journal of Cleaner Production, 251*, 119737. https://doi.org/10.1016/j.jclepro.2019.119737

Moldan, B., Janoušková, S., & Hák, T. (2012). How to understand and measure environmental sustainability: Indicators and targets. *Ecological Indicators, 17*. https://doi.org/10.1016/j.ecolind.2011.04.033

Morel, C. M., Acharya, T., Broun, D., Dangi, A., Elias, C., Ganguly, N. K., Gardner, C. A., Gupta, R. K., Haycock, J., Heher, A. D., Hotez, P. J., Kettler, H. E., Keusch, G. T., Krattiger, A. F., Kreutz, F. T., Lall, S., Lee, K., Mahoney, R., Martinez-Palomo, A., … Yun, M. (2005). Health innovation networks to help developing countries address neglected diseases. *Science, 309*(5733), 401–404. https://doi.org/10.1126/science.1115538

Morelli, J. (2011). Environmental sustainability: A definition for environmental professionals. *Journal of Environmental Sustainability, 1*(1). https://doi.org/10.14448/jes.01.0002

Moriña, A. (2017). Inclusive education in higher education: Challenges and opportunities. *European Journal of Special Needs Education, 32*(1). https://doi.org/10.1080/08856257.2016.1254964

Nagel, D.A., Naccarato, T.T., Philip, M.T., Ploszay, V.K., Winkler, J., Sanchez-Ramirez, D.C., & Penner, J. L. (2022). Understanding student-run health initiatives in the context of community-based services: A concept analysis and proposed definitions. *Journal of Primary Care & Community Health, 13*. https://doi.org/10.1177/21501319221126293

National Apprenticeship Promotion Scheme (NAPS) | Ministry of Skill Development and Entrepreneurship. (n.d.). Retrieved August 12, 2025, from https://www.msde.gov.in/offerings/schemes-and-services/details/national-apprenticeship-promotion-scheme-naps-YjM4ATMtQWa

NCS|Home: *National Career Service - Career guidance and Jobs in India and related services*. (n.d.). Retrieved August 12, 2025, from https://www.ncs.gov.in/

Niño-Amézquita, J., Legotin, F., & Barbakov, O. (2017). Economic success and sustainability in pharmaceutical sector: A case of Indian SMES. *Entrepreneurship and Sustainability Issues, 5*(1). https://doi.org/10.9770/jesi.2017.5.1(13)

Nouri, A. I., Hassali, M. A., & Hashmi, F. K. (2020). Contribution of pharmacy education to pharmaceutical research and development: Critical insights from educators. *Perspectives in Public Health, 140*(1). https://doi.org/10.1177/1757913919832927

Olawade, D. B., Popoola, T. T., Egbon, E., & David-Olawade, A. C. (2025). Sustainable healthcare practices: Pathways to a carbon-neutral future for the medical industry. *Sustainable Futures, 9*, 100783. https://doi.org/10.1016/j.sftr.2025.100783

Oliveira, M. C., & Proença, J. (2025). Sustainable campus operations in higher education institutions: A systematic literature review. *Sustainability, 17*(2), 607. https://doi.org/10.3390/su17020607

Palsokar, G., & Tajne, M. (2018). A study on the perceived gap in between industry and academia with reference to the curriculum of post-graduate courses in pharmaceutical sciences in India. *Indian Journal of Pharmaceutical Education and Research, 52*(1). https://doi.org/10.5530/ijper.52.1.2

Panchagnula, R., & Thomas, N. S. (2000). Biopharmaceutics and pharmacokinetics in drug research. *International Journal of Pharmaceutics, 201*(2). https://doi.org/10.1016/S0378-5173(00)00344-6

Pearson, M. L., & Hubball, H. T. (2012). Curricular integration in pharmacy education. *American Journal of Pharmaceutical Education, 76*(10). https://doi.org/10.5688/ajpe7610204

Pereira, L., & Cotas, J. (2024). Seaweed: A sustainable solution for greening drug manufacturing in the pursuit of sustainable healthcare. *Exploration of Drug Science, 2*(1), 50–84. https://doi.org/10.37349/eds.2024.00036

Persky, A. M. (2012). The impact of team-based learning on a foundational pharmacokinetics course. *American Journal of Pharmaceutical Education, 76*(2). https://doi.org/10.5688/ajpe76231

Pol, R. P., Somade, P. M., Chopade, A. R., Naikwade, N. S., & Dias, R. J. (2017). Current pharmacy curriculum in India and need for an update. *International Journal of Life-Sciences Scientific Research, 3*(6). https://doi.org/10.21276/ijlssr.2017.3.6.5

Pradhan Mantri Kaushal Vikas Yojana 4.0 (PMKVY 4.0) | Ministry of Skill Development and Entrepreneurship. (n.d.). Retrieved August 12, 2025, from https://www.msde.gov.in/offerings/schemes-and-services/details/pradhan-mantri-kaushal-vikas-yojana-4-0-pmkvy-4-0-2021-ITO3ATMtQWa

Pradhan, P., Joshi, S., Dahal, K., Hu, Y., Subedi, D. R., Putra, M. P. I. F., Vaidya, S., Pant, L. P., Dhakal, S., Hubacek, K., Rupakheti, M., Roberts, D. C., & van den Hurk, B. (2025). Policy relevance of IPCC reports for the Sustainable Development Goals and beyond. *Resources, Environment and Sustainability, 19*, 100192. https://doi.org/10.1016/J.RESENV.2025.100192

Prior, D. D., Seshadrinath, S. M., Zhang, M. (Yu), & McCormack, M. (2025). Measuring sustainable development goals (SDGs) in higher education through semantic matching. *Studies in Higher Education, 50*(7), 1556–1569. https://doi.org/10.1080/03075079.2024.2386625

Purvis, B., Mao, Y., & Robinson, D. (2019). Three pillars of sustainability: In search of conceptual origins. *Sustainability Science, 14*(3). https://doi.org/10.1007/s11625-018-0627-5

Pushpakom, S., Iorio, F., Eyers, P. A., Escott, K. J., Hopper, S., Wells, A., Doig, A., Guilliams, T., Latimer, J., McNamee, C., Norris, A., Sanseau, P., Cavalla, D., & Pirmohamed, M. (2019). Drug repurposing: Progress, challenges and recommendations. *Nature Reviews Drug Discovery, 18*(1), 41–58. https://doi.org/10.1038/nrd.2018.168

Ramísio, P. J., Pinto, L. M. C., Gouveia, N., Costa, H., & Arezes, D. (2019). Sustainability strategy in higher education institutions: Lessons learned from a nine-year case study. *Journal of Cleaner Production, 222*, 300–309. https://doi.org/10.1016/j.jclepro.2019.02.257

Rodríguez-Zurita, D., Jaya-Montalvo, M., Moreira-Arboleda, J., Raya-Diez, E., & Carrión-Mero, P. (2025). Sustainable development through service learning and community engagement in higher education: A systematic literature review. *International Journal of Sustainability in Higher Education, 26*(1), 158–201. https://doi.org/10.1108/IJSHE-10-2023-0461

Sakao, T., Bocken, N., Nasr, N., & Umeda, Y. (2024). Implementing circular economy activities in manufacturing for environmental sustainability. *CIRP Annals, 73*(2), 457–481. https://doi.org/10.1016/J.CIRP.2024.06.002

Salvia, A. L., Leal Filho, W., Brandli, L. L., & Griebeler, J. S. (2019). Assessing research trends related to sustainable development goals: Local and global issues. *Journal of Cleaner Production, 208*, 841–849. https://doi.org/10.1016/j.jclepro.2018.09.242

Schrogie, J. (2008). Estrogens and thrombosis. *Clinical Pharmacology & Therapeutics, 83*(4), 526–526. https://doi.org/10.1038/clpt.2008.17

Sector Skill Councils (SSC) | Ministry of Skill Development and Entrepreneurship | NSDC. (n.d.). Retrieved August 12, 2025, from https://nsdcindia.org/sector-skill-councils

Serrano-Bedia, A.-M., & Perez-Perez, M. (2022). Transition towards a circular economy: A review of the role of higher education as a key supporting stakeholder in Web of Science. *Sustainable Production and Consumption, 31*, 82–96. https://doi.org/10.1016/j.spc.2022.02.001

SETAC. (2020). Guidelines for social life cycle assessment of products. *Management, 15*(2), 12-138

Shin, H. Y., Kim, K. Y., & Kang, P. (2020). Concept analysis of community health outreach. *BMC Health Services Research, 20*(1), 417. https://doi.org/10.1186/s12913-020-05266-7

Shulman, L. S. (2005). Signature pedagogies in the professions. *Daedalus, 134*(3). https://doi.org/10.1162/0011526054622015

Škokić, V., Jelić, P., & Jerković, I. (2025). The role and contribution of sustainable development goals as a transformative framework in higher education: A case study of the University of Split. *World, 6*(1), 22. https://doi.org/10.3390/world6010022

Soini, K., Korhonen-Kurki, K., & Asikainen, H. (2019). Transactional learning and sustainability co-creation in a university – business collaboration. *International Journal of Sustainability in Higher Education, 20*(6), 965–984. https://doi.org/10.1108/IJSHE-11-2018-0215

Spelt, E. J. H., Biemans, H. J. A., Tobi, H., Luning, P. A., & Mulder, M. (2009). Teaching and learning in interdisciplinary higher education: A systematic review. *Educational Psychology Review, 21*(4). https://doi.org/10.1007/s10648-009-9113-z

Startup India. (n.d.). Retrieved August 12, 2025, from https://www.startupindia.gov.in/

Steenmeijer, M. A., Rodrigues, J. F. D., Zijp, M. C., & Waaijers-van der Loop, S. L. (2022). The environmental impact of the Dutch health-care sector beyond climate change: An input–output analysis. *The Lancet Planetary Health, 6*(12). https://doi.org/10.1016/S2542-5196(22)00244-3

Thakur, R., Chavan, M., Vasoya, A., Kasturiwale, H., Ghosh, S., & Mishra, S. (2024). Bridging academia and industry: A study on the skill development effects of internships and on-the-job training programs. *Educational Administration Theory and Practices.* https://doi.org/10.53555/kuey.v30i4.2276

Tralau-Stewart, C. J., Wyatt, C. A., Kleyn, D. E., & Ayad, A. (2009). Drug discovery: New models for industry-academic partnerships. *Drug Discovery Today, 14*(1–2). https://doi.org/10.1016/j.drudis.2008.10.003

Van Wilder, L., Boone, L., Ragas, A., Moermond, C., Pieters, L., Rechlin, A., Vidaurre, R., De Smedt, D., & Dewulf, J. (2024). A holistic framework for integrated sustainability assessment of pharmaceuticals. *Journal of Cleaner Production*, *467*, 142978. https://doi.org/10.1016/j.jclepro.2024.142978

Vora, L. K., Gholap, A. D., Jetha, K., Thakur, R. R. S., Solanki, H. K., & Chavda, V. P. (2023). Artificial intelligence in pharmaceutical technology and drug delivery design. *Pharmaceutics*, *15*(7), 1916. https://doi.org/10.3390/pharmaceutics15071916

Weaver, E., O'Hagan, C., & Lamprou, D. A. (2022). The sustainability of emerging technologies for use in pharmaceutical manufacturing. *Expert Opinion on Drug Delivery*, *19*(7). https://doi.org/10.1080/17425247.2022.2093857

Yarime, M., Trencher, G., Mino, T., Scholz, R. W., Olsson, L., Ness, B., Frantzeskaki, N., & Rotmans, J. (2012). Establishing sustainability science in higher education institutions: Towards an integration of academic development, institutionalization, and stakeholder collaborations. *Sustainability Science*, *7*(SUPPL. 1). https://doi.org/10.1007/s11625-012-0157-5

Yu, L. X. (2008). Pharmaceutical quality by design: Product and process development, understanding, and control. *Pharmaceutical Research*, *25*(4). https://doi.org/10.1007/s11095-007-9511-1

10 Low-Carbon Emission Models for Hospitals and Pharmaceutical Industries for a Clean and Green Environment

Mandeep Kumar Gupta, Kanupriya Chauhan, Geetanjali Mehara, and Rajnish Srivastava

1 Introduction

Climate change must be addressed promptly; thus, global initiatives to minimize carbon emissions have been developed. Carbon emissions, primarily from the burning of fossil fuels, have a significant impact on the worldwide economy, human well-being, and the environment (Lelieveld et al., 2019). A lot of businesses, like health and pharmaceuticals, need to lower their carbon footprints to be more environmentally friendly and last longer. Hospitals and the pharmaceutical industry are significant contributors of carbon emissions because they use a lot of energy, create a lot of medical waste, and ship things. To slow down climate change and build a sustainable future, we need to cut down on carbon emissions. Moving to a low-carbon economy is important for keeping global temperatures stable, encouraging technological progress, and slowly lowering energy costs. This change not only lessens the bad consequences of climate change, but it also creates opportunities for economic expansion through the creation of green technologies and eco-friendly ways of doing business. Pharmaceutical and healthcare industries are responsible for a large amount of worldwide carbon emissions, making up about 4.4% of all emissions. Hospitals make up about 39% of this sector's emissions, while the pharmaceutical business makes up 14% (Belkhir & Elmeligi, 2019). Some of the things that add to these companies' carbon footprints are the energy-intensive work they do, the way they manage their supply chains, and the way they get rid of waste. Hospitals, for instance, use a lot of energy to run their medical equipment and to heat, cool, and light their buildings. Getting rid of medicines and medical supplies adds to their carbon footprint. To solve these problems, we need to have a full understanding of how these companies are creating pollution. Low-carbon emissions models must be utilized to lower the amount of carbon that pharmaceutical and healthcare companies release into the air. These models aim to lower the health risks of air pollution, promote environmentally friendly activities, make sure that businesses follow global climate agreements, and cut down on emissions of greenhouse gases from all sectors. These models talk about many ways to do things, like making waste management better, using renewable energy sources, making energy use more efficient, and using green technologies in healthcare operations. By concentrating on these areas, hospitals and the pharmaceutical industry may

DOI: 10.4324/9781003640486-10

greatly reduce their carbon footprints while still providing high-quality service and making their products easy to get. Because they are always open and use a lot of energy, clinics are one of the most energy-intensive enterprises. Healthcare facilities consume a lot of water, make a lot of healthcare waste, and consume plenty of power; all of that adds to carbon emissions, according to research. Here are the main reasons why hospitals let out CO_2:

Hospitals consume an enormous amount of energy to run medical equipment, heat, chill, and light their buildings. The Environmental Protection Agency (EPA) says that hospitals in the US use about 10% of all commercial energy (Bawaneh et al., 2019). Using renewable energy sources like solar panels and wind turbines is a huge step in cutting down on carbon emissions. Hospitals make a lot of medical waste, such as used needles, disposable medical equipment, and packaging. When these materials are thrown away in the wrong way, they pollute the air and release greenhouse gases.

Reprocessing and recycling medical equipment are two sustainable waste management strategies that can mitigate this impact. The use of water in hospitals affects the environment as well. Hospitals require water for sterilization, sanitation, and patient care. Since wastewater treatment and disposal increase carbon emissions, water conservation measures and efficient wastewater treatment methods are essential (Vallée, 2024). The purchase and transportation of pharmaceuticals and medical supplies significantly increase the carbon footprints of hospitals. Purchasing drugs locally and optimizing supply chain processes can reduce transportation-related emissions. Hospital construction frequently overlooks energy efficiency. Remodeling older hospital buildings with energy-efficient architecture, insulation, and smart technologies can reduce energy use. Energy-efficient equipment, digital healthcare solutions like telemedicine, and green building certifications like LEED certification are just a few strategies hospitals may employ to reduce carbon emissions (Dion et al., 2023). Hospitals may also work with renewable energy providers to transition to sustainable energy sources. Hospitals that implemented energy-saving measures were able to reduce emissions by 30% without compromising the quality of care, according to a 2020 study published in The Lancet Planetary Health (Zikhathile et al., 2022).

2 Energy Consumption in Hospitals

Healthcare facilities are among the most energy-intensive structures due to the essential services they provide and their continuous operation. The primary explanation for energy consumption in hospitals is the use of lighting systems that operate continuously in patient rooms, hallways, and surgical areas, as well as heating, ventilation, and air-conditioning (HVAC) systems that maintain hygienic and temperature-regulated conditions (Mohammadpour et al., 2016).

Also, high-powered medical gadgets like MRI equipment, X-ray equipment, and life-support systems need a lot more energy. In addition, heated water sources used for cleaning, washing clothing, and sterilizing, as well as cooking and eating, added a lot to the facility's total consumption of energy (Figure 10.1). Information technology systems, such as servers, patient monitoring systems, and electronic medical records, contribute to the ongoing energy consumption. Numerous sources of greenhouse gas emissions manifest these energy requirements. Fossil-fuel-based infrastructure frequently generates electricity consumption as the primary source, leading to indirect carbon dioxide (CO_2) emissions. On-site fossil fuel combustion for furnaces, backup generators, or heating systems generates direct CO_2 emissions (Figure 10.1). Hospitals also generate emissions from transportation through activities such as ambulance operations and supply delivery. Medicinal gases, including nitrous oxide and anesthetic medicines, are another significant source of high global warming potential (Mofolasayo, 2023). Additionally, hospitals generate methane (CH_4) and nitrous oxide (N_2O) emissions during decommissioning or incineration, which includes food, biomedical refuse, and general trash (Figure 10.1). These activities also generate indirect emissions from water consumption and treatment systems, as well as from upstream supply chain operations, such as the manufacturing and transportation of medications, disposable medical instruments, and construction materials. The combination of these factors results in hospitals being significant contributors to institutional carbon footprints, necessitating targeted energy-efficient and sustainability initiatives (Dion & Evans, 2024) (Table 10.1).

Table 10.1 Sources of energy consumption and types of emissions in hospitals

Source	*Type of Emission*	*Examples*
Electricity consumption	Indirect CO_2	Lighting, equipment, and HVAC systems powered by grid electricity
On-site fossil fuel use	Direct CO_2	Boilers and generators using natural gas, diesel, or oil
Transportation	Direct CO_2	Ambulances, staff and patient transport, and supply deliveries
Waste generation	Methane (CH_4), CO_2, N_2O	Food waste, biomedical waste, and general landfill waste
Medical gases	High global warming potential (GWP) gases	Nitrous oxide, anesthetic gases (e.g., desflurane, sevoflurane)
Water treatment and use	Indirect emissions (Scope 3)	Emissions from heating water and sewage treatment
Procurement (supply chain)	Scope 3 emissions	Pharmaceuticals, single-use devices, instruments, and packaging
Construction and renovation	Embodied carbon	Materials like steel, cement, and plastics used in hospital infrastructure

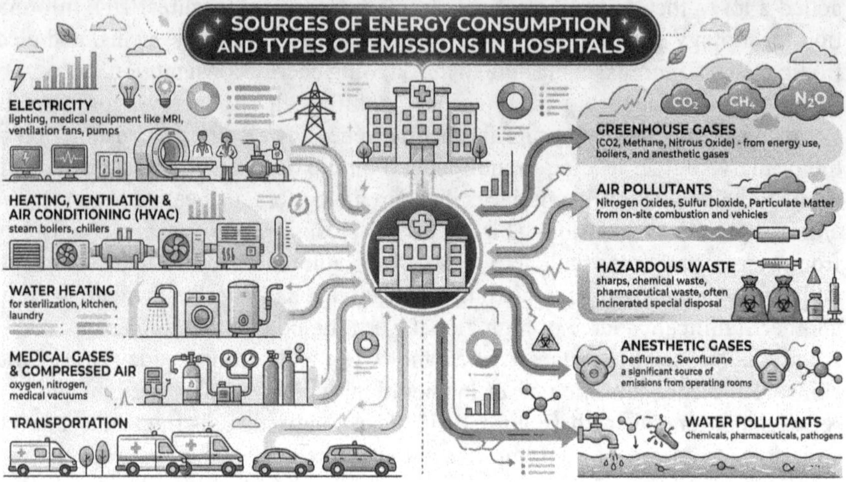

Figure 10.1 Sources of energy consumption and types of emission in hospitals.

2.1 Case Studies of High-Emission Hospitals

Due to their 24/7 operations, use of advanced medical equipment, and use of high-emission resources like anesthetic gases and pharmaceuticals, healthcare facilities are major contributors to global greenhouse gas (GHG) emissions. The case studies that follow show the pollution levels of hospitals that release a lot of pollutants, in addition to the systemic variables that make their environmental impact worse. Hospitals make up most of the National Health Service's (NHS) carbon emissions, which is about 5% of the UK's overall carbon emissions (Tudor et al., 2015). Often depending on natural gas, many NHS hospitals still run with antiquated infrastructure and ineffective heating systems, according to a 2019 assessment. Furthermore, greatly affecting direct (Scope 1) emissions is the usage of volatile anesthetic drugs like desflurane. Many NHS buildings still have high emitters despite recent sustainability projects because of ingrained legacy systems and underfunded retrofitting projects (Rodríguez-Jiménez et al., 2023). Driven by continuous HVAC operation, diagnostic imaging, and surgical suites, the Cleveland Clinic—a large academic medical center—has always had a high per-square-foot energy usage. Before sustainability projects, the hospital's carbon intensity per bed ranked among the highest in the nation. An energy audit turned up significant lighting system and air-handling unit inefficiencies. While attempts at retrofitting resulted in a 30% decrease in emissions, the original footprint shows the emissions difficulty of big, sophisticated hospitals in wealthy countries. The modern academic hospital, University of California San Francisco Medical Center, is highly advanced. Its significant carbon footprint—mostly from energy-intensive research labs, clinical imaging, and a sizable fleet of vehicles—has drawn attention, though. Early evaluations of its sustainability performance revealed less than ideal energy-to-outcome efficiency, which led to a strategy redesigning green building certifications and clean energy purchases.

Still, its past emissions levels offer a useful benchmark for emissions from big, highly technologically advanced medical facilities. Leading public hospital in India, AIIMS, emphasizes the emissions problem in fast-urbanizing countries. With more than 2 million outpatient visits a year, the hospital has a significant power consumption largely from coal-dominated grids. Attributed to ineffective infrastructure, diesel generators, and medical waste incineration, a 2021 projection of AIIMS's yearly carbon emissions exceeds 40,000,000 CO_2e (Zhong & Huang, 2019). AIIMS started trial projects in solar panel installations and biological waste separation despite financial restrictions.

2.2 Low-Carbon Emission Strategies for Hospitals

By their very nature, hospitals are heavy consumers of materials, water, drugs, and energy, so they contribute greatly to national and worldwide GHG emissions. Turning toward low-carbon operations calls for a multi-tiered strategy including behavior modification, procurement, clinical practice, and infrastructure. Key tactics arranged by region of intervention follow below:

2.2.1 Infrastructure and Energy Efficiency

- High-efficiency HVAC systems, insulation material, and LED lighting retrofitting current structures.
- Constructing new hospitals with solar shading and natural ventilation toward green certifications (such as LEED and BREEAM).
- Small-scale wind, solar thermal, and solar PV on-site renewable energy projects.
- Real-time monitoring, control, and optimization of energy usage with smart energy management platforms (Gershenfeld et al., 2010).

2.2.2 Sustainable Medical Gases Management

- Changing from desflurane and nitrous oxide (great global warming potential) to lower-emission substitutes like sevoflurane or total intravenous anesthesia (TIVA).
- Systems for scavenging gases used in waste anesthetic treatment to catch and neutralize them.
- Tracking volatile agents in real time to decrease unneeded emissions (Gómez-Chaparro et al., 2018).

2.2.3 Low-Carbon Procurement and Supply Chains

- Green procurement rules favoring low-carbon, recyclable, or reused medical supplies and equipment.
- Local food and medicine procurement helps to lower emissions connected to transportation.
- Vendor involvement initiatives requiring eco-certifications and emissions openness (Du et al., 2017).

2.2.4 *Waste Reduction and Circularity*

- Strict control over inventory and end product management helps to minimize biomedical waste; replace disposables with reusable fabrics, such as surgical gowns and drapes (Tomić & Schneider, 2018).

2.2.5 *Renewable Transport and Fleet Management*

- Turning now to hybrid and electric hospital move fleets (ambulances and supply vehicles).
- Using rewards, bike racks, or shuttle services helps staff and patients use public transportation.
- Telemedicine helps to lower emissions linked to travel for outpatient visits (Škrinjar et al., 2020).

2.2.6 *Water and Heating Innovations*

- Greywater recycling and rainwater collecting systems help to lower the use of potable water.
- Solar-assisted hot water systems help to reduce dependency on heating derived from coal or electricity.
- To cut needless water heating, low-flow fixtures and automated faucets help (De Freitas Melo et al., 2017).

2.2.7 *Sustainable Food Services*

- In cafeterias, plant-forward meals help to lower emissions from diets rich in meat.
- Food waste composting and procurement from organic or regenerative farms.
- Meal-prep strategies and energy-efficient kitchen appliances (L. Wang, 2014).

2.2.8 *Behavioral and Administrative Strategies*

- To monitor climate projects, green teams, or sustainability committees.
- Programs on energy saving, trash separation, and environmentally friendly behaviors, including staff awareness-raising campaigns on these topics.
- Environmental audits and reporting systems, including the Global Green and Healthy Hospitals (GGHH) network (Pandiyan et al., 2023).

2.2.9 *Digital and Smart Technologies*

- Telehealth systems cut paper use and patient travel.
- Electronic medical records (EMRs) will help to simplify procedures and replace paper charts.
- Internet of Things (IoT)-based control of lights, energy systems, and temperature-sensitive storage (Bibri & Krogstie, 2020).

3 Energy Efficiency Measures

3.1 HVAC System Optimization

Theoretically, HVAC system optimization is the strategic use of thermodynamic concepts, control systems, and energy modeling to raise the performance and efficiency of HVAC systems. Fundamentally, it integrates the laws of thermodynamics to regulate energy flow, thereby ensuring efficient transmission and conservation of heat with minimal losses. Grounded in fluid physics, the design maximizes air and fluid flow to lower resistance and pressure drops in pipes and ducts. Concurrent with this is the application of heat transfer theories to improve the efficiency of coils and heat exchangers. By means of feedback mechanisms including sensors and PID (proportional–integral–derivative) controllers, control systems significantly help to sustain interior thermal conditions dynamically. Using predictive algorithms and real-time data, advanced methods such as model predictive control (MPC) change system performance preemptively, hence increasing responsiveness and lowering wasteful energy use. Accurate building thermal load calculations—which are affected by occupancy, insulation, and outside temperature—are also rather important for the optimizing process. Using building simulation technologies such as EnergyPlus, DesignBuilder, and CFD tools helps model and assess theoretical performance, thereby allowing engineers to virtually test and improve system strategies. The most effective balance of comfort, affordability, and energy use is found by means of mathematical optimization methods like linear programming, genetic algorithms, and multi-objective analysis. Exergy analysis also helps one understand where energy quality is compromised, thereby driving additional improvements. In theory, HVAC system optimization is a multidisciplinary technique combining physics, engineering, and computational modeling to produce sustainable, high-efficiency temperature control solutions (Taheri et al., 2022).

3.2 Energy-Efficient Lighting

Sustainable infrastructure in hospitals and pharmaceutical enterprises relies on energy-efficient lighting to reduce energy use and carbon emissions. Traditional lighting systems like incandescent and fluorescent lights use a lot of electricity and generate heat, which strains HVAC systems. In contrast, energy-efficient lighting solutions, such as LEDs, use less power, last longer, and emit less heat. LEDs use 70% less energy than conventional lighting, making them perfect for 24/7 hospitals and labs (Montoya et al., 2017). Adding smart lighting controls to LEDs boosts energy savings. Occupancy sensors, daylight harvesting sensors, and timers adjust lighting to real-time needs, saving energy in unoccupied or naturally lit areas. In halls, patient rooms, and storage spaces, lights can fade or turn off when no movement is detected. BMS- or AEMS-based centralized lighting management offers planned lighting control, maintenance warnings, and performance tracking. Energy-efficient lighting provides steady, glare-free, and controlled illumination in pharmaceutical plants, ensuring environmental sustainability and regulatory compliance (Nethravathi & Murali, 2022). In temperature-sensitive situations, low-heat LEDs protect materials. Hospitals and pharmaceutical companies can reduce their carbon footprint, improve lighting, and improve environmental performance by employing energy-efficient lighting. This advances the goal of low-carbon emission models for green and clean environments.

3.3 Advanced Energy Management Systems

Advanced Energy Management Systems (AEMS) reduce hospital and pharmaceutical carbon emissions by optimizing energy use, waste, and renewable sources. These technologies evolve from reactive energy to smart, data-driven, automated energy control. AEMS analyzes hospital and pharmaceutical energy use using smart sensors, IoT, real-time monitoring, and predictive analytics. This data helps facility managers identify inefficiencies, set benchmarks, and respond aggressively. AEMS reduces energy waste by controlling light, HVAC, healthcare devices, and laboratory systems dependent on usage, time of day, or surroundings. Integration with BMS and cloud-based platforms improves AEMS capabilities through online control and monitoring, power forecasting, and demand-side response program participation. Scheduling with on-site energy sources like sunlight from solar panels or wind turbines can favor clean energy and reduce fossil fuel consumption. To ensure sustainability and production standards, AEMS tracks highly energy-intensive pharmaceutical procedures like sterilization, freezing, and chemical synthesis. Lowering manufacturing energy use and reclaiming power from unused heat or process outputs reduces carbon emissions. AEMS assist hospitals in achieving ecological and carbon neutrality goals while improving efficiency and cost. Modern, greener, healthier healthcare infrastructure needs these systems (Onu et al., 2023; Alevizos et al., 2023).

3.4 Renewable Energy Integration and Solar and Wind Energy

Solar and wind energy are essential for low-carbon hospitals and pharmaceutical enterprises. This technique reduces energy insecurity, GHG emissions, and fossil fuel use by integrating renewable and sustainable energy sources into the power system. Photovoltaic (PV) panels generate scalable, affordable solar energy for healthcare. Hospital and pharmacy HVAC, medical equipment, and lights are powered by solar. Pharmaceutical firms use solar thermal systems to heat water and steam for industrial operations and sterilization. Solar battery storage devices can store daylight energy during grid disruptions or peak load times, ensuring important services run. Wind energy is another great renewable resource, especially in open or rural areas with room for small to medium-sized turbines. Hybrid renewable systems can use wind energy to supplement solar power at night or on overcast days. Combining solar and wind energy requires smart grid interfaces, energy storage, and AEMS that dynamically adjust energy flows based on supply and demand. High initial investment, variability of renewable output, and space constraints exist, but the long-term benefits—lowered operational costs, increased energy independence, and environmental sustainability—make renewable energy integration essential to clean and green healthcare and pharmaceutical infrastructure (Talaat et al., 2019).

3.5 Cogeneration Systems and Waste Management Strategies

From natural gas or biogas, advanced energy solutions, including cogeneration systems, also referred to as combined heat and power (CHP) systems, generate electricity and heat. Over usual systems that generate heat and electricity individually, this dual-output technology increases fuel economy by 70–80%. Reducing energy reliance, cogeneration can run hospitals and pharmaceutical plants on extra heat for sterilization, water heating, and space heating as well as power. These systems minimize energy expenditure and GHG emissions and provide stable energy for continuous operations. Strategies for managing healthcare waste help to lower health and environmental hazards. Effective solutions are separating trash at the source, recycling, and properly disposing of sharps, infectious waste, and chemical byproducts. Autoclaving, hands-on controlled burning, and advanced plasma gasification handle medical waste. Zero-waste rules and circular economy projects, including composting organic waste and recycling packaging, help to maximize resource economy. Integrated waste management helps to lower methane emissions, landfill stress, and contamination. Strategic waste management and cogeneration help to assist sustainable development by encouraging resource economy, emission control, and ecological responsibility in healthcare (Onovwiona & Ugursal, 2006).

3.6 Recycling Programs and Medical Waste Disposal

Building a sustainable, low-carbon healthcare environment requires comprehensive recycling and medical waste disposal initiatives. Hospitals and pharmaceutical firms start recycling with a waste audit to identify recyclables and waste sources. Schools can use a multi-stream waste segregation system to separate non-recyclable or hazardous materials from recyclables. Clear signs, color-coded containers, and recycling places reduce contamination and promote compliance. Staff training programs are essential for administrative and clinical staff to understand and follow recycling regulations. Procurement guidelines can promote sustainability by prioritizing recyclable or recycled products. Advanced sorting and compacting tools boost recycling production and reduce storage space. Legal, low-emission, eco-friendly medical waste disposal strategies are needed. Waste should be sorted into sharps, infectious, pathological, pharmaceutical, and chemical categories at generation. This allows proper treatment and reduces cross-contamination. Innovative treatment methods involving autoclaving (steam sterilization), microwave irradiation, and chemical disinfection can safely eliminate infectious waste without burning. Burning should be done with modern scrubbers and filters to reduce air pollution. Pharmaceuticals can be regulated to prevent environmental contamination through reverse distribution and take-back. Promoting reusable surgical instruments and linens, digitizing medical records to reduce paper waste, and reducing single-use plastics to reduce waste volumes. Policy modifications, performance reviews, and constant monitoring keep trash disposal and recycling systems sustainable and efficient. These methods protect the environment and public health while reducing GHG emissions and achieving hospital carbon neutrality (Ordway et al., 2020).

4 Energy Consumption and Emission Sources

Energy-intensive and a major contributor to GHG emissions and environmental degradation, the pharmaceutical industry is crucial to the improvement of global health (Ogbuagu et al., n.d.). Operations include the synthesis of active pharmaceutical ingredients (APIs), formulation, sterilization, HVAC systems, and waste management, which account for most energy use in pharmaceutical production (Baumann & Baxendale, 2015). Large volumes of carbon dioxide (CO_2), methane (CH_4), and nitrous oxide (N_2O) are emitted into the atmosphere from the considerable power and thermal energy required for these processes—which are generally derived from fossil fuels such as coal, natural gas, and oil (Filonchyk et al., 2024). Pharmaceutical companies also release hazardous wastes, hazardous air pollutants (HAPs), and volatile organic compounds (VOCs) in addition to emissions from energy production (W. Wang et al., 2023). Apart from aggravating localized degradation of air and water quality, these contaminants seriously affect the ecology. High GHG levels aggravate the greenhouse effect, harming ecosystems and human civilizations with rising sea levels, changing global temperatures, and more severe weather patterns (Saxena, 2025). Pharmaceutical effluents dumped into water sources run the danger of bioaccumulating in aquatic life, disturbing ecosystems, and maybe fostering the development of antibiotic-resistant bacterial strains in the interim (Kayode-Afolayan et al., 2022). Additionally helping to create smog, acid rain, and direct toxicity to plants and animals are emissions of VOCs and harmful byproducts. Notable case studies have helped to expose these environmental hazards (Zhou et al., 2023). For instance, the pharmaceutical manufacturing centers of Hyderabad, India, have been found to be pollution hotspots where untreated waste releases, including strong concentrations of APIs and other chemicals, have contaminated local water systems and multiplied multi-drug-resistant bacteria, thus endangering public health (*Hyderabad's Pharmaceutical Pollution Crisis Changing Markets*, n.d.). Like this, many companies in Puerto Rico, a key global center for producing drugs, have been exposed to legal action for surpassing allowed VOC emissions, therefore affecting the public health and air quality in the nearby areas. These pictures show how urgently the entire industry must adopt sustainable methods to reduce emissions (*Full List of Pharmaceutical Companies in Puerto Rico (2025)*, n.d.). Many pharmaceutical companies have reacted by giving low-carbon projects top attention to reducing their environmental effect (Booth et al., 2023). These steps include upgrading to energy-efficient equipment, like variable frequency drives, high-efficiency HVAC systems, and LED lighting, in addition to adopting continuous manufacturing techniques, which simplify production and consume less energy than conventional batch methods (Kashinath et al., 2025). To reduce their reliance on fossil fuels, pharmaceutical companies are progressively including renewable energy sources, particularly solar and wind power (*Pharmaceutical Facilities Are Increasingly Integrating Renewable Energy Sources, Especially Solar and Wind Power, to Reduce Their Dependency on Fossil Fuels—Yahoo India Search Results*, n.d.). While developments in green chemistry aim to reduce solvent use and the generation of hazardous waste, solvent recovery systems and carbon capture technologies are also being investigated to help to further limit emissions (Aboagye et al., 2021). Following recommendations offered by environmental management systems such as ISO 14001 helps businesses to improve their environmental performance (*ISO 14005—Environmental Management Systems—Guidelines for a Flexible Approach to Phased Implementation*, n.d.). Reducing the whole carbon footprint of pharmaceuticals also depends on using sustainable packaging materials and collaborating with suppliers to lower upstream emissions. These integrated low-carbon solutions not only fulfill corporate responsibility and regulatory compliance but also safeguard the environment and public health and ensure that pharmaceutical production advances in line with ideas of sustainable development (Mudgal et al., 2024).

5 Green Chemistry Principles

A major component of the pharmaceutical sector's attempts to support sustainability is green chemistry ideas, which lower environmental consequences while maintaining output and efficiency (Ahmad et al., 2024). One of the primary principles of green chemistry is using sustainable raw materials—that are less toxic, renewable, and biodegradable feedstocks—instead of petroleum-based or environmentally dangerous ones (Slootweg, 2024). For example, the use of plant-derived solvents, biobased reagents, and renewable catalysts is rising to minimize the environmental effect of pharmaceutical products and their dependence on few resources (Dkhar et al., 2025). Another essential component is process optimization tactics, which aim to maximize reaction conditions, decrease waste, and raise product yields. Solvent-less or aqueous-phase synthesis, catalytic processes over stoichiometric ones, high atom economy reactions, and process intensification are among the techniques lowering energy usage and harmful byproducts (Taylor et al., 2023). In the manufacture of green drugs, the change from batch processing to continuous manufacturing marks a radical turn (Kashinath et al., 2025). Continuous production combines synthesis, purification, and formulation into one effective process. This gives you better control over the reaction parameters, more consistent product quality, less energy use, and less waste of materials (Domokos et al., 2021). This method not only increases output, but it also automates and monitors in real time, which cuts down on the need to reprocess and waste resources (Ajiga et al., 2024). Energy-efficient equipment, such as new heat recovery systems, energy-optimized reactors, variable-speed drives, and high-efficiency HVAC systems, balances these process improvements by lowering the amount of energy the facility uses overall (Asim et al., 2022). These improvements help businesses meet legal and environmental standards while also cutting costs and carbon emissions by a large amount

(Ayush Singh, 2024). One of the most important tools for these green chemistry projects is the life cycle assessment (LCA). This is a detailed method for looking at the environmental impact of an item or process over its entire life cycle, from getting the raw materials to making it, distributing it, using it, and finally getting rid of it or recycling it (Curran, 2013). LCA helps the pharmaceutical industry figure out which manufacturing activities, such as energy use during API synthesis or large emissions from solvent use, are the worst for the environment (Chen et al., 2024). Pharmaceutical businesses can utilize LCA to measure these effects and choose materials, create procedures, and come up with end-of-life disposal plans that help reduce their impact on the environment (Chen et al., 2024). Using LCA also encourages transparent reporting to stakeholders and compliance with environmental requirements such as ISO 14040 and ISO 14044 (Ingwersen & EPA Amir Safaei, n.d.). A full approach to sustainable pharmaceutical manufacture includes using green chemistry ideas in advanced process optimization, continuous manufacturing technology, energy-efficient infrastructure, viable raw material sourcing, and detailed life cycle analysis (Ahmad et al., 2024). These tactics lower production costs, raise the level of social responsibility, and eliminate waste, energy use, and emissions. This makes sure that the pharmaceutical industry grows in line with aims for protecting the environment and promoting sustainable development (Milanesi et al., 2020).

6 Role of Policymakers

Scientists, people in the pharmaceutical industry, and lawmakers all need to work together to make the pharmaceutical industry more environmentally friendly (Chaturvedi et al., 2017) (Table 10.2). Policymakers oversee creating laws and standards for businesses to follow to encourage them to be more environmentally friendly (*Principles of Effective Regulation: A Summary Guide for Regulators and Policymakers*, 2021). Legislative action may make people want to do things, like giving tax advantages and subsidies to green technologies, and it can also punish people who don't obey the rules. This can assist the industry in evolving toward using responsible waste management, production practices that are good for the environment, and technology that uses less energy (*Tax Incentives Can Help Enhance Adoption of Sustainability Manufacturing: Experts—The Economic Times*, n.d.). Also, setting clear and internationally acknowledged norms regarding continuous production, LCA, and green chemistry encourages creativity and long-term investment in sustainable technologies by making sure that markets are consistent and predictable. Pharmaceutical businesses, suppliers, and investors are some of the most important players in the industry who need to be involved in making these sustainability initiatives happen in the local area (Toniolo et al., 2021). They have the power and tools to invest in renewable energy, streamline supply chains, and use greener manufacturing methods (Qadir et al., 2021). Corporate leadership's commitment to environmental, social, and governance (ESG) goals substantially affects how thoroughly sustainable practices are integrated into organizational operations (de Souza Barbosa et al., 2023). Many organizations

Table 10.2 Role of Policymakers in promoting sustainable development, environmental protection, and industrial innovation Naruetharadhol et al. (2024); The Role of Public Policy in Promoting Sustainable Development (2017)

Aspect	*Role of Policymakers*	*Examples*
Policy formulation	Develop and implement laws, regulations, and standards	Environmental laws, emission caps, and carbon pricing
Financial incentives	Provide subsidies, tax benefits, and grants to encourage sustainable practices	Renewable energy subsidies, R&D funding
Regulatory oversight	Monitor and enforce compliance with environmental and safety regulations	Inspections, penalties for violations
Public awareness and education	Promote awareness about sustainability among industries and citizens	Green campaigns, environmental education programs
Stakeholder engagement	Facilitate dialogue and collaboration between government, industry, and the public	Public–private partnerships, industry forums
Support for innovation	Invest in research and innovation to drive green technologies	Support for clean tech and sustainable manufacturing
International cooperation	Collaborate on global treaties and agreements for sustainability	Paris Agreement, SDGs alignment
Risk management and adaptation	Develop strategies to manage climate risks and industrial challenges	Climate adaptation plans, disaster risk policies
Infrastructure development	Build and upgrade infrastructure to support sustainable growth	Smart grids, public transport, and waste management
Market regulation	Set market rules to favor sustainable products and discourage harmful practices	Eco-labeling, banning single-use plastics

are beginning to recognize that in addition to minimizing ecological footprints, environmentally aware methods can have financial advantages by lowering energy and raw material costs, boosting process efficiency, and enhancing brand recognition (Salim Ba Awain et al., 2021). Green technologies, including solvent recovery systems, waste valorization methods, and biodegradable excipients, may also be developed more quickly if the sector actively participates in open innovation platforms, collaborative research, and public–private partnerships (Chang, 2020). Academic institutions, research teams, and technical experts comprise the scientific community, which contributes by promoting innovation through the development of advanced biotechnological tools, process optimization, computational models, and green chemistry ideas (PDF; *Innovation through Collaboration: Advancing Higher Education Research*, n.d.). Researchers look at process intensification techniques, alternative raw materials, and novel catalysts to reduce energy use and waste generation (Sai Bharadwaj et al., 2025). By collaborating, scientists and business executives can ensure that laboratory results are translated into practical, scalable, and lucrative solutions (Abi Saad & Agogué, 2024). Furthermore, LCA approaches are improved by the scientific community to accurately estimate the environmental consequences of pharmaceutical goods and to influence business practices and regulatory choices (Liu et al., 2024). Even with these chances to work together, development is taking longer than it should because of several issues. The high upfront costs are a major barrier to the use of sustainable technology, which may hinder small and medium-sized businesses (SMEs) from using it because they don't have a lot of money (Baig et al., 2020). Adoption of new methods may also be hampered by an absence of technical skills and opposition to change within current business cultures (Warrick, 2023). Different environmental standards and rules in different nations make it harder to put global plans into action (Islam et al., 2023). Also, if academics and industry don't work together, there may be a gap between scientific advancement and its use in the real world. Problems with intellectual property, competition, and rules about sharing data may make it much harder for scientists to share information freely (Bansal et al., 2019). Removing these barriers would need concerted efforts to help SMEs financially and technically, encourage cross-sectoral cooperation, and standardize regulatory regimes globally (Abu et al., 2025). Only via such collaborative and well-supported efforts can the pharmaceutical business achieve its sustainability objectives by striking a balance between environmental stewardship, economic development, and public health imperatives (Bade et al., 2024).

7 Technical Challenges

Several technological, financial, and regulatory barriers, each with its own set of challenges, severely restrict the widespread adoption of innovative and sustainable technologies across a range of industries, including manufacturing, energy, and medicine (Xiao et al., 2024). Technical challenges are often caused by the need for advanced infrastructure and technologies that can seamlessly integrate into existing production systems without compromising operational safety or product quality (Haber & Carmeli, 2023). The substantial research, technical expertise, and process reengineering required to create and scale up green technologies such as waste reduction strategies, biobased raw materials, and energy-efficient manufacturing processes are currently beyond the capabilities of many enterprises (İncekara, 2022). Additionally, these new technologies' lack of standardization limits their widespread acceptance and makes integrating them with current systems more challenging (Haber & Carmeli, 2023). Financial limitations are a major obstacle in addition to these technical ones because, especially for small and medium-sized enterprises (SMEs), adopting sustainable practices—like updating production lines, replacing antiquated equipment, and training staff—can be prohibitively expensive (D. Hu et al., 2023). These companies usually have low profit margins and are ill-prepared to take on the risk and delayed benefits of large capital investments in sustainability-focused technologies. If even bigger companies are hesitant to invest in green technology due to worries about long-term profitability and consumer acceptability, progress might be further halted. Absence of enough financial incentives, subsidies, or low-interest loans aimed to support long-term economic growth aggravates the problem (*Why Do P&C Companies Usually Have Low Profit Margins? Does It Pose Risk to P&C Actuaries/Careers/Salaries? : R/Actuary*, n.d.). Furthermore, important in delaying the introduction of creative sustainability ideas and technologies are regulatory challenges (Sharma et al., 2023). Given the fast development of technology and the often antiquated or out-of-date present regulatory systems, businesses may find it challenging to secure timely permission for new materials or technologies (Akpobome, 2024). Divergent national and international regulations can complicate matters for businesses operating overseas by requiring them to follow various, often contradictory compliance paths (*Legal Challenges in Enforcing Competition Law in the Global Economy—Attorney Aaron Hall*, n.d.). This raises administrative load and hinders the introduction of environmentally friendly technologies. Regulatory uncertainty may hinder companies from launching creative ideas if there is no clear path to clearance or if non-compliance is deemed to have too great implications (Wu & Tham, 2023). Industries may address these linked difficulties using a range of techniques (*The Future of Industrial Strategies: Five Grand Challenges for Resilient Manufacturing*, 2023). Encouragement of cooperation among stakeholders, including legislators, business leaders, academic institutions, and non-governmental organizations, guarantees that technological innovation closely fits changing societal needs and regulatory expectations (Kujala et al., 2022). Public policy programs such as tax credits, subsidies, or subsidized financing options could help to lower financial demands, particularly for small businesses trying to switch to greener options (*Subsidy: Subsidy Solutions: Complementing Price Ceilings in Public Policy—FasterCapital*, n.d.). Investors may be more secure in their decisions if regulatory procedures were simplified, worldwide standards were unified, and clear, forward-looking ideas for sustainable technology certification were offered (*Simpler, More Streamlined and Smarter Regulations Are Required to Address Evolving Policy Challenges*, n.d.). Using internal modular or phased implementation strategies helps companies progressively increase their capacity for sustainability and distribute risks and expenses over time (Zopounidis & Lemonakis, 2024). Staff training and upskilling are also crucial to guarantee that technical proficiency remains current with advances in technology (*The Growing Importance Of Upskilling In The Tech Era*, n.d.). As customer knowledge and demand for sustainable goods rise, market forces may eventually drive companies toward greener methods, providing early adopters with a competitive advantage, improved reputation, and long-term profitability (Yadav et al., 2024). The combined effect of financial aid, regulatory change, technical innovation, and strategic planning may thereby remove the main barriers to sustained industrial transformation that exist today (C. Wang et al., 2024).

8 Future Directions and Innovations

Since the healthcare sector globally is expanding, its green footprint, especially in carbon emissions, is also increasing (Or & Seppänen, 2024). The hospital and pharmaceutical industries, being major energy users and waste producers, are pivotal in steering the sectors in the direction of sustainability (Table 10.3). The future of low-carbon emission models for these industries is to incorporate cutting-edge technologies, policy paradigm shifts, and the integration of circular economic values (Olawade et al., 2025). Among the primary future directions is the use of solar, wind, and geothermal energy as a source of renewable energy in hospital and pharmaceutical operations. The use of smart grids, energy-efficient HVAC systems, and LED lights can reduce energy usage even further. Green building design innovations such as the incorporation of sustainable building materials, rainwater harvesting systems, and natural ventilation will play a role in carbon neutrality (Aadya Sharma, 2024; J.-L. Hu & Bui, 2024; Reddy et al., 2024). In the pharmaceutical industry, intensification processes and green chemistry practices are set to transform drug production. Continuous manufacturing methods that are waste-minimizing, solvent recovery systems, and substitution of harmful chemicals with safer chemicals are becoming increasingly popular. Digitalization and application of artificial intelligence (AI) can be used to increase resource optimization, predictive maintenance, and online monitoring of emissions (Achieng M, 2025; Cravotto, 2025). Another area of great potential is the creation of low-emission models of transportation for medical supply chains, e.g., electric and hybrid delivery trucks, drone last-mile delivery, and consolidated logistics (Ferreira & Esperança, 2025). In waste management, technologies like on-site treatment of waste, biodegradable packaging, and enhanced recycling practices will be critical (Hajam et al., 2023). Adding ESG standards to institutional policies can help hold people accountable and encourage them to keep getting better. To come up with solutions that can be used on a large scale and last, stakeholders like government agencies, industry leaders, research institutions, and non-governmental organizations will need to work together (Sklavos et al., 2024). Teaching healthcare and industrial workers about sustainable practices will help create a culture of caring for the environment. Also, using blockchain and IoT technologies can make carbon tracking and reporting more open, which will make it easier to follow the rules and international climate agreements (Hariyani et al., 2025). The adoption of low-carbon technologies must be encouraged by governments and regulatory agencies through grants, tax benefits, and strict environmental regulations. Global collaboration and information exchange will hasten the shift to more environmentally friendly pharmaceutical and healthcare systems (Rissman et al., 2020). Future studies should look at lifecycle assessments, the carbon footprint of drugs, and patient-centered models that connect health outcomes with environmental sustainability (Asperti et al., 2025; Olawade et al., 2025). As people become more aware of the environment and the need for eco-friendly healthcare services and medicines, the industry will also change to meet this demand (Montesinos et al., 2024; Scholz et al., 2024). In conclusion, an integrated, multidisciplinary strategy that incorporates technological innovation, policy support, stakeholder engagement, and educational initiatives

Table 10.3 Future direction and innovation in hospitals and pharmaceutical industries Aadya Sharma (2024); Achieng M (2025); Asperti et al. (2025); Cravotto (2025); Hajam et al. (2023); J.-L. Hu and Bui (2024); Montesinos et al. (2024); Olawade et al. (2025); Or and Seppänen (2024); Rissman et al. (2020); Sklavos et al. (2024)

S. No.	*Future Direction/Innovation*	*Description*
1	Integration of renewable energy sources	Implementation of solar, wind, and bioenergy systems in hospitals and pharma industries to reduce reliance on fossil fuels
2	Green building design and retrofitting	Adoption of LEED-certified infrastructure and energy-efficient retrofitting techniques for existing buildings
3	Circular economy practices	Encouraging waste minimization, reuse, recycling, and upcycling processes to close the resource loop
4	Carbon capture and storage (CCS) technologies	Adoption of CCS systems in pharma manufacturing units to trap and store CO_2 emissions
5	Smart energy management systems	Use of AI and IoT-based smart grids and sensors to monitor and optimize energy usage in real time
6	Sustainable supply chain management	Promotion of green logistics, eco-friendly packaging, and local sourcing to minimize transportation-related emissions
7	Adoption of green chemistry principles	Designing chemical processes that reduce or eliminate the use and generation of hazardous substances
8	Electrification of transport and logistics systems	Transition to electric ambulances, delivery vans, and other vehicles within hospitals and pharma logistics
9	Environmental performance metrics and carbon auditing	Regular carbon footprint audits and implementation of Key Environmental Performance Indicators (KEPIs)
10	Policy framework and incentive mechanisms	Development of government policies and financial incentives to encourage investment in low-carbon infrastructure and technologies
11	Research and development in green technologies	Investment in R&D for emerging low-emission technologies and biodegradable materials for pharmaceutical use
12	Workforce training and environmental awareness	Capacity-building programs to train staff in sustainability practices and promote environmental responsibility
13	Digital health solutions and telemedicine	Reducing patient travel emissions by promoting virtual consultations and remote diagnostics
14	Water and energy co-optimization strategies	Designing systems that optimize both water and energy use simultaneously to minimize environmental impact
15	Carbon-neutral pharmaceutical manufacturing models	Long-term goal of creating net-zero carbon-emitting pharma production facilities using integrated sustainable approaches

is essential for the future of low-carbon emission models in the healthcare and pharmaceutical industries. The pharmaceutical and healthcare industries can set an example for the global fight against climate change and lessen their carbon footprint by investing in these future directions. This will ensure a cleaner, healthier, and more sustainable environment for future generations.

9 Conclusion

In the quest for a sustainable world, the need to lower carbon emissions from the healthcare and pharmaceutical industries has never been stronger. Pharmaceutical industries and hospitals are among the greatest sources of GHG emissions globally because they are among the greatest energy consumers, use fossil fuels as their source of power, have intricate supply chains, and use more resources to run. This chapter has discussed a variety of low-carbon emission models that show practical ways toward environmental responsibility without compromising the best in patient care and drug quality. With energy-efficient buildings, renewable energy integration, minimizing waste, water conservation, and green procurement practices, healthcare and pharma facilities can significantly lower their carbon footprint. In addition to this, the use of digital technologies, AI-driven energy monitoring, and eco-friendly logistics is crucial for maximizing resource efficiency and operational performance. This green transition has been facilitated by regulatory frameworks, green certifications, and public–private partnerships, which promote accountability and innovation. Crucially, the long-term success of these initiatives still depends on a cultural shift toward environmental consciousness among all stakeholders, from upper management to entry-level workers. Educational campaigns, incentives, and transparent sustainability reporting can all help people feel like they are all responsible. The models and case studies show that environmental sustainability and economic viability can work together through careful planning and investment. Climate change is still a threat to health and the environment, so hospitals and the pharmaceutical industry need to set an example by using and promoting sustainable practices. The future of healthcare needs to do more than just help people get better; it also needs to protect the Earth. So, using low-carbon strategies is not just a choice; it is a necessary step toward making the world a cleaner, greener, and healthier world. In order to enhance and broaden these models, this chapter concludes by promoting the implementation of additional research, innovative concepts, and multidisciplinary collaboration. This will help make being environmentally responsible a routine element of healthcare and pharmaceutical operations worldwide.

Bibliography

Abi Saad, E., & Agogué, M. (2024). Living Labs in science-industry collaborations: Roles, design, and application patterns. *Technovation*, *135*, 103066. https://doi.org/10.1016/J.TECHNOVATION.2024.103066

Aboagye, E. A., Chea, J. D., & Yenkie, K. M. (2021). Systems level roadmap for solvent recovery and reuse in industries. *IScience*, *24*(10), 103114. https://doi.org/10.1016/J.ISCI.2021.103114

Abu, N., da Silva, F. P., & Vieira, P. R. (2025). Government support for SMEs in the Fintech Era: Enhancing access to finance, survival, and performance. *Digital Business*, *5*(1), 100099. https://doi.org/10.1016/J.DIGBUS.2024.100099

Achieng M, N. (2025). Green chemistry in pharmaceuticals: Reducing environmental impact. *Newport International Journal of Public Health and Pharmacy*, *6*(2), 36–41. https://doi.org/10.59298/NIJPP/2025/623641

Ahmad, S., Jaiswal, R., Yadav, R., & Verma, S. (2024). Recent advances in green chemistry approaches for pharmaceutical synthesis. *Sustainable Chemistry One World*, *4*, 100029. https://doi.org/10.1016/J.SCOWO.2024.100029

Ajiga, D., Okeleke, P. A., Folorunsho, S. O., & Ezeigweneme, C. (2024). The role of software automation in improving industrial operations and efficiency. *International Journal of Engineering Research Updates*, *7*(1), 022–035. https://doi.org/10.53430/IJERU.2024.7.1.0031

Akpobome, O. (2024). The impact of emerging technologies on legal frameworks: A model for adaptive regulation. *International Journal of Research Publication and Reviews Journal Homepage: Www.Ijrpr.Com*, *5*(7), 5046–5060. www.ijrpr.com

Alevizos, V., Georgousis, I., & Kapodistria, A. (2023). Toward climate neutrality: A comprehensive overview of sustainable operations management, optimization, and wastewater treatment methods. *Pollutants*, *3*(4). https://doi.org/10.3390/pollutants3040036

Asim, N., Badiei, M., Mohammad, M., Razali, H., Rajabi, A., Chin Haw, L., & Jameelah Ghazali, M. (2022). Sustainability of heating, ventilation and air-conditioning (HVAC) systems in buildings—An overview. *International Journal of Environmental Research and Public Health*, *19*(2), 1016. https://doi.org/10.3390/IJERPH19021016

Asperti, F., Cannavacciuolo, L., Foglia, E., Garagiola, E., Gheduzzi, E., & Manetti, S. (2025). Seventy-two shades of environmental sustainability in healthcare: A holistic framework proposal. *Journal of Cleaner Production*, *493*, 144850. https://doi.org/10.1016/j.jclepro.2025.144850

Ayush Singh. (2024). Sustainability practices in business operations. *International Journal for Research Publication and Seminar*, *15*(3), 18–34. https://doi.org/10.36676/JRPS.V15.I3.1424

Bade, C., Olsacher, A., Boehme, P., Truebel, H., Bürger, L., & Fehring, L. (2024). Sustainability in the pharmaceutical industry—An assessment of sustainability maturity and effects of sustainability measure implementation on supply chain security. *Corporate Social Responsibility and Environmental Management*, *31*(1), 224–242. https://doi.org/10.1002/CSR.2564

Baig, S. A., Abrar, M., Batool, A., Hashim, M., & Shabbir, R. (2020). Barriers to the adoption of sustainable supply chain management practices: Moderating role of firm size. *Cogent Business and Management*, *7*(1), 1841525. https://doi.org/10.1080/23311975.2020.1841525

Bansal, S., Mahendiratta, S., Kumar, S., Sarma, P., Prakash, A., & Medhi, B. (2019). Collaborative research in modern era: Need and challenges. *Indian Journal of Pharmacology*, *51*(3), 137. https://doi.org/10.4103/IJP.IJP_394_19

Baumann, M., & Baxendale, I. R. (2015). The synthesis of active pharmaceutical ingredients (APIs) using continuous flow chemistry. *Beilstein Journal of Organic Chemistry*, *11*, 1194–1219. https://doi.org/10.3762/BJOC.11.134

Bawaneh, K., Nezami, F. G., Rasheduzzaman, M., & Deken, B. (2019). Energy consumption analysis and characterization of healthcare facilities in the United States. *Energies*, *12*(19). https://doi.org/10.3390/en12193775

Belkhir, L., & Elmeligi, A. (2019). Carbon footprint of the global pharmaceutical industry and relative impact of its major players. *Journal of Cleaner Production*, *214*. https://doi.org/10.1016/j.jclepro.2018.11.204

Bibri, S. E., & Krogstie, J. (2020). Environmentally data-driven smart sustainable cities: Applied innovative solutions for energy efficiency, pollution reduction, and urban metabolism. *Energy Informatics*, *3*(1). https://doi.org/10.1186/s42162-020-00130-8

Bilgen, S. (2014). Structure and environmental impact of global energy consumption. *Renewable and Sustainable Energy Reviews*, *38*. https://doi.org/10.1016/j.rser.2014.07.004

Booth, A., Jager, A., Faulkner, S. D., Winchester, C. C., & Shaw, S. E. (2023). Pharmaceutical company targets and strategies to address climate change: Content analysis of public reports from 20 pharmaceutical companies. *International Journal of Environmental Research and Public Health*, *20*(4), 3206. doi: 10.3390/ijerph20043206

Carmona, M., Feria, J., Golpe, A. A., & Iglesias, J. (2017). Energy consumption in the US reconsidered. Evidence across sources and economic sectors. *Renewable and Sustainable Energy Reviews*, *77*. https://doi.org/10.1016/j.rser.2016.11.227

Chang, S. H. (2020). Utilization of green organic solvents in solvent extraction and liquid membrane for sustainable wastewater treatment and resource recovery—A review. *Environmental Science and Pollution Research 2020 27:26*, *27*(26), 32371–32388. https://doi.org/10.1007/S11356-020-09639-7

Chaturvedi, U., Sharma, M., Dangayach, G. S., & Sarkar, P. (2017). Evolution and adoption of sustainable practices in the pharmaceutical industry: An overview with an Indian perspective. *Journal of Cleaner Production*, *168*, 1358–1369. https://doi.org/10.1016/J.JCLEPRO.2017.08.184

Chen, Z., Lian, J. Z., Zhu, H., Zhang, J., Zhang, Y., Xiang, X., Huang, D., Tjokro, K., Barbarossa, V., Cucurachi, S., & Dong, B. (2024). Application of life cycle assessment in the pharmaceutical industry: A critical review. *Journal of Cleaner Production*, *459*, 142550. https://doi.org/10.1016/J.JCLEPRO.2024.142550

Cravotto, G. (2025). Reshaping chemical manufacturing towards green process intensification: Recent findings and perspectives. *Processes*, *13*(2), 459. https://doi.org/10.3390/pr13020459

Curran, M. A. (2013). Life cycle assessment: A review of the methodology and its application to sustainability. *Current Opinion in Chemical Engineering*, *2*(3), 273–277. https://doi.org/10.1016/J.COCHE.2013.02.002

De Freitas Melo, D., De Souza Lage, E., Rocha, A. V., & De Jesus Cardoso, B. (2017). Improving the consumption and water heating efficiency in smart buildings. *2017 13th International Conference and Expo on Emerging Technologies for a Smarter World, CEWIT 2017*, *2018-January*. Stony Brook, NY, USA. https://doi.org/10.1109/CEWIT.2017.8263304

de Souza Barbosa, A., da Silva, M. C. B. C., da Silva, L. B., Morioka, S. N., & de Souza, V. F. (2023). Integration of Environmental, Social, and Governance (ESG) criteria: Their impacts on corporate sustainability performance. *Humanities and Social Sciences Communications 2023 10:1*, *10*(1), 1–18. https://doi.org/10.1057/s41599-023-01919-0

Dion, H., & Evans, M. (2024). Strategic frameworks for sustainability and corporate governance in healthcare facilities; approaches to energy-efficient hospital management. *Benchmarking*, *31*(2). https://doi.org/10.1108/BIJ-04-2022-0219

Dion, H., Evans, M., & Farrell, P. (2023). Hospitals management transformative initiatives; towards energy efficiency and environmental sustainability in healthcare facilities. *Journal of Engineering, Design and Technology*, *21*(2). https://doi.org/10.1108/JEDT-04-2022-0200

Dkhar, D. S., Swain, R. P., Dubey, R., Patel, G. K., & Chandra, P. (2025). Plant-derived enzymes as sustainable biocatalysts for biosensing and industrial applications. *Industrial Crops and Products*, *233*, 121336. https://doi.org/10.1016/J.INDCROP.2025.121336

Domokos, A., Nagy, B., Szilágyi, B., Marosi, G., & Nagy, Z. K. (2021). Integrated continuous pharmaceutical technologies-A review. *Organic Process Research & Development*, *25*(4), 721–739. https://doi.org/10.1021/ACS.OPRD.0C00504

Du, S., Hu, L., & Wang, L. (2017). Low-carbon supply policies and supply chain performance with carbon concerned demand. *Annals of Operations Research*, 255(1–2). https://doi.org/10.1007/s10479-015-1988-0

Ferreira, J. C., & Esperança, M. (2025). Enhancing sustainable last-mile delivery: The impact of electric vehicles and AI optimization on urban logistics. *World Electric Vehicle Journal*, *16*(5), 242. https://doi.org/10.3390/wevj16050242

Filonchyk, M., Peterson, M. P., Zhang, L., Hurynovich, V., & He, Y. (2024). Greenhouse gases emissions and global climate change: Examining the influence of CO2, CH4, and N2O. *Science of the Total Environment*, *935*, 173359. https://doi.org/10.1016/J.SCITOTENV.2024.173359

Full List of Pharmaceutical Companies in Puerto Rico (2025). (n.d.). Retrieved June 14, 2025, from https://pharmchoices.com/biotech-pharmaceutical-companies-in-puerto-rico/

Gershenfeld, N., Samouhos, S., & Nordman, B. (2010). Intelligent infrastructure for energy efficiency. *Science*, *327*(5969). https://doi.org/10.1126/science.1174082

Gómez-Chaparro, M., García-Sanz-Calcedo, J., & Márquez, L. A. (2018). Analytical determination of medical gases consumption and their impact on hospital sustainability. *Sustainability (Switzerland)*, *10*(8). https://doi.org/10.3390/su10082948

Gunningham N, Sinclair D. (1999) Integrative regulation: A principle-based approach to environmental policy. *Law & Social Inquiry*. *24*(4), 853–96.

Haber, L., & Carmeli, A. (2023). Leading the challenges of implementing new technologies in organizations. *Technology in Society*, *74*, 102300. https://doi.org/10.1016/J.TECHSOC.2023.102300

Hajam, Y. A., Kumar, R., & Kumar, A. (2023). Environmental waste management strategies and vermi transformation for sustainable development. *Environmental Challenges*, *13*, 100747. https://doi.org/10.1016/j.envc.2023.100747

Hariyani, D., Hariyani, P., Mishra, S., & Sharma, M. K. (2025). A literature review on transformative impacts of blockchain technology on manufacturing management and industrial engineering practices. *Green Technologies and Sustainability*, *3*(3), 100169. https://doi.org/10.1016/j.grets.2025.100169

Hu, D., Fang, X., & DiGiovanni, Y. M. (2023). Technological progress, financial constrains, and digital financial inclusion. *Small Business Economics*, *61*(4), 1693–1721. https://doi.org/10.1007/s11187-023-00745-7

Hu, J.-L., & Bui, N. H. B. (2024). The future design of smart energy systems with energy flexumers: A constructive literature review. *Energies*, *17*(9), 2039. https://doi.org/10.3390/en17092039

Hyderabad's Pharmaceutical Pollution Crisis Changing Markets. (n.d.). Retrieved June 14, 2025, from https://changingmarkets.org/report/hyderabads-pharmaceutical-pollution-crisis/

İncekara, M. (2022). Determinants of process reengineering and waste management as resource efficiency practices and their impact on production cost performance of Small and Medium Enterprises in the manufacturing sector. *Journal of Cleaner Production*, *356*, 131712. https://doi.org/10.1016/J.JCLEPRO.2022.131712

Ingwersen, W., & EPA Amir Safaei, U. (n.d.). *Workshop on carbon LCA of vehicles Introduction to Life Cycle Assessment methodology and Standards*.

Islam, M., Wattoo, O. M., & Saleem, S. (2023). Environmental regulations and their implications for global sustainability. *Pakistan Journal of Humanities and Social Sciences*, *11*(3). https://doi.org/10.52131/PJHSS.2023.1103.0665

ISO 14005 - Environmental management systems – Guidelines for a flexible approach to phased implementation. (n.d.). Retrieved June 14, 2025, from https://committee.iso.org/sites/tc207sc1/home/projects/published/iso-14005---environmental-manage.html

Kashinath, K. P., Sanjay, L. R., Ashokbhai, M. K., Roy, S., Sardar, M. S., & Kaity, S. (2025). Continuous manufacturing based paradigm shift in pharmaceuticals production and current regulatory framework. *Chemical Engineering Research and Design, 215*, 1–22. https://doi.org/10.1016/J.CHERD.2025.01.003

Kayode-Afolayan, S. D., Ahuekwe, E. F., & Nwinyi, O. C. (2022). Impacts of pharmaceutical effluents on aquatic ecosystems. *Scientific African, 17*, e01288. https://doi.org/10.1016/J.SCIAF.2022.E01288

Kujala, J., Sachs, S., Leinonen, H., Heikkinen, A., & Laude, D. (2022). Stakeholder engagement: Past, present, and future. *Business and Society, 61*(5), 1136–1196. https://doi.org/10.1177/00076503211066595/ASSET/4E32B04D-993D-4E1C-844E-83B669D35A46/ASSETS/IMAGES/LARGE/10.1177_00076503211066595-FIG2.JPG

Legal Challenges in Enforcing Competition Law in the Global Economy - Attorney Aaron Hall. (n.d.). Retrieved June 14, 2025, from https://aaronhall.com/legal-challenges-in-enforcing-competition-law-in-the-global-economy/

Lelieveld, J., Klingmüller, K., Pozzer, A., Burnett, R. T., Haines, A., & Ramanathan, V. (2019). Effects of fossil fuel and total anthropogenic emission removal on public health and climate. *Proceedings of the National Academy of Sciences of the United States of America, 116*(15). https://doi.org/10.1073/pnas.1819989116

Liu, M., Zhu, G., & Tian, Y. (2024). The historical evolution and research trends of life cycle assessment. *Green Carbon, 2*(4), 425–437. https://doi.org/10.1016/J.GREENCA.2024.08.003

Milanesi, M., Runfola, A., & Guercini, S. (2020). Pharmaceutical industry riding the wave of sustainability: Review and opportunities for future research. *Journal of Cleaner Production, 261*, 121204. https://doi.org/10.1016/J.JCLEPRO.2020.121204

Mofolasayo, A. (2023). Assessing and managing the direct and indirect emissions from electric and fossil-powered vehicles. *Sustainability (Switzerland), 15*(2). https://doi.org/10.3390/su15021138

Mohammadpour, A., Anumba, C. J., & Messner, J. I. (2016). Integrated framework for patient safety and energy efficiency in healthcare facilities retrofit projects. *Health Environments Research and Design Journal, 9*(4). https://doi.org/10.1177/1937586716639903

Montesinos, L., Checa Rifá, P., Rifá Fabregat, M., Maldonado-Romo, J., Capacci, S., Maccaro, A., & Piaggio, D. (2024). Sustainability across the medical device lifecycle: A scoping review. *Sustainability, 16*(4), 1433. https://doi.org/10.3390/su16041433

Montoya, F. G., Peña-García, A., Juaidi, A., & Manzano-Agugliaro, F. (2017). Indoor lighting techniques: An overview of evolution and new trends for energy saving. *Energy and Buildings, 140*. https://doi.org/10.1016/j.enbuild.2017.01.028

Mudgal, D., Pagone, E., & Salonitis, K. (2024). Selecting sustainable packaging materials and strategies: A holistic approach considering whole life cycle and customer preferences. *Journal of Cleaner Production, 481*, 144133. https://doi.org/10.1016/J.JCLEPRO.2024.144133

Naruetharadhol, P., ConwayLenihan, A., & McGuirk, H. (2024). Assessing the role of public policy in fostering global eco-innovation. *Journal of Open Innovation: Technology, Market, and Complexity, 10*(2), 100294. https://doi.org/10.1016/J.JOITMC.2024.100294

Nethravathi, S., & Murali, V. (2022). A novel residential energy management system based on sequential Whale optimization algorithm and Fuzzy logic. *Distributed Generation and Alternative Energy Journal, 37*(3). https://doi.org/10.13052/dgaej2156-3306.3739

Ogbuagu, O., Mbata, A., Balogun, O., Journals, O. O.-I., & 2024, undefined. (n.d.). Sustainable pharmaceutical supply chains: Green chemistry approaches to drug production and distribution. *Researchgate.Net*. Retrieved June 13, 2025, from https://www.researchgate.net/profile/Oluchukwu-Ogbuagu/publication/390388281_Sustainable_Pharmaceutical_Supply_Chains_Green_Chemistry_Approaches_to_Drug_Production_and_Distribution/links/67ec298f9b1c6c48776d25ad/Sustainable-Pharmaceutical-Supply-Chains-Green-Chemistry-Approaches-to-Drug-Production-and-Distribution.pdf

Olawade, D. B., Popoola, T. T., Egbon, E., & David-Olawade, A. C. (2025). Sustainable healthcare practices: Pathways to a carbon-neutral future for the medical industry. *Sustainable Futures*, *9*, 100783. https://doi.org/10.1016/j.sftr.2025.100783

Onovwiona, H. I., & Ugursal, V. I. (2006). Residential cogeneration systems: Review of the current technology. *Renewable and Sustainable Energy Reviews*, *10*(5). https://doi.org/10.1016/j.rser.2004.07.005

Onu, P., Pradhan, A., & Mbohwa, C. (2023). EcoMechatronics: Advancing Sustainable Production Through Mechatronic Systems. *2023 IEEE International Conference on Industrial Engineering and Engineering Management, IEEM 2023*. https://doi.org/10.1109/IEEM58616.2023.10406694

Or, Z., & Seppänen, A.-V. (2024). The role of the health sector in tackling climate change: A narrative review. *Health Policy*, *143*, 105053. https://doi.org/10.1016/j.healthpol.2024.105053

Ordway, A., Pitonyak, J. S., & Johnson, K. L. (2020). Durable medical equipment reuse and recycling: Uncovering hidden opportunities for reducing medical waste. *Disability and Rehabilitation: Assistive Technology*, *15*(1). https://doi.org/10.1080/17483107.2018.1508516

Pandiyan, P., Saravanan, S., Usha, K., Kannadasan, R., Alsharif, M. H., & Kim, M. K. (2023). Technological advancements toward smart energy management in smart cities. *Energy Reports*, *10*. https://doi.org/10.1016/j.egyr.2023.07.021

(PDF) Innovation through Collaboration: Advancing Higher Education Research. (n.d.). Retrieved June 14, 2025, from https://www.researchgate.net/publication/375422779_Innovation_through_Collaboration_Advancing_Higher_Education_Research

Pharmaceutical facilities are increasingly integrating renewable energy sources, especially solar and wind power, to reduce their dependency on fossil fuels. - Yahoo India Search Results. (n.d.). Retrieved June 14, 2025, from https://in.search.yahoo.com/search?fr=mcafee&type=E210IN826G0&p=Pharmaceutical+facilities+are+increasingly+integrating+renewable+energy+sources%2C+especially+solar+and+wind+power%2C+to+reduce+their+dependency+on+fossil+fuels

Qadir, S. A., Al-Motairi, H., Tahir, F., & Al-Fagih, L. (2021). Incentives and strategies for financing the renewable energy transition: A review. *Energy Reports*, *7*, 3590–3606. https://doi.org/10.1016/J.EGYR.2021.06.041

Reddy, V. J., Hariram, N. P., Ghazali, M. F., & Kumarasamy, S. (2024). Pathway to sustainability: An overview of renewable energy integration in building systems. *Sustainability*, *16*(2), 638. https://doi.org/10.3390/su16020638

Rissman, J., Bataille, C., Masanet, E., Aden, N., Morrow, W. R., Zhou, N., Elliott, N., Dell, R., Heeren, N., Huckestein, B., Cresko, J., Miller, S. A., Roy, J., Fennell, P., Cremmins, B., Koch Blank, T., Hone, D., Williams, E. D., de la Rue du Can, S., … Helseth, J. (2020). Technologies and policies to decarbonize global industry: Review and assessment of mitigation drivers through 2070. *Applied Energy*, *266*, 114848. https://doi.org/10.1016/j.apenergy.2020.114848

Rodríguez-Jiménez, L., Romero-Martín, M., Spruell, T., Steley, Z., & Gómez-Salgado, J. (2023). The carbon footprint of healthcare settings: A systematic review. *Journal of Advanced Nursing, 79*(8). https://doi.org/10.1111/jan.15671

Sai Bharadwaj, A. V. S. L., Nayak, R. R., Koteswararao, J., Sampath, C., Gaddala, B., Pawar, B. G., & Gupta, N. K. (2025). Environmental life-cycle assessment and green principles in process intensification: A review of novel catalysts from solid waste. *Chemical Engineering and Processing - Process Intensification, 211*, 110208. https://doi.org/10.1016/J.CEP.2025.110208

Salim Ba Awain, A. M., Jantan, M. D., & Sukati, I. (2021). Assessing the effect of integration in logistics sector on economic growth: Evidence from sultanate of Oman. *International Business Research, 15*(1), 35. https://doi.org/10.5539/IBR.V15N1P35

Saxena, V. (2025). Water quality, air pollution, and climate change: Investigating the environmental impacts of industrialization and urbanization. *Water, Air, and Soil Pollution, 236*(2), 1–40. https://doi.org/10.1007/s11270-024-07702-4

Scholz, F., Börner, N., Schust, S. A., Schardey, J., Kühn, F., Renz, B., Angele, M., Werner, J., Guba, M., & Jacob, S. (2024). Focus on patient perspectives in climate action policies for healthcare. A German survey analysis on what patients are willing to do. *Frontiers in Public Health, 12*. https://doi.org/10.3389/fpubh.2024.1477313

Sharma, A. (2024). Current trends and future directions in renewable energy systems. *International Journal for Research Publication and Seminar, 15*(2), 186–198. https://doi.org/10.36676/jrps.v15.i2.1408

Sharma, B., Gurung, A., Pradhan, P., Darjee, D., & Kotla, N. K. (2023). Navigating the regulatory landscape: Key trends shaping today's regulatory affairs environment. *International Journal of Drug Regulatory Affairs, 11*(4), 87–92. https://doi.org/10.22270/IJDRA.V11I4.639

Simpler, more streamlined and smarter regulations are required to address evolving policy challenges. (n.d.). Retrieved June 14, 2025, from https://www.oecd.org/en/about/news/press-releases/2025/04/simpler-more-streamlined-and-smarter-regulations-are-required-to-address-evolving-policy-challenges.html

Sitaraman G. (2020). A Grand Strategy of Resilience. *Foreign Affairs, 99*(5), 165–74.

Sklavos, G., Theodossiou, G., Papanikolaou, Z., Karelakis, C., & Ragazou, K. (2024). Environmental, social, and governance-based artificial intelligence governance: Digitalizing firms' leadership and human resources management. *Sustainability, 16*(16), 7154. https://doi.org/10.3390/su16167154

Škrinjar, J. P., Abramović, B., Bukvić, L., & Marušić, Ž. (2020). Managing fuel consumption and emissions in the renewed fleet of a transport company. *Sustainability (Switzerland), 12*(12). https://doi.org/10.3390/su12125047

Slootweg, J. C. (2024). Sustainable chemistry: Green, circular, and safe-by-design. *One Earth, 7*(5), 754–758. https://doi.org/10.1016/J.ONEEAR.2024.04.006

Subsidy: Subsidy Solutions: Complementing Price Ceilings in Public Policy - FasterCapital. (n.d.). Retrieved June 14, 2025, from https://fastercapital.com/content/Subsidy--Subsidy-Solutions--Complementing-Price-Ceilings-in-Public-Policy.html

Taheri, S., Hosseini, P., & Razban, A. (2022). Model predictive control of heating, ventilation, and air conditioning (HVAC) systems: A state-of-the-art review. *Journal of Building Engineering, 60*. https://doi.org/10.1016/j.jobe.2022.105067

Talaat, M., Farahat, M. A., & Elkholy, M. H. (2019). Renewable power integration: Experimental and simulation study to investigate the ability of integrating wave, solar and wind energies. *Energy, 170*. https://doi.org/10.1016/j.energy.2018.12.171

Tax incentives can help enhance adoption of sustainability manufacturing: Experts - The Economic Times. (n.d.). Retrieved June 14, 2025, from https://economictimes.indiatimes.com/news/economy/policy/tax-incentives-can-help-enhance-adoption-of-sustainability-manufacturing-experts/articleshow/110115593.cms

Taylor, C. J., Pomberger, A., Felton, K. C., Grainger, R., Barecka, M., Chamberlain, T. W., Bourne, R. A., Johnson, C. N., & Lapkin, A. A. (2023). A brief introduction to chemical reaction optimization. *Chemical Reviews, 123*(6), 3089–3126. https://doi.org/10.1021/acs.chemrev.2c00798

The Growing Importance Of Upskilling In The Tech Era. (n.d.). Retrieved June 14, 2025, from https://www.forbes.com/councils/forbeshumanresourcescouncil/2025/05/02/the-growing-importance-of-upskilling-in-the-tech-era/

The Role of Public Policy in Promoting Sustainable Development. (2017). www.ijrar.org

Tomić, T., & Schneider, D. R. (2018). The role of energy from waste in circular economy and closing the loop concept – Energy analysis approach. *Renewable and Sustainable Energy Reviews, 98*. https://doi.org/10.1016/j.rser.2018.09.029

Toniolo, S., Borsoi, L., & Camana, D. (2021). Life cycle assessment: Methods, limitations, and illustrations. *Methods in Sustainability Science: Assessment, Prioritization, Improvement, Design and Optimization*, 105–118. https://doi.org/10.1016/B978-0-12-823987-2.00007-6

Tudor, T., Baddley, J., & Mayhew-Manchón, L. (2015). Examining the uptake of low-carbon approaches within the healthcare sector: Case studies from the National Health Service in England. *International Journal of Healthcare, 1*(1). https://doi.org/10.5430/ijh.v1n1p61

Vallée, A. (2024). Green hospitals face to climate change: Between sobriety and resilience. *Heliyon, 10*(2). https://doi.org/10.1016/j.heliyon.2024.e24769

Wang, C., Deng, X., Wang, D., & Pan, X. (2024). Financial regulation, financing constraints, and enterprise innovation performance. *International Review of Financial Analysis, 95*, 103387. https://doi.org/10.1016/J.IRFA.2024.103387

Wang, L. (2014). Energy efficiency technologies for sustainable food processing. *Energy Efficiency, 7*(5). https://doi.org/10.1007/s12053-014-9256-8

Wang, W., Yan, Y., Fang, H., Li, J., Zha, S., & Wu, T. (2023). Volatile organic compound emissions from typical industries: Implications for the importance of oxygenated volatile organic compounds. *Atmospheric Pollution Research, 14*(1), 101640. https://doi.org/10.1016/J.APR.2022.101640

Warrick, D. D. (2023). Revisiting resistance to change and how to manage it: What has been learned and what organizations need to do. *Business Horizons, 66*(4), 433–441. https://doi.org/10.1016/J.BUSHOR.2022.09.001

Why do P&C companies usually have low profit margins? Does it pose risk to P&C actuaries/careers/salaries? : r/actuary. (n.d.). Retrieved June 14, 2025, from https://www.reddit.com/r/actuary/comments/ovkhz9/why_do_pc_companies_usually_have_low_profit/

Wu, Y., & Tham, J. (2023). The impact of environmental regulation, environment, social and government performance, and technological innovation on enterprise resilience under a green recovery. *Heliyon, 9*(10), e20278. https://doi.org/10.1016/J.HELIYON.2023.E20278

Xiao, J., Xu, Z., Xiao, A., Wang, X., & Skare, M. (2024). Overcoming barriers and seizing opportunities in the innovative adoption of next-generation digital technologies. *Journal of Innovation & Knowledge, 9*(4), 100622. https://doi.org/10.1016/J.JIK.2024.100622

Yadav, M., Gupta, R., & Nair, K. (2024). Time for sustainable marketing to build a green conscience in consumers: Evidence from a hybrid review. *Journal of Cleaner Production, 443*, 141188. https://doi.org/10.1016/J.JCLEPRO.2024.141188

Zhong, S., & Huang, C. (2019). Climate change and human health: Risks and responses. *Kexue Tongbao/Chinese Science Bulletin*, *64*(19). https://doi.org/10.1360/N972018-00898

Zhou, X., Zhou, X., Wang, C., & Zhou, H. (2023). Environmental and human health impacts of volatile organic compounds: A perspective review. *Chemosphere*, *313*, 137489. https://doi.org/10.1016/J.CHEMOSPHERE.2022.137489

Zikhathile, T., Atagana, H., Bwapwa, J., & Sawtell, D. (2022). A review of the impact that healthcare risk waste treatment technologies have on the environment. *International Journal of Environmental Research and Public Health*, *19*(19). https://doi.org/10.3390/ijerph191911967

Zopounidis, C., & Lemonakis, C. (2024). The company of the future: Integrating sustainability, growth, and profitability in contemporary business models. *Development and Sustainability in Economics and Finance*, *1*, 100003. https://doi.org/10.1016/J.DSEF.2024.100003

www.ingramcontent.com/pod-product-compliance
Lightning Source LLC
LaVergne TN
LVHW010650300926
849161LV00005B/1080
* 9 7 8 1 0 4 1 0 7 4 3 2 8 *